AF684117

ANSI®
Z136.1 – 2007
Revision of
ANSI Z136.1-2000

American National Standard for Safe Use of Lasers

Secretariat
Laser Institute of America

Approved March 16, 2007
American National Standards Institute, Inc.

American National Standard

An American National Standard implies a consensus of those substantially concerned with its scope and provisions. An American National Standard is intended as a guide to aid the manufacturer, the consumer and the general public. The existence of an American National Standard does not in any respect preclude anyone, whether he or she has approved the standard or not, from manufacturing, marketing, purchasing, or using products, processes or procedures not conforming to the standard. American National Standards are subject to periodic review and users are cautioned to obtain the latest editions.

CAUTION NOTICE: This American National Standard may be revised or withdrawn at any time. The procedures of the American National Standards Institute require that action be taken periodically to reaffirm, revise, or withdraw this standard no later than five years from the date of publication. Purchasers of American National Standards may receive current information on all standards by calling or writing the American National Standards Institute.

Published by

Laser Institute of America
13501 Ingenuity Drive, Suite 128
Orlando, FL 32826

ISBN-13: 978-0-912035-65-9 & ISBN-10: 0-912035-65-X

Printed in the United States of America

Foreword (This introduction is not a normative part of ANSI Z136.1-2007, American National Standard for Safe Use of Lasers.)

In 1968, the American National Standards Institute (ANSI) approved the initiation of the Safe Use of Lasers Standards Project under the sponsorship of the Telephone Group.

Prior to 1985, Z136 standards were developed by ANSI Committee Z136 and submitted for approval and issuance as ANSI Z136 standards. Since 1985, Z136 standards are developed by the ANSI Accredited Standards Committee (ASC) Z136. A copy of the procedures for development of these standards can be obtained from the secretariat, the Laser Institute of America, 13501 Ingenuity Drive, Suite 128, Orlando, FL 32826 or viewed at www.z136.org.

The present scope of ASC Z136 covers protection against hazards associated with the use of lasers, laser diodes and certain diodes used in optical fiber communication systems.

ASC Z136 is responsible for the development and maintenance of this standard. In addition to the consensus body, ASC Z136 is composed of standards subcommittees (SSC) and technical subcommittees (TSC) involved in Z136 standards development and an editorial working group. At the time of this printing, the following standards and technical subcommittees were active:

SSC-1	Safe Use of Lasers (parent document)
SSC-2	Safe Use of Lasers and LEDs in Telecommunications Applications
SSC-3	Safe Use of Lasers in Health Care Facilities
SSC-4	Measurements and Instrumentation
SSC-5	Safe Use of Lasers in Educational Institutions
SSC-6	Safe Use of Lasers Outdoors
SSC-7	Eyewear and Protective Barriers
SSC-8	Safe Use of Lasers in Research, Development and Testing
SSC-9	Safe Use of Lasers in Manufacturing Environments
SSC-10	Safe Use of Lasers in Entertainment, Displays and Exhibitions
TSC-1	Biological Effects and Medical Surveillance
TSC-2	Hazard Evaluation and Classification
TSC-4	Control Measures and Training
TSC-5	Non-Beam Hazards
TSC-7	Analysis and Applications
EWG	Editorial Working Group

The six standards currently issued are:

ANSI Z136.1-2007, American National Standard for Safe Use of Lasers (replaces ANSI Z136.1-2000)

ANSI Z136.2-1997, American National Standard for Safe Use of Optical Fiber Communication Systems Utilizing Laser Diode and LED Sources (replaces ANSI Z136.2-1989)

ANSI Z136.3-2005, American National Standard for Safe Use of Lasers in Health Care Facilities (replaces ANSI Z136.3-1996)

ANSI Z136.4-2005, Recommended Practice for Laser Safety Measurements for Hazard Evaluation (first edition)

ANSI Z136.5-2000, American National Standard for Safe Use of Lasers in Educational Institutions (first edition)

ANSI Z136.6-2005, American National Standard for Safe Use of Lasers Outdoors (replaces ANSI Z136.6-2000)

This American National Standard provides guidance for the safe use of lasers and laser systems by defining control measures for each of four laser hazard classifications. Once a laser or laser system is properly classified, there should be no need to carry out tedious measurements or calculations to meet the provisions of this standard. However, technical information on masurements, calculations and biological effects is also provided within the standard and its appendixes.

It is expected that this standard will be periodically revised as new information and experience in the use of lasers are gained. Future revisions may have modified methodology, and use of the most current document is highly recommended.

While there is considerable compatibility among existing laser safety standards, some requirements differ among state, federal, and international standards. These differences may have an effect on the particulars of the applicable control measures.

Suggestions for improvements of the standard are welcome. They should be sent to ASC Z136 Secretariat, Laser Institute of America, 13501 Ingenuity Drive, Suite 128, Orlando, FL 32826.

This standard was processed and approved for submittal to ANSI by Accredited Standards Committee Z136 on the Safe Use of Lasers. Committee approval of the standard does not necessarily imply that all members voted for its approval.

Ron Petersen, Committee Chair
Sheldon Zimmerman, Committee Vice-Chair
Robert Thomas, Committee Secretary

Notice (This notice is not a normative part of ANSI Z136.1-2007, American National Standard for Safe Use of Lasers.)

Z136 standards and recommended practices are developed through a consensus standards development process approved by the American National Standards Institute. The process brings together volunteers representing varied viewpoints and interests to achieve consensus on laser safety related issues. As secretariat to ASC Z136, the Laser Institute of America (LIA) administers the process and provides financial and clerical support to the committee.

The LIA and its directors, officers, employees, members, affiliates and sponsors, expressly disclaim liability for any personal injury, property or other damages of any nature whatsoever, whether special, indirect, consequential or compensatory, directly or indirectly resulting from the publication, use of, or reliance on this document or these standards. The LIA's service as secretariat does not constitute, and LIA does not make any endorsement, warranty or referral of any particular standards, practices, goods, or services that may be referenced in this document. The LIA also makes no guarantee or warranty as to the accuracy or completeness of any information published herein. The LIA has no power, nor does it undertake to police or enforce compliance with the contents of this document.

In issuing and making this document available, the LIA is not undertaking to render professional or other services for or on behalf of any person or entity. Nor is the LIA undertaking to perform any duty owed by any person or entity to someone else. Anyone using this document should rely on his or her own independent judgment or, as appropriate, seek the advice of a competent professional in determining the exercise of reasonable care in any given circumstances.

Participants At the time it approved this standard, ASC Z136 had the following members:

Organization Represented	*Name of Representative*
Academy of Laser Dentistry	Joel White
American College of Obstetricians & Gynecologists	Ira Horowitz
American Dental Association	Douglas Dederich
American Glaucoma Society	Michael Berlin
American Industrial Hygiene Association	R. Timothy Hitchcock
American Society for Laser Medicine & Surgery	Jerome Garden Roy Geronemus (Alt)
American Society of Safety Engineers	Thomas V. Fleming Walter Nickens (Alt)
American Veterinary Medical Association	Kenneth Bartels
American Welding Society	Mark McLear William Arthur (Alt)
Association of periOperative Registered Nurses	Penny J. Smalley
Camden County College	Fred Seeber
Cincinnati State Technical & Community College	Prem Batra
Corning, Inc.	C. Eugene Moss
Delphi Corporation	Paul Daniel Jr.
Health Physics Society	Thomas Johnson David Sliney (Alt)
High-Rez Diagnostics, Inc.	Richard Hughes
Institute of Electrical and Electronics Engineers, Inc. (SCC-39)	Ron Petersen
International Imaging Industry Association (I3A)	Joseph Greco
L*A*I International	Thomas Lieb
Laser and Electro-Optic Manufacturers Association	Breck Hitz
Laser Institute of America	Richard Greene
LFI International	Roberta McHatton
Laser Safety Consulting, LLC.	Darrell Seeley
Lawrence Berkeley National Laboratory	Lawrence McLouth
Lawrence Livermore National Laboratory	Ken Barat
Los Alamos National Laboratory	Connon Odom
National Aeronautics and Space Administration	Guy Camomilli Randall Scott (Alt)
National Institute of Standards and Technology (NIST)	John Lehman
Optical Society of America	James Zavislan

Organization Represented	*Name of Representative*
Power Technology, Inc.	William Burgess
Rockwell Laser Industries	William Ertle
Terabeam	John Bell
Underwriters Laboratories, Inc.	Peter Boden David Dubiel (Alt)
University of Texas, Southwestern Medical Center	John Hoopman
US Department of Health and Human Services, Center for Devices and Radiological Health	Jerome Dennis
US Department of Labor, Occupational Safety & Health Administration	Robert Curtis
US Department of the Air Force, Air Force Research Laboratory	Benjamin Rockwell Robert Thomas (Alt)
US Department of the Air Force, Surgeon General's Office	Steven Rademacher
US Department of the Army, Medical Research & Materiel Command	Bruce Stuck
US Department of the Army, US Army CHPPM	Jeffrey Pfoutz Penelope Galoff (Alt)
US Department of the Navy, Naval Sea Systems Command	Sheldon Zimmerman Mary Gorschboth (Alt)
US Department of the Navy, Space & Naval Warfare System Command	James Sheehy
Individual Members	Robert Aldrich Richard Crowson Ben Edwards Robert Handren, Jr. Ami Kestenbaum David J. Lund Wesley Marshall Jay Parkinson Randolph Paura Frank Rainer William P. Roach David Sliney James Smith Nikolay Stoev Paul Testagrossa Stephen Trokel Robert Weiner Myron Wolbarsht Anthony Zmorenski

The various subcommittees that participated in developing this standard had the following members:

Safe Use of Lasers SSC-1

William P. Roach, Chair
Benjamin Rockwell, Vice-Chair
Kristy Hayes, Secretary

Robert Aldrich
Will Arthur
Ken Barat
John Bell
Michael Berlin
William Burgess
Guy Camomilli
Richard Crowson
Paul Daniel
Jerome Dennis
Jane Ehrgott
William Ertle
Robert Faaland
Don Farrer
Thomas Fleming
James Franks
Penelope Galoff
Jerome Garden
Terence Garrison
Mary Gorschboth
Andy Hagel
Rebecca Hall
Robert Handren
R. Timothy Hitchcock
John Hoopman
Thomas Johnson
Kimberly Kantner
James Kenney
Ami Kestenbaum
John Lehman
Susan Lohr
David Lund

Leon McLin
Wesley Marshall
Kim Merritt
C. Eugene Moss
Walter Nickens
John O'Donnell
John O'Hagan
Jay Parkinson
Mary Payton
Ron Petersen
Frank Rainer
Fred Seeber
Darrell Seeley
James Sheehy
David Sliney
Penny J. Smalley
James Smith
Dale Smith
Dadi Song
Nikolay Stoev
Emily Stoler
Bruce Stuck
Robert Thomas
Dan Thomas
Stephen Trokel
Robert Weiner
Jamaal Whitmore
Mike Wolbarsht
James Zavislan
Gary Zeman
Sheldon Zimmerman
Anthony Zmorenski

Laser Bioeffects, TSC-1

Bruce Stuck, Chair
Myron Wolbarsht, Vice-Chair
Russell McCally, Secretary

Robert Aldrich
Kenneth Bartels
Alan Blatterman
Jeremiah Brown, Jr.
Clarence Cain
Francois Delori
Jerome Dennis
William Ertle

Donald Farrer
Penelope Galoff
Mary Gorschboth
Thomas Johnson
Maurice Landers
Charles Lin
David J. Lund
Martin Mainster

Laser Bioeffects, TSC-1 (cont.)

Wesley Marshall
Don McDuffie
Leon McLin
C. Eugene Moss
John O'Hagan
Ron Petersen
William P. Roach
Benjamin Rockwell
James Sheehy
David Sliney
Robert Thomas
Stephen Trokel
Robert Weiner
James Zavislan
Sheldon Zimmerman
Joseph Zuclich
Harry Zwick

Hazard Evaluation & Classification, TSC-2

David Sliney, Chair
James Franks, Vice-Chair
Robert Thomas, Secretary

Robert Aldrich
Jerome Dennis
Howard Donovan
Robert Faaland
Jerome Garden
R. Timothy Hitchcock
Kimberly Kantner
Martin Langlois
David J. Lund
Wesley Marshall
Leon McLin
John O'Donnell
Connon Odom
Jay Parkinson
Mary G. Payton
Ron Petersen
William P. Roach
Benjamin Rockwell
Dale Smith
Gregory Smith
Nikolay Stoev
Bruce Stuck
Bill Triplett
Stephen Trokel
Robert Weiner
James Zavislan
Sheldon Zimmerman

Control Measures & Training, TSC-4

William Ertle, Chair
R. Timothy Hitchcock, Vice-Chair
Anthony Zmorenski, Secretary

Robert Aldrich
William Arthur
Mary Baker
Ken Barat
Clarence Cain
Richard Crowson
Paul Daniel, Jr.
Jerome Dennis
Howard Donovan
Robert Faaland
Thomas Fleming
Penelope Galoff
Terence Garrison
Richard Greene
Patrick Hancock
Robert Handren
Joel Harrington
John Hoopman
Kimberly Kantner
Thomas Lieb
Susan Lohr
Tom MacMullin
Wesley Marshall
Mark McLear
C. Eugene Moss
John O'Donnell
John O'Hagan
Jay Parkinson
Mary G. Payton
Ron Petersen
Frank Rainer
William P. Roach
Benjamin Rockwell
Darrell Seeley
James Sheehy
David Sliney

Control Measures & Training, TSC-4 (cont.)

Penny J. Smalley
James Smith
Dale Smith
Casey Stack
Nikolay Stoev
Bruce Stuck
Paul Testagrossa
Robert Thomas
Stephen Trokel
Robert Tucker
Robert Weiner
Jamaal Whitmore
Myron Wolbarsht
Sheldon Zimmerman

Non-Beam Hazards, TSC-5

C. Eugene Moss, Chair
R. Timothy Hitchcock, Vice-Chair

Ken Barat
Ben Edwards
Joseph Greco
Stephen Hemperly
Richard Hughes
Betty Minor
Benjamin Rockwell
Penny J. Smalley
Robert Thomas
Dan Thomas
Arthur Varenelli

Analysis and Applications, TSC-7

Wesley Marshall, Chair
Robert Thomas, Vice-Chair
Mark Webb, Secretary

Robert Aldrich
James Franks
Mary Gorschboth
R. Timothy Hitchcock
Jay Parkinson
Ron Petersen
Benjamin Rockwell
Dale Smith
Nikolay Stoev
Dan Thomas
Robert Weiner
Sheldon Zimmerman
Anthony Zmorenski

Editorial Working Group, EWG

Ami Kestenbaum, Chair

Richard Hughes
Bill Janssen
Thomas Johnson
Barbara Sams
Darrell Seeley
Nikolay Stoev
Sheldon Zimmerman

CONTENTS

SECTION PAGE

Tables

Figures

SECTION PAGE

American National Standard for Safe Use of Lasers

1. General

1.1 Scope.

This standard provides recommendations for the safe use of lasers and laser systems that operate at wavelengths between 0.18 μm and 1 mm.

1.2 Application.

The objective of this standard is to provide reasonable and adequate guidance for the safe use of lasers and laser systems. A practical means for accomplishing this is first to (1) classify lasers and laser systems according to their relative hazards and then to (2) specify appropriate controls for each classification.

Other special application standards within the Z136 series may deviate from the requirements of this standard. Each deviation is valid only for applications within the scope of the standard in which it appears.

The basis of the hazard classification scheme in Section 3 of this standard is the ability of the laser beam to cause biological damage to the eye or skin during use. For example:

A Class 1 laser system is:

- Considered to be incapable of producing damaging radiation levels during operation, and
- Exempt from any control measures or other forms of surveillance.

Note: For the purposes of this standard, products which have been classified previously as Class IIa under the Federal Laser Product Performance Standard (FLPPS) should be treated the same as Class 1.

A Class 1M laser system is:

- Considered to be incapable of producing hazardous exposure conditions during normal operation unless the beam is viewed with an optical instrument such as an eye-loupe (diverging beam) or a telescope (collimated beam), and
- Exempt from any control measures other than to prevent potentially hazardous optically aided viewing; and is exempt from other forms of surveillance.

A Class 2 laser system:

- Emits in the visible portion of the spectrum (0.4 to 0.7 μm), and
- Eye protection is normally afforded by the aversion response.

A Class 2M laser system:

- Emits in the visible portion of the spectrum (0.4 to 0.7 μm), and

- Eye protection is normally afforded by the aversion response for unaided viewing.
- However, Class 2M is potentially hazardous if viewed with certain optical aids.

A Class 3 laser system (medium-power):

- May be hazardous under direct and specular reflection viewing conditions, but is normally not a diffuse reflection or fire hazard.

There are two subclasses:

- A Class 3R laser system is potentially hazardous under some direct and specular reflection viewing condition if the eye is appropriately focused and stable, but the probability of an actual injury is small. This laser will not pose either a fire hazard or diffuse-reflection hazard.
- A Class 3B laser system may be hazardous under direct and specular reflection viewing conditions, but is normally not a diffuse reflection or fire hazard.

Note: For lasers classified as Class IIIa see Appendix H for guidance.

A Class 4 laser system (high-power):

- Is a hazard to the eye or skin from the direct beam, and
- May pose a diffuse reflection or fire hazard
- May also produce laser generated air contaminants (LGAC) and hazardous plasma radiation (see Section 7).

Lasers or laser systems designated for a specific class by a manufacturer in accordance with the Federal Laser Product Performance Standard (FLLPS) (or latest revision thereof) or International Electrotechnical Commission (IEC) 60825-1 (or latest revision thereof) may be considered as fulfilling all classification requirements of this standard. In cases where the laser or laser system classification is not provided, or where the class level may change because of the addition or deletion of engineering control measures (see Section 4.3), the laser or laser system shall be classified by the Laser Safety Officer (LSO) in accordance with the descriptions given in Section 3, the methods described in Section 9, or both.

The recommended step-by-step procedure for using this standard is as follows:

1) Determine the appropriate class of the laser or laser system.
2) Comply with the measures specified for that class of laser or laser system, using Table 1 as a guide. This procedure will in most cases eliminate the need for measurement of laser radiation, quantitative analysis of hazard potential, or use of the Maximum Permissible Exposures (MPEs) as given in Section 8 and Tables 5a and 5b of this standard.

Table 1. Requirements by Laser Classification

Class	Procedural & Administrative Controls	Training	Medical Surveillance	LSO
1	Not Required	Not Required	Not Required	Not Required
1M	Required	Application Dependent (2)	Application Dependent (2)	Application Dependent (2)
2	Not Required (1)	Not Required (1)	Not Required	Not Required
2M	Required	Application Dependent (2)	Application Dependent (2)	Application Dependent (2)
3R	Not Required (1)	Not Required (1)	Not Required	Not Required (1)
3B	Required	Required	Suggested	Required
4	Required	Required	Suggested	Required

Note: During maintenance and service the classification associated with the maximum level of accessible laser radiation shall be used to determine the applicable control measures.

1) *Not required except for conditions of intentional intrabeam exposure applications.*
2) *Certain uses of Class 1M or 2M lasers or laser systems that exceed Class 1 or Class 2 because they do not satisfy Measurement Condition 1 may require hazard evaluation and/or manufacturer's information (see Section 4.1.1.3).*

Sections 8 and 9 should be consulted for quantitative evaluation of the hazard associated with a given laser or laser system. To use the ocular MPEs for the retinal hazard region (provided in Tables 5a and 5b), determine whether the source is a point source or whether extended source viewing conditions apply (see Figures B1, B3, and B4 in Appendix B for illustrated viewing conditions).

For the purposes of this standard, except for short-distance viewing of small diameter or focused Class 3B lasers (see Section 3.3.3), only Class 4 lasers are capable of producing hazardous diffuse reflections; hence calculations for viewing diffuse reflections are normally only necessary for Class 4 lasers.

The laser hazard classification system is based entirely on the laser radiation emission. Non-beam hazards must be dealt with separately and are addressed in Section 7.

1.3 Laser Safety Programs.

1.3.1 General. Management (employer) has the fundamental responsibility for the assurance of the safe use of lasers owned and/or operated in facilities under its control. Management (employer) shall establish and maintain an adequate program for the control of laser hazards. Employer and/or facility safety programs and employee training programs shall be provided for Class 3B or Class 4 lasers and laser systems. Employer and/or facility safety programs and employee training should be provided for laser systems containing embedded Class 3B and Class 4 lasers. Employer and/or facility safety programs and employee training programs are not required for Class 1 lasers and laser systems that do not contain embedded Class 3B and Class 4 lasers (see Section 3.1 and Table 1).

The following guidelines for laser safety programs contain requirements (designated by *shall*) and recommendations (designated by *should*). In the case of a recommendation it may be useful for the employer to review Section 3 of this standard and perform a hazard evaluation, with particular emphasis on the total foreseen risk based on consideration of the laser, laser system and application, as well as the environment in which it is used and the personnel using the laser. The evaluation would include considerations such as the likelihood of the use of viewing optics, and the intentional or unintentional misuse of a laser that, under normal conditions, would not be considered to be hazardous. In many situations the implementation of a recommendation may not be necessary. In other situations, it may be useful or prudent to implement the recommendation in order to assure the safe use of lasers for a specific application.

1.3.2 Laser Safety Program Provisions. The laser safety program established by the employer shall include provisions for the following:

1) Designation of an individual as the Laser Safety Officer (LSO) with the authority and responsibility to effect the knowledgeable evaluation and control of laser hazards, and the implementation of appropriate control measures, as well as to monitor and enforce compliance with required standards and regulations. The specific duties and responsibilities of the LSO are designated in normative Appendix A. *(Note: A normative appendix is an extension of the standard, and as such is an integral part of the standard.)* Throughout the body of this standard, it shall be understood that wherever duties or responsibilities of the LSO are specified, it will mean that the LSO either performs the stated task or assures that the task is performed by qualified individual(s).

2) Education of authorized personnel (LSOs, operators, service personnel and others) in the safe use of lasers and laser systems and as applicable, the assessment and control of laser hazards. This may be accomplished through training programs. Employers should consider the benefits of initiating awareness training for employees working with and around lasers and laser systems greater than Class 1. If training is warranted for embedded lasers it shall extend to those routinely around the systems, who will be present when maintenance requiring beam access or service occurs (see Section 5 and Appendix D).

3) Application of adequate protective measures for the control of laser hazards as required in Section 4.

4) Incident investigation, including reporting of alleged accidents to the LSO, and preparation of action plans for the prevention of future accidents following a known or suspected incident.

5) An appropriate medical examination and medical surveillance program in accordance with Section 6.

6) Formation of a Laser Safety Committee when the number, hazards, complexity and/or diversity of laser activities warrants. The structure and responsibilities for a Laser Safety Committee are presented in Appendix A.

1.3.3 Personnel Responsibilities. Employees who work with lasers or laser systems and their supervisors have responsibilities for establishing their safe use. Suggested responsibilities for these individuals are provided in Appendix A.

Individuals involved in purchasing lasers and laser systems should contact the LSO to aid in the implementation of the laser safety program. Suggested actions are provided in Appendix A, Section A3.

Individuals fabricating, altering or installing a Class 3B or 4 laser or laser system should contact the LSO to aid in the implementation of the laser safety program.

2. Definitions

The definitions of the terms listed below are based on a pragmatic rather than a basic approach. Therefore, the terms defined are limited to those actually used in this standard and its appendixes and are in no way intended to constitute a dictionary of terms used in the laser field as a whole.

absorption. Transformation of radiant energy to a different form of energy by interaction with matter.

accessible emission limit (AEL). The maximum accessible emission level permitted within a particular laser hazard class.

accessible optical radiation. Optical radiation to which the human eye or skin may be exposed for the condition (operation, maintenance, or service) specified.

alpha max. The angular subtense of an extended source beyond which additional subtense does not contribute to the hazard and need not be considered. This value is 100 mrad for retinal thermal effects and 110 mrad for the retinal photochemical effects. Symbol: α_{max}

alpha min. The angular subtense of a source below which the source can be effectively considered as a point source. The value of alpha min is1.5 mrad. Symbol: α_{min}

aperture. An opening, window, or lens through which optical radiation can pass.

apparent visual angle. The angular subtense (α) of the source as calculated from source size and distance from the eye. It is not the beam divergence of the source (see Section 8.1 and Figure B4 for criteria).

attenuation. The decrease in the radiant flux as it passes through an absorbing or scattering medium.

authorized personnel. Individuals approved by management to operate, maintain, service, or install laser equipment.

average power. The total energy in an exposure or emission divided by the duration of the exposure or emission.

aversion response. Closure of the eyelid, eye movement, pupillary constriction, or movement of the head to avoid an exposure to a noxious or bright light stimulant. In this standard, the aversion response to an exposure from a bright, visible, laser source is assumed to limit the exposure of a specific retinal area to 0.25 s or less.

beam. A collection of light/photonic rays characterized by direction, diameter (or dimensions), and divergence (or convergence).

beam diameter. The distance between diametrically opposed points in that cross-section of a beam where the power per unit area is $1/e$ (0.368) times that of the peak power per unit area.

blink reflex. The blink reflex is the involuntary closure of the eyes as a result of stimulation by an external event such as an irritation of the cornea or conjunctiva, a bright flash, the rapid approach of an object, an auditory stimulus or with facial movements. In this standard the ocular aversion response for a bright flash of light is assumed to limit the exposure of a specific retinal area to 0.25 s or less.

C_A. Correction factor which increases the MPE in the near infrared (IR-A) spectral band (0.7-1.4 μm) based upon reduced absorption properties of melanin pigment granules found in the skin and in the retinal pigment epithelium.

C_B. Correction factor which increases the MPE in the red end of the visible spectrum (0.45-0.60 μm), because of greatly reduced photochemical hazards.

C_C. Correction factor which increases the MPE for ocular exposure because of pre-retinal absorption of radiant energy in the spectral region between 1.15 and 1.40 μm.

C_E. Correction factor used for calculating the extended source MPE for the eye from the point source MPE, when the laser source subtends a visual angle exceeding α_{min}.

C_P. Correction factor which reduces the MPE for repetitive-pulse exposure of the eye.

carcinogen. An agent potentially capable of causing cancer.

coagulation. The process of congealing by an increase in viscosity characterized by a condensation of material from a liquid to a gelatinous or solid state.

coherent. A beam of light characterized by a fixed phase relationship (spatial coherence) or single wavelength, i.e., monochromatic (temporal coherence).

collateral radiation. Any electromagnetic radiation, except laser radiation, emitted by a laser or laser system which is physically necessary for its operation.

collecting optics. Lenses or optical instruments having magnification and thereby producing an increase in energy or power density. Such devices may include telescopes, binoculars, microscopes, or loupes.

collimated beam. Effectively, a "parallel" beam of light with very low divergence or convergence.

Condition 1. Pertains to optically aided viewing of collimated beams through telescopes or binoculars.

Condition 2. Pertains to optically aided viewing of sources with highly divergent beams through magnifiers or eye loupes or unaided viewing with or without strong accommodation (Condition 2 has slightly different measurement conditions in IEC 60825-1).

continuous wave (CW). In this standard, a laser operating with a continuous output for a period $\geq$ 0.25 s is regarded as a CW laser.

controlled area (laser). An area where the occupancy and activity of those within is subject to control and supervision for the purpose of protection from laser radiation hazards.

cornea. The transparent outer layer of the human eye which covers the iris and the crystalline lens. The cornea is the main refracting element of the eye.

critical frequency. The pulse repetition frequency above which the laser output is considered continuous wave (CW). For example, for a short unintentional exposure (0.25 s to 10 s) to nanosecond (or longer) pulses, the critical frequency is 55 kHz for wavelengths between 0.40 and 1.05 μm, and 20 kHz for wavelengths between 1.05 and 1.40 μm.

diffuse reflection. Change of the spatial distribution of a beam of radiation when it is reflected in many directions by a surface or by a medium.

divergence. In this standard, the divergence is the increase in the diameter of the laser beam with distance from the exit aperture, based on the full angle at the point where the irradiance (or radiant exposure for pulsed lasers) is $1/e$ times the maximum value. Symbol: ϕ

effective energy. Energy, in joules, through the applicable measurement aperture. Symbol: Q_{eff}

effective power. Power, in watts, through the applicable measurement aperture. Symbol: Φ_{eff}

electromagnetic radiation. The flow of energy consisting of orthogonally vibrating electric and magnetic fields lying transverse to the direction of propagation. Gamma rays, X-ray, ultraviolet, visible, infrared, and radio waves occupy various portions of the electromagnetic spectrum and differ only in frequency, wavelength, and photon energy.

embedded laser. An enclosed laser that has a higher classification than the laser system in which it is incorporated, where the system's lower classification is appropriate due to the engineering features limiting accessible emission.

enclosed laser. A laser that is contained within a protective housing of itself or of the laser or laser system in which it is incorporated. Opening or removing of the protective housing provides additional access to laser radiation above the applicable MPE than possible with the protective housing in place (an embedded laser is an example of one type of enclosed laser).

energy. The capacity for doing work. Energy content is commonly used to characterize the output from pulsed lasers, and is generally expressed in joules (J).

epithelium (of the cornea). The layer of cells forming the outer surface of the cornea.

erythema. For the purposes of the standard, redness of the skin due to exposure from laser radiation.

extended source. A source of optical radiation with an angular subtense at the cornea larger than α_{min}. See *point source.*

eye-safe laser. A Class 1 laser product. Because of the frequent misuse of the term "eye-safe wavelength" to mean "retina-safe," (e.g., at 1.5-1.6 μm) and *eye-safe laser* to refer to a laser emitting at wavelengths outside the retinal-hazard region, the term "eye-safe" can be a misnomer. Hence, the use of *eye-safe laser* is discouraged.

fail-safe interlock. An interlock where the failure of a single mechanical or electrical component of the interlock will cause the system to go into, or remain in, a safe mode.

field of view. The full solid angle from which a detector's active area receives radiation.

focal length. The distance from the secondary nodal point of a lens to the secondary focal point. For a thin lens imaging a distant source, the focal length is the distance between the lens and the focal point.

focal point. The point toward which radiation converges or from which radiation diverges or appears to diverge.

half-power point. The time on either the leading or trailing edge of a laser pulse at which the power is one-half of its maximum value.

hertz (Hz). The unit which expresses the frequency of a periodic oscillation in cycles per second.

infrared. In this standard, the region of the electromagnetic spectrum between the long-wavelength extreme of the visible spectrum (about 0.7 μm) and the shortest microwaves (about 1 mm).

infrared radiation. Electromagnetic radiation with wavelengths which lie within the range 0.7 μm to 1 mm.

installation. Placement and connection of laser equipment at the appropriate site to enable intended operation.

integrated radiance. The integral of the radiance over the exposure duration, expressed in joules-per-centimeter-squared per-steradian ($J{\cdot}cm^{-2}{\cdot}sr^{-1}$).

intrabeam viewing. The viewing condition whereby the eye is exposed to all or part of a laser beam.

iris. The circular pigmented structure which lies behind the cornea of the human eye. The iris is perforated by the pupil.

irradiance. Radiant power incident per unit area upon a surface, expressed in watts-per-centimeter-squared ($W{\cdot}cm^{-2}$). Symbol: E

joule. A unit of energy. 1 joule = 1 N·m; 1 joule = 1 watt • second.

Lambertian surface. An ideal (diffuse) surface whose emitted or reflected radiance is independent of the viewing angle.

laser. A device that produces radiant energy predominantly by stimulated emission. Laser radiation may be highly coherent temporally, or spatially, or both. An acronym for **L**ight **A**mplification by **S**timulated **E**mission of **R**adiation.

laser barrier. A device used to block or attenuate incident direct or diffuse laser radiation. Laser barriers are frequently used during times of service to the laser system when it is desirable to establish a boundary for a controlled laser area.

laser classification. An indication of the beam hazard level of a laser or laser system during normal operation or the determination thereof. The hazard level of a laser or laser system is represented by a number or a numbered capital letter. The laser classifications are Class 1, Class 1M, Class 2, Class 2M, Class 3R, Class 3B and Class 4. In general, the potential beam hazard level increases in the same order.

laser diode. A laser employing a forward-biased semiconductor junction as the active medium.

laser personnel. Persons who routinely work around hazardous laser beams. This standard requires such persons to be protected by engineering controls, administrative procedures, or both.

laser pointer. A laser product that is usually hand held that emits a low-divergence visible beam and is intended for designating specific objects or images during discussions, lectures or presentations as well as for the aiming of firearms or other visual targeting practice. These products are normally Class 1, Class 2 or Class 3R.

laser safety officer (LSO). One who has authority and responsibility to monitor and enforce the control of laser hazards and effect the knowledgeable evaluation and control of laser hazards.

laser system. An assembly of electrical, mechanical, and optical components which includes a laser.

lesion. An abnormal change in the structure of an organ or part due to injury or disease.

limiting angular subtense. See *alpha min.*

limiting aperture diameter. The diameter of a circle over which irradiance or radiant exposure is averaged for purposes of hazard evaluation and classification. Symbol: D_f

limiting cone angle. The cone angle through which radiance or integrated radiance is averaged when photochemical effects are considered in hazard evaluation and classification. Symbol: γ

limiting exposure duration. An exposure duration which is specifically limited by the design or intended use(s). Symbol: T_{max}

macula. The small uniquely pigmented specialized area of the retina of the eye, which, in normal individuals, is predominantly employed for acute central vision (i.e., area of best visual acuity).

magnified viewing. Viewing a small object through an optical system that increases the apparent object size. This type of optical system can make a diverging laser beam more hazardous (e.g., using a magnifying optic to view an optical fiber with a laser beam emitted).

maintenance. Performance of those adjustments or procedures (specified in the user information provided by the manufacturer and considered preventative, to maintain optimal performance of the laser system), which are to be carried out by the user to ensure the intended performance of the product. It does not include *operation* or *service* as defined in this section.

maximum permissible exposure (MPE). The level of laser radiation to which an unprotected person may be exposed without adverse biological changes in the eye or skin.

measurement aperture. The aperture used for classification of a laser to determine the effective power or energy that is compared with the AEL for each laser hazard class.

meter. A unit of length in the international system of units; currently defined as the length of a path traversed in vacuum by light during a period of 1/299792458 seconds. Typically, the meter is subdivided into the following units:

centimeter (cm)	=	10^{-2} m
millimeter (mm)	=	10^{-3} m
micrometer (μm)	=	10^{-6} m
nanometer (nm)	=	10^{-9} m

minimum viewing distance. The minimum distance at which the eye can produce a focused image of a diffuse source, usually assumed to be 10 cm.

monochromatic light. Having or consisting of one color or wavelength.

nominal hazard zone (NHZ). The space within which the level of the direct, reflected, or scattered radiation may exceed the applicable MPE. Exposure levels beyond the boundary of the NHZ are below the appropriate MPE.

nominal ocular hazard distance (NOHD). The distance along the axis of the unobstructed beam from a laser, fiber end, or connector to the human eye beyond which the irradiance or radiant exposure is not expected to exceed the applicable MPE.

non-beam hazard. A class of hazards that result from factors other than direct human exposure to a laser beam.

normative appendix. Conforming to or based on norms of an authoritative standard; a principle of right action binding upon the members of a group and serving to guide, control, or regulate proper and acceptable behavior.

ocular fundus. The interior posterior surface of the eye (the retina), as seen upon ophthalmoscopic examination.

operation. The performance of the laser or laser system over the full range of its intended functions (normal operation). It does not include *maintenance* or *service* as defined in this section.

ophthalmoscope. An instrument for examining the interior of the eye.

optically aided viewing. Viewing with a telescopic (binocular) or magnifying optic. Under certain circumstances, viewing with an optical aid can increase the hazard from a laser beam (see *telescopic viewing* or *magnified viewing*).

optical density. The logarithm to the base ten of the reciprocal of the transmittance at a particular wavelength:

$$D_\lambda = \log_{10} (1/\tau_\lambda)$$

where τ_λ is the transmittance at the wavelength of interest. Symbol: $D(\lambda)$, D_λ or OD

photochemical effect. A biological effect produced by a chemical action brought about by the absorption of photons by molecules that directly alter the molecule.

photosensitizers. Substances which increase the sensitivity of a material to exposure by optical radiation.

pigment epithelium (of the retina). The layer of cells which contain brown or black pigment granules next to and behind the rods and cones.

plasma radiation. Black-body radiation generated by luminescence of matter in a laser generated plume.

point source. For purposes of this standard, a source with an angular subtense at the cornea equal to or less than alpha-min (α_{min}), i.e., ≤ 1.5 mrad.

point source viewing. The viewing condition whereby the angular subtense of the source, α, is equal to or less than the limiting angular subtense, α_{min}.

power. The rate at which energy is emitted, transferred, or received. Unit: watts (W) (joules per second).

protective housing. An enclosure that surrounds the laser or laser system and prevents access to laser radiation above the applicable MPE. The aperture through which the useful beam is emitted is not part of the protective housing. The protective housing limits access to other associated radiant energy emissions and to electrical hazards associated with components and terminals, and may enclose associated optics and a workstation.

pulse duration. The duration of a laser pulse, usually measured as the time interval between the half-power points on the leading and trailing edges of the pulse. Typical units:

microsecond (μs)	=	10^{-6} s
nanosecond (ns)	=	10^{-9} s
picosecond (ps)	=	10^{-12} s
femtosecond (fs)	=	10^{-15} s

Symbol: *t*

pulse-repetition frequency (PRF). The number of pulses occurring per second, expressed in hertz. Symbol: *F*.

pulsed laser. A laser which delivers its energy in the form of a single pulse or a train of pulses. In this standard, the duration of a pulse is less than 0.25 s.

pupil. The variable aperture in the iris through which light travels to the interior of the eye.

Q-switch. A device for producing very short (~10-250 ns), intense laser pulses by enhancing the storage and dumping of electronic energy in and out of the lasing medium, respectively.

Q-switched laser. A laser that emits short (~10-250 ns), high-power pulses by means of a Q-switch.

radian (rad). A unit of angular measure equal to the angle subtended at the center of a circle by an arc whose length is equal to the radius of the circle. 1 radian ~ 57.3 degrees; 2π radians = 360 degrees.

radiance. Radiant flux or power output per unit solid angle per unit area expressed in watts-per-centimeter squared per-steradian ($W \cdot cm^{-2} \cdot sr^{-1}$). Symbol: *L*

radiant energy. Energy emitted, transferred, or received in the form of radiation. Unit: joules (J). Symbol: *Q*

radiant exposure. Surface density of the radiant energy received, expressed in units of joules-per-centimeter squared ($J{\cdot}cm^{-2}$). Symbol: *H*

radiant flux. Power emitted, transferred, or received in the form of radiation. Unit: watts (W). Also called *radiant power*. Symbol: Φ

radiant power. Power emitted, transferred, or received in the form of radiation, expressed in watts (W). Synonym: *radiant flux*.

radiometry. For the purposes of this standard, the measurement of infrared, visible, and ultraviolet radiation.

reflectance. The ratio of total reflected radiant power to total incident power. Also called "reflectivity."

reflection. Deviation of radiation following incidence on a surface.

refraction. The bending of a beam of light in transmission through an interface between two dissimilar media or in a medium whose refractive index is a continuous function of position (graded index medium).

refractive index (of a medium). Denoted by *n*, the ratio of the velocity of light in a vacuum to the phase velocity in the medium. Synonym: *index of refraction*.

repetitive pulse laser. A laser with multiple pulses of radiant energy occurring in a sequence.

retina. The sensory tissue that receives the incident image formed by the cornea and lens of the human eye.

retinal hazard region. Optical radiation with wavelengths between 0.4 and 1.4 μm, where the principal hazard is usually to the retina.

safety latch. A mechanical device designed to require a conscious decision to override the latch to gain entry into a controlled area.

scanning laser. A laser having a time-varying direction, origin, or pattern of propagation with respect to a stationary frame of reference.

scintillation. The rapid changes in irradiance levels in a cross-section of a laser beam.

secured enclosure. An enclosure to which casual access is impeded by an appropriate means, e.g., a door secured by a magnetically or electrically operated lock or latch, or by fasteners that need a tool to remove.

service. The performance of procedures, typically defined as repair, to bring the laser or laser system or laser product back to full and normal operational status. It does not include *operation* or *maintenance* as defined in this section.

shall. The word *shall* is to be understood as mandatory.

should. The word *should* is to be understood as advisory.

solid angle. The three-dimensional angular spread at the vertex of a cone measured by the area intercepted by the cone on a unit sphere whose center is the vertex of the cone. Solid angle is expressed in steradians (sr).

source. A laser or a laser-illuminated reflecting surface.

spectator. An individual who wishes to observe or watch a laser or laser system in operation, and who may lack the appropriate laser safety training.

specular reflection. A mirror-like reflection.

steradian (sr). The unit of measure for a solid angle. There are 4π steradians about any point in space.

standard operating procedure (SOP). Formal written description of the safety and administrative procedures to be followed in performing a specific task.

T_1. The exposure duration (time) at which MPEs based upon thermal injury are replaced by MPEs based upon photochemical injury to the retina.

T_2. The exposure duration (time) beyond which extended source MPEs based upon thermal injury are expressed as a constant irradiance.

T_{max}. The total expected or anticipated exposure duration (see Section 3 for classification; see Section 8 for intended use determination). T_{max} may differ depending upon its use.

telescopic viewing. Viewing an object from a long distance with the aid of an optical system that increases the visual size of the image. The system (e.g., binoculars) generally collects light through a large aperture thus magnifying hazards from large-beam, collimated lasers.

thermal effect. An effect brought about by the temperature elevation of a substance due to laser exposure.

threshold limit (TL). The term is applied to laser protective eyewear filters, protective windows, and barriers. The TL is an expression of the "resistance factor" for beam penetration of a laser protective device. This is generally related by the Threshold Limit (TL) of the protective device, expressed in $W{\cdot}cm^{-2}$ or $J{\cdot}cm^{-2}$. It is the maximum average irradiance or radiant exposure at a given beam diameter for which a laser protective device provides adequate beam resistance. Thus, laser exposures delivered on the protective device at or below the TL will limit beam penetration to levels at or below the applicable MPE.

t_{min}. For a pulsed laser, the maximum duration for which the MPE is the same as the MPE for a 1 ns exposure. For thermal biological effects, this corresponds to the "thermal confinement duration" during which heat flow does not significantly change the absorbed energy content of the thermal relaxation volume of the irradiated tissue.

transmission. Passage of radiation through a medium.

transmittance. The ratio of transmitted power (energy) to incident power (energy).

ultraviolet radiation. In this standard, electromagnetic radiation with wavelengths between 0.18 and 0.40 μm (shorter than those of visible radiation).

uncontrolled area. An area where the occupancy and activity of those within is not subject to control and supervision for the purpose of protection from radiation hazards.

viewing window. A visually transparent part of an enclosure that contains a laser process. It may be possible to observe the laser processes through the viewing windows.

visible radiation (light). The term is used to describe electromagnetic radiation which can be detected by the human eye. In this standard, this term is used to describe wavelengths which lie in the range 0.4 to 0.7 μm. Derivative standards may legitimately use 0.38 – 0.78 μm for the visible radiation range.

watt (W). The unit of power or radiant flux. 1 watt = 1 joule-per-second.

wavelength. The distance in the line of advance of a sinusoidal wave from any one point to the next point of corresponding phase (e.g., the distance from one peak to the next).

work practices. Procedures used to accomplish a task.

3. Hazard Evaluation and Classification

3.1 General.

Several aspects of the application of a laser or laser system influence the total laser hazard evaluation and, thereby, influence the application of control measures:

(1) The laser or laser system's capability of injuring personnel or interfering with task performance

(2) The environment in which the laser is used, including access to the beam path (considering enclosures, baffle, beam, etc.)

(3) The personnel who may use or be exposed to laser radiation

Note: See also Section 7 Non-Beam Hazards such as those resulting from interactions with the beam during its intended operation.

The laser hazard class is based on the laser's capability of injuring personnel (first half of aspect (1) above). Any laser or laser system shall be classified according to its accessible radiation during operation. Lasers and laser systems classified in accordance with this standard shall be labeled with the appropriate hazard classification (see Section 3.3). Classification labeling used in conformance with the Federal Laser Product Performance

Standard may be used to satisfy this labeling requirement. It should be noted that in some cases there may be differences between this standard and the Federal Laser Product Performance Standard (see Appendix C for references). Under the Center for Devices and Radiological Health (CDRH) Laser Notice 50, some products may also be labeled with the explanatory labels specified in IEC 60825-1 Ed. 1.2 (or latest revision thereof); these products are also considered as meeting the classification labeling requirement of this standard. However, if the laser has been modified subsequent to classification by the manufacturer, the laser may have to be re-classified (see Section 4.1.2).

Aspects (2) and (3) vary with each laser application and cannot be readily standardized. The total hazard evaluation procedure shall consider all aspects, although in most cases only aspect (1) influences the control measures which are applicable.

Only personnel trained in laser safety, optical engineering, physics or a related field are suited to perform the detailed hazard evaluation computations or the classification determinations of a laser or laser system as outlined in this section. In some instances, the LSO may not possess these qualifications, and may choose to delegate (effect) this responsibility. When this occurs, such evaluations are to be performed only by individuals who, as a result of training or experience, can provide knowledgeable technical assistance. Only then can the LSO be assured that the calculations and risk determinations will be accomplished correctly. Note that errors in such analysis could result in the specification of inadequate controls and present potentially hazardous conditions to personnel in the laser area.

3.2 Laser Considerations.

The LSO or knowledgeable individual responsible for laser classification shall ensure that laser output data are valid in accordance with Section 9 (Measurements). Classification shall be based on the maximum output power or radiant energy available for the intended use.

Note: The LSO would normally rely on the manufacturer's information for most commercial laser products and not need to perform measurements (see Section 1.2).

3.2.1 Multiwavelength Lasers. The classification of lasers or laser systems capable of emitting numerous wavelengths shall be based on the most hazardous possible operation (see Section 8.2.1).

3.2.1.1 A multiwavelength laser which by design can operate only as a single-wavelength laser shall be classified as a single-wavelength laser.

3.2.1.2 A multiwavelength laser which by design can operate over two or more wavelength regions (as defined in Section 8.2.3) shall require the classification to be determined in each region of operation. The classification of the laser shall be that of the most hazardous region. The appropriate control measures for each region shall be applied.

3.2.2 Repetitive-Pulse Lasers. The evaluation of repetitive-pulse lasers or exposures requires the use of certain correction factors (see Section 8). Within any time T, the AEL for multiple pulses or temporal variation shall not exceed the AEL for a single exposure of duration T.

3.2.3 Radiometric Parameters of the Laser Required for Determining Laser Hazard Classification.

3.2.3.1 Classification of essentially all lasers requires the following parameters:

(1) Wavelength(s) or wavelength range

(2) For CW or repetitive-pulse lasers: average power output within specified limiting apertures (effective power) and limiting exposure duration T_{max} inherent in the design or intended use of the laser or laser system

(3) For pulsed lasers: total energy per pulse (or peak power) within specified limiting apertures (effective energy), pulse duration, pulse repetition frequency, and emergent beam radiant exposure

3.2.3.2 Classification of extended source lasers or laser systems (such as laser arrays, injection laser diodes, and lasers having a permanent diffuser within the output optics) requires, in addition to the parameters listed in Section 3.2.3.1, knowledge of the apparent visual angle subtended by the source. However, evaluating these laser sources as point sources will provide conservative results.

3.2.3.3 Classification of highly diverging beam lasers (e.g., many laser diode emitters) requires determination of effective power or energy at the specified distance (see Section 9). This determination is made at the distance indicating the greatest hazard, but no closer than 10 cm from the closest point of human access (Condition 2). Determinations of hazards from optically aided viewing (i.e., telescopes and binoculars) should be made at the distance indicating the greatest hazard, but no closer than 2 m from the laser exit port, for all wavelengths (0.302 to 2.8 μm) that transmit through common optics (Condition 1). When determining hazards from optically aided viewing, the correct measurement aperture and measurement distance should be chosen from Table 9.

Note: See Appendix H for differences between the classification scheme of this standard and previous editions of this standard.

3.2.3.4 To determine the laser's potential for producing injury, it is necessary to consider not only if the laser output irradiance or radiant exposure exceeds the MPE for the unaided eye (treated by the measurement Condition 2) at 10 cm, but also whether a hazard would exist if the laser beam power or pulse energy were concentrated by optics and confined to the area of the limiting aperture from Tables 8a and 8b for the applicable MPE for the unaided eye. Table 9 provides the measurement apertures for the measurement of the AEL energy or power. The AEL for Class 1 is the identical energy for Class 1M, but measurement conditions differ (see Table 9).

Class 1M or 2M laser output shall be limited to the AEL for Class 3B under aided viewing measurement conditions (treated by the measurement Condition 1).

3.2.3.4.1 Most lasers can be considered point sources. For such lasers, the Class 1 AELs shall be determined by the product of two factors:

(1) The MPE for the unaided eye (see Tables 5a and 5b) for limiting exposure duration T_{max}

(2) The area of the limiting aperture for the unaided eye from Table 8b, i.e., the Class 1 AEL = MPE × (area of limiting aperture)

3.2.3.4.2 For lasers or laser systems which are extended sources and emit in the spectral range 0.4 µm to 1.4 µm, the MPE to be used in calculating the Class 1 AELs shall be determined from Table 5b. However, using Table 5a for evaluation of laser sources will provide conservative results. For thermal effects, the MPEs for extended sources include a correction factor C_E and often differ from the point source MPEs listed in Table 5a. The value of C_E is subject to the following conditions:

(1) For classification when telescopes will not be used, C_E is computed for the angle subtended by the source at the evaluation distance (see Table 9). The evaluation distance is the minimum accessible distance that creates the maximum hazard, but no closer than 10 cm from the laser exit port (Condition 2).

Note: For focused beams, the laser beam is generally most hazardous near the external beam waist or focal point.

(2) For classification considering the use of telescopes, C_E is computed for the angles subtended by the source through the optics at the evaluation distance (see Table 9). The standard optic used for classification is a 7-power optic with a 50 mm entrance aperture (Condition 1). The angular subtense through the optics is the angular subtense for unaided viewing multiplied by the power of the optics. The evaluation distance for optics is the distance which creates the maximum hazard, but no closer than 2 m (Condition 1) from the laser exit port.

Note: For beams that have an external beam waist or focal point farther than 2 m from the laser, the laser beam is generally most hazardous near the external beam waist or focal point.

(3) Photochemical effects are based on radiance and integrated radiance averaged over the limiting cone angle (γ). For photochemical hazards, no corrections are necessary when optics are used to view extended sources larger than 11 mrad.

(4) For optically aided viewing of sources having a potential photochemical viewing hazard and an angular subtense smaller than 11 mrad, only the emitted power or energy contained within a cone angle of 11 mrad from the magnified image is used to compute the irradiance or radiant exposure that is compared to the MPE.

Note: If this determination is difficult to apply, point source MPEs from Table 5a may be used and will result in a conservative Class 1 AEL.

3.2.3.5 The AELs for Class 2 and 2M shall be determined in the same manner as Class 1 AELs, except the MPEs are based on an exposure duration of 0.25 s (aversion response). For CW point source conditions, the MPE is 2.5 $mW \cdot cm^{-2}$, and the AEL is 1.0 mW.

3.3 Laser and Laser System Hazard Classification Definitions.

Tables C1 and C2 in Appendix C offer summaries of levels for laser and laser system classification: Table C1 for CW lasers with emission duration $\geq$ 0.25 s; and Table C2 for pulsed lasers with an emission duration < 0.25 s.

3.3.1 Classes 1 and 1M Lasers and Laser Systems.

3.3.1.1 Any laser, or laser system containing a laser, that cannot emit accessible laser radiation levels during operation in excess of the applicable Class 1 AEL for any emission duration within the maximum duration inherent in the design or intended use of the laser or laser system is a Class 1 laser or laser system during operation. The maximum exposure duration is assumed to be no more than 30,000 s except for infrared systems ($\lambda > 0.7$ µm) , where 100 s shall be used. The exemption strictly applies to emitted laser radiation hazards and not to other potential hazards (see Section 7).

3.3.1.2 Lasers or laser systems intended for a specific use may be designated Class 1 by the LSO on the basis that use for a limiting exposure duration of T_{max} is less than 100 s, provided that the accessible laser radiation does not exceed the corresponding Class 1 AEL for any emission duration within the maximum duration inherent in that specific use.

3.3.1.3 Any laser or laser system that cannot emit during operation, accessible laser radiation levels in excess of the applicable Class 1 AEL under the conditions of measurement for the unaided eye, but exceeds the Class 1 AEL for telescopic viewing (Condition 1 in Table 9) and does not exceed the Class 3B AEL, for any emission duration within the maximum duration inherent in the design or intended use of the laser or laser system is a Class 1M laser or laser system. The maximum exposure duration is assumed to be no more than 30,000 s.

3.3.2 Classes 2 and 2M Visible Lasers and Laser Systems. Classes 2 and 2M lasers and laser systems are visible (0.4 to 0.7 µm) CW and repetitive-pulse lasers and laser systems which can emit accessible radiant energy exceeding the appropriate Class 1 AEL for the maximum duration inherent in the design or intended use of the laser or laser system, but not exceeding the Class 1 AEL for any applicable pulse (emission) duration < 0.25 s and not exceeding an accessible average radiant power of 1 mW. Class 2M lasers and laser systems pose the same ocular hazards to the unaided eye as Class 2, but are potentially hazardous when viewed with optical aids.

3.3.2.1 Any laser or laser system that cannot emit during operation accessible laser radiation levels in excess of the applicable Class 2 AEL under the conditions of measurement for the unaided eye, but exceeds the Class 2 AEL for telescopic viewing (Condition 1 in Table 9) and does not exceed the Class 3B AEL, for any emission duration within the maximum duration inherent in the design or intended use of the laser or laser system is a Class 2M laser or laser system. The maximum exposure duration is assumed to be no more than 0.25 s.

3.3.3 Classes 3R and 3B Lasers and Laser Systems

3.3.3.1 Class 3R lasers and laser systems include lasers and laser systems which have an accessible output between 1 and 5 times the Class 1 AEL for wavelengths shorter than 0.4 µm or longer than 0.7 µm, or less than 5 times the Class 2 AEL for wavelengths between 0.4 and 0.7 µm.

Note: Products can be classified as Class 1M and Class 2M even if their output exceeds Class 3R.

3.3.3.2 Class 3B lasers and laser systems include:

(1) Lasers and laser systems operating outside the retinal hazard region (i.e. < 0.4 µm or > 1.4 µm) which can emit accessible radiant power in excess of the Class 3R AEL

during any emission duration within the maximum duration inherent in the design of the laser or laser system, but which (a) cannot emit an average radiant power in excess of 0.5 W for $T \geq 0.25$ s or (b) cannot produce a radiant energy greater than 0.125 J within an exposure time $T < 0.25$ s.

(2) Visible (0.4 to 0.7 μm) and near infrared (0.7 to 1.4 μm) lasers and laser systems which emit in excess of the AEL of Class 3R but which (a) cannot emit an average radiant power in excess of 0.5 W for $T \geq 0.25$ s and (b) cannot emit a radiant energy greater than 0.03 C_A J per pulse. For this limit, pulses separated by less than t_{min} are to be considered one pulse.

3.3.4 Class 4 Lasers and Laser Systems. Class 4 lasers and laser systems are those that emit radiation that exceed the Class 3B AEL.

3.4 Environment in Which the Laser is Used.

Following laser or laser system classification, environmental factors require consideration. Their importance in the total hazard evaluation depends on the laser classification. The decision by the LSO to employ additional control measures not specifically required in Section 4 of this standard (or eliminate some that are, see Section 4.2), is influenced by environmental considerations principally for Class 3B and Class 4 lasers or laser systems.

The probability of personnel exposure to hazardous laser radiation shall be considered. This may be influenced by whether the laser is used indoors or outdoors. Examples of indoor applications include laser use in classrooms, machine shops, closed research laboratories or factory production lines. Examples of outdoor applications include laser use in laser light shows, highway construction sites, military laser ranges, the atmosphere above occupied areas, pipeline construction trenches, mining tunnels, free-space communications, or in outer space. Other environmental hazards (see Section 7) shall also be considered.

If exposure of unprotected personnel to the primary or specularly reflected beam is possible, the LSO shall determine the irradiance or radiant exposure for the primary or specularly reflected beam or the radiance of an extended source (see Appendix B) at the location(s) of possible exposure.

3.4.1 Nominal Hazard Zones. Where applicable, e.g., in the presence of unenclosed Class 3B and Class 4 beam paths, the LSO may specify the Nominal Hazard Zone (NHZ). If the beam of an unenclosed Class 3B or Class 4 laser or laser system is contained within a region having adequate control measures to protect personnel from exposure to levels of radiation above the appropriate MPE, that region may be considered to contain the NHZ. The NHZ may be determined by information supplied by the laser or laser system manufacturer, by measurement, or by using the appropriate laser range equation or other equivalent assessment as described in this section and Appendix B.

The LSO shall assure that consideration is given to direct, reflected and scattered radiation in the establishment of boundaries for the laser controlled area. The LSO may declare the laser use area as the NHZ in lieu of calculating all possible NHZ distances, such as in the case of a dedicated laser use room. Control measures are required within the NHZ and may fully enclose the NHZ when this area is limited in size (see Section 4.3.10). Viewing the main beam or a specular laser target with an optical instrument is potentially hazardous due to the instrument's light-gathering capability (see Section 4.3.5.2; Appendixes B4.2, B6.4.3 and B6.6.3; and Examples 22-24, 45, and 53). Therefore, use of such optical systems may effectively increase the NHZ boundaries and must be considered in the overall hazard analysis.

3.4.2 Indoor Laser Operations. In general, only the laser is considered in evaluating an indoor laser operation if the beam is enclosed or is operated in a controlled area. The step-by-step procedure described below in Steps 1 through 7 is recommended for evaluation of the NHZ of laser and laser systems when used indoors if there is a potential for exposure of unprotected personnel. In this evaluation, consider all optics (lenses, mirrors, fiber optics, etc.) which are a permanent part of the laser beam path.

Step 1. Determine and evaluate the NHZ of all possible beam paths. Include multiple beam paths due to lack of fixed positioning and unintended beam paths due to unstable mounts, bearing wear, vibration, etc.

Step 2. Determine the NHZ for specular reflections (as from optical surfaces).

Step 3. Determine the extent of hazardous diffuse reflections if the emergent laser beam is focused. Hazardous diffuse reflections are possible from a focused or small-diameter beam of a Class 3B laser. However, the angular subtense of the source is normally sufficiently small at all practical viewing distances that point source MPEs apply. Determine the NHZ.

Step 4. Determine the likelihood for operation or maintenance personnel being within the NHZ during operation.

Step 5. Determine whether optical aids such as eye loupes or hand magnifiers will be used within 10 cm of a highly diverging beam.

Step 6. Determine whether other hazards exist (see Section 7).

3.4.3 Outdoor Laser Operations. The total hazard evaluation of a particular laser system depends on defining the extent of several potentially hazardous conditions. In this evaluation, consider all optics (lenses, mirrors, fiber optics, etc.) which are a permanent part of the laser beam path. This may be done in a step-by-step manner, as given below in Steps 1 through 7.

Note: For normal optics, a maximum transmission that would be expected is 90% in the wavelength range 0.4 to 0.7 μm, and 70% in the wavelength range of 0.302 to 0.400 μm and 0.7 to 2.8. μm.

Step 1. Determine the NHZ of the laser. Calculations of radiant exposure or beam irradiance as a function of range can be made with the range equation (see Appendix B6.3).

These calculated ranges are only estimates beyond a few hundred meters, since uncertainties arise from atmospheric effects (for example, scintillation due to turbulence).

Step 2. Evaluate potential hazards from transmission through windows and specular reflections. Specular surfaces ordinarily encountered (for example, windows and mirrors in vehicles and windows in buildings) are oriented vertically and will usually reflect a horizontal beam in a horizontal plane.

Note: As much as 8% of the beam's original irradiance or radiant exposure can be reflected toward the laser from a clear glass window which is oriented perpendicular to the beam. If the beam strikes a flat, specular surface at an angle, a much greater percentage of the beam can be reflected beyond, or to the side of, the target area. If the beam strikes a still pond or other similar surface at a grazing angle, effective reflectivity also may be high. Specular reflective surfaces, such as raindrops, wet leaves, and most other shiny natural objects, seldom reflect hazardous radiant intensities beyond one meter from these reflectors.

Step 3. Determine whether hazardous diffuse reflections exist (see Table 3 and Examples 47 - 55 in Appendix B6.6). Determine the corresponding NHZ.

Step 4. Determine whether the beam will visually interfere with critical tasks. Refer to ANSI Z136.6 for more information on operation of visible laser systems outdoors at night.

Step 5. Evaluate the stability of the laser platform to determine the extent of lateral range control and the lateral constraints that should be placed on the beam traverse. Determine the corresponding NHZ during operation.

Step 6. Consider the likelihood of people being in the NHZ.

Step 7. Determine whether optical aids such as telescopes or binoculars could be used within or near the beam path.

Step 8. Determine if visible lasers will be used near airports at night. Levels of laser irradiance as low as 50 $nW \cdot cm^{-2}$ may be of concern. Refer to FAA Order 7400.2 (or latest revision thereof) and to ANSI Z136.6-2005 (or latest revision thereof) for additional guidance.

3.5 Personnel.

The personnel who may be in the vicinity of a laser and its emitted beam(s), including maintenance personnel, service personnel, visitors and operators, can influence the total hazard evaluation and, hence, influence the decision to adopt additional control measures.

3.5.1 If children or others unable to read or understand warning labels may be exposed to potentially hazardous laser radiation, the evaluation of the hazard is affected and control measures may require appropriate modification.

3.5.2. For certain lasers or laser systems (for example, lasers in a research setting, military laser rangefinders and some lasers used in the construction industry), the principal hazard control rests with the operator, whose responsibility is to avoid aiming the laser at personnel or flat mirror-like surfaces.

The following are considerations regarding operating personnel and those who may be exposed:

(1) Maturity of judgment of the laser user(s)

(2) General level of safety training and experience of laser user(s) (that is, whether high school students, military personnel, production line operators, scientists, etc.)

(3) Awareness on the part of onlookers that potentially hazardous laser radiation may be present and awareness of the relevant safety precautions

(4) Degree of training in laser safety of all individuals involved in laser operation

(5) Reliability of individuals to follow standard operating procedures (SOPs) and recommended control procedures

(6) Number of individuals and their locations relative to the primary beam or reflections, and potential for accidental exposure

(7) Other hazards not due to laser radiation which may cause the individuals to react unexpectedly or which influence the choice of personal protective equipment

Note: Examples of typical lasers classified in accordance with this standard are given in Table C1 and Table C2 of Appendix C. Examples of calculations which may be useful in applying this standard are given in Appendix B.

4. Control Measures

4.1 General Considerations.

Control measures shall be devised to reduce the possibility of exposure of the eye and skin to hazardous levels of laser radiation and other hazards associated with laser devices during operation and maintenance (see Section 7).

The LSO shall have the authority to monitor and enforce the control of laser hazards and effect the knowledgeable evaluation and control of laser hazards (see Sections 1.3.2 (1) and Appendix A1.1) and conduct surveillance of the appropriate control measures. The LSO may, at times, delegate specific responsibilities to a Deputy LSO or other responsible person (see Appendix A1.1).

For all uses of lasers and laser systems, it is recommended that the minimum laser radiation required for the application be used. Also, it is recommended that the beam height be maintained at a level other than the normal position of the eye of a person in the standing or seated positions.

Review of reported incidents has demonstrated that accidental eye and skin exposures to laser radiation, and accidents related to the non-beam hazards of a laser or laser system, are most often associated with the following conditions:

(1) Unanticipated eye exposure during alignment

(2) Misaligned optics and upwardly directed beams

(3) Available eye protection not used

(4) Equipment malfunction

(5) Improper methods of handling high voltage

(6) Intentional exposure of unprotected personnel

(7) Operators unfamiliar with laser equipment

(8) Lack of protection for non-beam hazards

(9) Improper restoration of equipment following service

(10) Eyewear worn not appropriate for laser in use

(11) Unanticipated eye/skin exposure during laser usage

(12) Inhalation of laser generated air contaminants and/or viewing laser generated plasmas

(13) Fires resulting from the ignition of materials

(14) Eye or skin injury of photochemical origin

(15) Failure to follow standard operating procedures (SOPs)

The thorough understanding of the scope of laser hazards can facilitate the choice of the most appropriate and/or required control measures. This can be implemented with training programs (see Section 5).

Engineering controls (items incorporated into the laser or laser system or designed into the installation by the user) shall be given primary consideration in instituting a control measure program for limiting access to laser radiation (see Section 4.3).

Enclosure of the laser equipment or beam path is the preferred method of control, since the enclosure will isolate or minimize the hazard.

If engineering controls are impractical or inadequate (see Sections 4.1.1 and 4.1.2), administrative and procedural controls (see Sections 4.4 and 4.5) and personal protective equipment (see Section 4.6) shall be used. The limits of any type of control measure (for example, failure modes of enclosures and eye protection, or the inability of some personnel to understand written warnings) shall be considered in developing a laser hazard control program.

Engineering, administrative, and procedural controls are summarized in Table 10.

4.1.1 Applicability of Control Measures. The purpose of control measures is to reduce the possibility of human exposure to hazardous laser radiation (see Section 3) and to non-beam hazards (see Section 7).

In some cases, more than one control measure may be specified. In such cases, more than one control measure which accomplishes the same purpose shall not be required.

4.1.1.1 Operation, Maintenance, and Service. Important in the implementation of control measures is the distinction between the functions of *operation*, *maintenance*, and *service*. First, lasers and laser systems are classified on the basis of the level of the laser radiation accessible during intended use (operation). Operation is detailed in the user operation instructions. Maintenance is a task specified in the maintenance instructions for assuring routine performance of the laser or laser system. This may include such frequently required tasks as cleaning and replenishment of expendables. Maintenance may or may not require beam access. Service functions are usually performed with far less frequency than maintenance functions (these may include replacing the laser resonator mirrors or repair of faulty components) and may require access to the laser beam by those performing the service functions. Service functions are delineated in the service manuals of the laser or laser system.

During periods of service or maintenance, control measures appropriate to the class of the embedded laser shall be implemented when the beam enclosures are removed and beam access is possible (see Sections 4.3.12 and 4.4.7).

The fact that beam access is possible during maintenance or service procedures will *not alter* the classification of the laser system which is based upon beam access conditions during operation.

Instructions for the safe operation of lasers and laser systems are provided by the manufacturer. However, under some conditions, such instructions may not be sufficiently detailed for specific application due to special use conditions. In this case, the LSO shall provide additional safety instructions.

> *Note: The applicability of the various control measures as related to class is summarized in Table 10. The classes to which the following sections apply are designated in parentheses in the title of each section title.*

The control measures described in the following subparagraphs of this section shall apply when a laser or laser system is in operation.

4.1.1.2 Supervised Laser Operation (Class 3B and Class 4). Class 3B and Class 4 lasers or laser systems shall be operated at all times under the direct supervision or control of an experienced, trained operator who shall maintain visual surveillance of conditions for safe use and terminate laser emission in the event of equipment malfunction or any other condition of unsafe use. The operator shall maintain visual access to the entire laser controlled area during all conditions of operation (see Section 4.3.10).

4.1.1.3 Unattended Laser Operation (All Classes). Only Class 1 lasers or laser systems shall be used for unattended operation in unsupervised areas without the implementation of additional control measures requirements as detailed below.

If a Class 1M, Class 2, Class 2M, or Class 3R laser or laser system is not operated at all times under the direct supervision or control of an experienced, trained operator, the laser or laser system shall be provided with a clearly visible label that includes the applicable information specified in Section 4.7.5.

If a Class 3B or Class 4 laser or laser system is not operated at all times under the direct supervision or control of an experienced, trained operator, the laser radiation levels to which access can be gained shall be limited by control measures such as beam traps, barriers, windows, or other means of area control so that unprotected spectators in the area shall not be exposed to levels that exceed the applicable MPE limits in any space in the area that they may occupy.

The unattended use of Class 3B or Class 4 lasers or laser systems shall be permitted only when the LSO has implemented appropriate control measures that provide adequate protection and laser safety training to those who may enter the laser controlled area during times of unattended use.

All areas where unattended Class 3B or Class 4 lasers and laser systems operate shall be provided with standard laser safety warning area signs containing the "Danger" signal word and appropriate instructions regarding the hazards of entry into the space when no operator is present (see Section 4.7.4).

4.1.2 Laser System Modifications (All Classes). The LSO may reclassify, using the provisions and requirements of this standard, a given laser or laser system which has been modified. However, one should note that lasers and laser systems which have been altered may necessitate recertification, reclassification, and compliance reporting under the requirements of the Federal Laser Product Performance Standard (FLPPS).

4.1.3 Lasers or Laser Systems for Health Care Use (All Classes). The control measures outlined herein shall not be considered to restrict or limit in any way the use of laser radiation of any type which may be intentionally administered to an individual for diagnostic, therapeutic, or medical research purposes, by or under the direction of qualified professionals engaged in health care. However, those administering and assisting in the administering of the laser radiation, as well as the patient where applicable, shall be protected by the control measures as outlined herein, and, as applicable, to the requirements as specified in the American National Standard for Safe Use of Lasers in Health Care Facilities, ANSI Z136.3-2005 (or latest revision thereof).

4.1.4 Electrical, Beam Interaction, and Other Associated Hazards. See Section 7.

4.1.5 Laser Pointers. It is recommended that the power of a laser pointer should not exceed 1 mW for most conventional uses.

The FDA includes laser pointers under the definition of a surveying, leveling, and alignment laser products. This is included in the U.S. Federal Laser Product Performance Standard (21 CFR Part 1040.11) for Specific Purpose Laser Products (latest revision). That section indicates that each such laser product shall comply with all of the applicable requirements of 1040.10 for a Class I, II, or IIIa laser product and shall not permit human access to laser radiation in excess of the accessible emission limits of Class I and, if applicable, Class II, or Class IIIa (CDRH classifications). Hence, by this definition, laser pointers are technically limited to the maximum Class 3R (5 mW) output.

Note: The FDA has issued a warning to parents and school officials about the possibility of eye damage to children from hand-held laser pointers which indicated that such devices are generally safe when used as intended by teachers and lecturers to highlight areas on a chart or screen. However, they are not to be considered as children's toys. They note that the light energy that laser pointers can aim into the eye can be more damaging than staring directly into the sun. Federal law requires a warning on the product label about this potential hazard to the eyes and the FDA suggests they should be used by children only with adequate supervision (www.fda.gov/bbs/topics/NEWS/NEW00609.html).

Laser pointers should be covered by an administrative control and not be given to children. It is of importance that users be aware that some communities have adopted local ordinances which impose limitations on laser pointer use and/or purchase.

Users of these products need to be alerted to the potential hazards and be encouraged to follow the recommended appropriate safety procedures. The key approach in safety programs for laser pointers is to recommend education and training to all involved with these products. The area posting recommendation in Section 4.3.9.1 (Class 3R) is not needed for laser pointers (see Appendix D1.2.3).

4.2 Substitution of Alternate Control Measures (Class 3B or Class 4).

Upon review and approval by the LSO, the engineering control measures specified in 4.3 and administrative controls specified in 4.4 for Class 3B and Class 4 lasers or laser systems, may be replaced by procedural, administrative (see Section 4.4), or other alternate engineering controls which provide equivalent protection. This situation could occur, for example, in medical or research and development environments.

Accordingly, if alternate control measures are instituted, then those personnel directly affected by the measures shall be provided the appropriate laser safety and operational training (see Sections 5 and 7).

4.3 Engineering Controls.

The engineering controls for a laser or laser system are as specified in Sections 4.3.1 to 4.3.14 and are summarized in Table 10.

Commercial laser products manufactured in compliance with the Federal Laser Product Performance Standard (FLPPS) will be certified by the manufacturer and will incorporate those engineering controls required by the FLPPS or the IEC 60825-1 standard (or latest revision thereof). The LSO shall effect any additional engineering control measures that are required as outlined in Section 4.

The use of the additional controls outlined in this section shall be considered in order to reduce the potential for hazard associated with some applications of lasers and laser systems.

Engineering controls (performance features) which are supplied by the manufacturer of certified products and are used in this document are described in Sections 4.3.1, 4.3.2, 4.3.3, 4.3.4, 4.3.5.1, 4.3.7, 4.3.8, and 4.3.14.

4.3.1 Protective Housings (All Classes). A protective housing shall be provided for all classes of lasers or laser systems (except as noted in Section 4.3.1.1). The protective housing may require interlocks (Section 4.3.2) and labels (Section 4.7).

Special safety procedures may be required when protective housings are removed, e.g., for alignment, (see temporary control area in Section 4.4.7). The use of appropriate eyewear is recommended at such times (see Section 4.6.2).

If a user-created enclosure does not meet the requirements of a protective housing (e.g., a non-interlocked cover), it shall be considered as a barrier or curtain and other controls are required per Section 4.3.1.1.

4.3.1.1 Operating a Laser without Protective Housing (Class 3B or 4). In some circumstances, such as research and development and during the manufacture or servicing of lasers, operation of lasers or laser systems without a protective housing may become necessary. In such cases the LSO shall effect a hazard analysis and ensure that control measures are instituted appropriate to the class of maximum accessible emission level to assure safe operation. These controls may include, but not be limited to:

(1) Laser controlled area (see Sections 4.3.10 and 4.3.11)

(2) Eye protection (see Section 4.6.2)

(3) Appropriate barriers, shrouds, beam stops, etc. (see Sections 4.3.8 and 4.6.4)

(4) Administrative and procedural controls (see Section 4.4)

(5) Education and training (see Section 5)

4.3.1.2 Walk-in Protective Housing (Embedded Class 3B or Class 4). Class 1 lasers or laser systems which contain embedded Class 3B or Class 4 lasers with protective housings which are of sufficient size to allow personnel within the working space (walk-in protective housings) shall be provided with an area warning system (floor mats, IR sensors, etc.) which is activated upon entry by personnel into the protective housing. The sensors shall be designed to interlock with the laser power supply or laser beam shutter so as to prevent access to laser radiation above the applicable MPE. Only authorized personnel shall be provided means to override the sensors for alignment or testing procedures if beam access is required for beam diagnostic purposes. If overridden, an appropriate warning (light, electronic tone, etc.) shall be activated. All appropriate control measures shall be implemented within the enclosure during such testing periods (see Sections 4.3.1.1, 4.3.12 and 4.6).

Note: Engineering controls are preferred over administrative controls.

4.3.2 Interlocks on Removable Protective Housings (All Classes with Embedded Class 3B or 4). Protective housings which enclose Class 3B or Class 4 lasers or laser systems shall be provided with an interlock system which is activated when the protective housing is opened or removed during operation and maintenance. The interlock or interlock system shall be designed to prevent access to laser radiation above the applicable MPE. The interlock may, for example, be electrically or mechanically interfaced to a shutter which interrupts the beam when the protective housing is opened or removed (see Section 7.2 for electrical hazards).

Fail-safe interlocks shall be provided for any portion of the protective housing which, by design, can be removed or displaced during operation and maintenance, and thereby allows access to Class 3B or Class 4 laser radiation. One method to fulfill the fail-safe requirement is the use of redundant electrical series connected interlocks.

The protective housing interlock shall not be defeated or overridden during operation unless the provisions of Section 4.3.1.1 have been fully implemented.

The LSO or designee should effect the regular inspection of the protective housing interlocks and verify they are functioning.

Adjustments or procedures during service on lasers or laser systems containing interlocks shall not cause the interlocks to be inoperative when the equipment is restored to its operational condition, except as noted in Section 4.3.1.1.

4.3.3 Service Access Panels (All Classes). Portions of the protective housing that are only intended to be removed from any laser or laser system by service personnel, which then permit direct access to laser radiation associated with a Class 3B or Class 4 laser or laser system, shall either:

(1) Be interlocked (fail-safe interlock not required), or

(2) Require a tool for removal and shall have an appropriate warning label (see Section 4.7) on the panel.

If the interlock can be bypassed or defeated, a warning label with the appropriate indications shall be located on the protective housing near the interlock (see Section 4.7). The label shall include language appropriate to the laser hazard. The interlock design shall not permit the service access panel to be replaced with the interlock remaining bypassed or defeated.

4.3.4 Key Control (Class 3B or Class 4). A Class 3B or Class 4 laser or laser system should be provided with a master switch. This master switch shall effect beam termination and/or system shutoff and shall be operated by a key, or by a coded access (such as a computer code). The authority for access to the master switch shall be vested in the appropriate supervisory personnel.

As an alternative, the master switch can be designed to allow system activation using a momentary switch action (or alternative) that initiates system operation with the option that the key (or alternative) can be removed after operation commences. In this mode, if the system ceases to operate, the key switch (or alternative) must again be used to restart the laser or laser system.

During periods of prolonged non-use (e.g., laser storage), the master switch should be left in a disabled condition (key removed or equivalent).

A single master switch on a main control unit shall be acceptable for multiple laser installations where the operational controls have been integrated.

All energy sources associated with Class 3B or Class 4 lasers or laser systems shall be designed to permit lockout/tagout procedures required by the Occupational Safety and Health Administration (OSHA) of the U.S. Department of Labor (see Section 10 for reference).

4.3.5 Viewing Windows, Display Screens, and Collecting Optics. In order to adequately address additional protection requirements, it is sometimes necessary to utilize a number of various protective devices such as viewing windows, display screens, and laser barriers as defined in Section 2.

4.3.5.1 Viewing Windows and Diffuse Display Screens (All Classes). All viewing windows and diffuse (reflective or transmitted) display screens included as an integral part of a laser or laser system shall incorporate a suitable means (such as interlocks, filters, attenuators) to maintain the laser radiation at the viewing position at or below the applicable MPE as determined by the LSO (see Section 4.6.2.5.2).

Important in the selection of window and display screen material are the factors of flammability and decomposition products of the material. It is essential that the material used for viewing windows and diffuse display screens does not support combustion or release laser generated airborne contaminants (LGAC) above the current occupational limits following exposure to laser radiation unless the proper safeguards are in place to ensure personnel safety (see Section 7).

4.3.5.2 Collecting Optics (All Classes). All collecting optics (such as lenses, telescopes, microscopes, endoscopes, eye-loupes, etc.) that integrate the use of a laser or laser system shall incorporate suitable means (such as interlocks, filters, attenuators) to maintain the laser radiation transmitted through the collecting optics to levels at or below the appropriate MPE, as determined by the LSO (see Section 4.6.2.5.2). Collecting optics filter housings shall be labeled in accordance with Section 4.6.5.3.

Note: Normal or prescription eyewear are not considered collecting optics.

4.3.6 Beam Paths (Class 3B or Class 4). Control of the laser beam path shall be accomplished as described in the following (see also Appendix B).

4.3.6.1 Fully Open Beam Path (Class 3B or Class 4). In applications of Class 3B or Class 4 lasers or laser systems where a beam path is unenclosed a laser hazard evaluation shall be effected by the LSO.

In some cases, the total hazard assessment may be dependent upon the nature of the environment, the geometry of the application or the spatial limitations of other hazards associated with the laser use. This may include, for example, localized fume or radiant exposure hazards produced during laser material processing or surgery, robotic working envelopes, location of walls, barriers, or other equipment in the laser environment (see Section 4.1.4 and Section 7).

4.3.6.2 Limited Open Beam Path (Class 3B or Class 4). In applications of Class 3B or Class 4 lasers or laser systems where the beam path is confined by design to significantly limit the degree of accessibility of the open beam, a hazard analysis shall be effected by the LSO. The analysis will define the area where laser radiation is accessible at levels above the appropriate MPE and will define the appropriate control measures in that area. The LSO shall establish controls appropriate to the magnitude and extent of the accessible radiation.

4.3.6.2.1 Class 1 Conditions. Frequently the hazard analysis will define an extremely limited NHZ and procedural controls can provide adequate protection. Class 1 conditions shall be considered as fulfilled for those limited open beam path lasers or laser systems where analysis, including measurements when necessary, confirms that the accessible levels during operation are at or below applicable MPE levels.

4.3.6.3 Enclosed Beam Path (All Classes). In applications of lasers or laser systems where the entire beam path is enclosed, and the enclosure fulfills all requirements of a protective housing (i.e., limits the laser radiation exposure at or below the applicable MPE; see Sections 4.3.1 and 4.3.2), the requirements of Class 1 are fulfilled and no further controls are required.

When the protective housing requirements are temporarily relaxed, such as during service, the LSO shall effect the appropriate controls. These may include a temporary laser control area (see Section 4.3.12) and administrative and procedural controls (see Section 4.4).

Protective housings which are of sufficient size to allow personnel within the enclosure (walk-in protective housings) require special interlocking (see Section 4.3.1.2).

4.3.7 Remote Interlock Connector (Class 3B or Class 4). A Class 3B laser or laser system should and Class 4 laser or laser system shall be provided with a remote interlock connector. The interlock connector facilitates electrical connections to an emergency master disconnector interlock, or to a room, entryway, floor, or area interlock, as may be required for a Class 4 controlled area (see Section 4.3.10.2).

When the terminals of the connector are open-circuited, the accessible radiation shall not exceed the applicable MPE.

4.3.8 Beam Stop or Attenuator (Class 3B or Class 4). A Class 3B laser or laser system should be provided with a permanently attached beam stop or attenuator (see Table 10).

A Class 4 laser or laser system shall be provided with a permanently attached beam stop or attenuator.

The beam stop or attenuator shall be capable of preventing access to laser radiation in excess of the applicable MPE when the laser or laser system output is not required, as in warm up procedures.

There may be a few instances, such as during service, when a temporary beam attenuator placed over the beam aperture can reduce the level of accessible laser radiation to levels at or below the applicable MPE. In this case, the LSO may deem that laser eye protection is not required.

Note: For those lasers or laser systems that do not require a warm-up time, the main power switch may be substituted for the requirement of a beam stop or attenuator.

4.3.9 Laser Area Warning Signs and Activation Warnings (Class 3R, Class 3B, or Class 4).

4.3.9.1 Warning Signs – Posting (Class 3R, Class 3B or Class 4).

Class 3R Laser Area: An area which contains a Class 3R laser or laser system should be posted with the appropriate sign as described in Section 4.7, except as excluded by Sections 4.5.1.10 and 4.1.5 (laser pointer).

Class 3B or Class 4 Laser Area: An area which contains a Class 3B or Class 4 laser or laser system shall be posted as described in Sections 4.3.10.1, 4.3.10.2, and 4.3.11.1 with the appropriate sign described in Section 4.7, except as excluded by Section 4.5.1.10.

Temporary Laser Controlled Area (Class 3B and Class 4): The exterior boundary of a temporary laser controlled area (see Section 4.3.12) shall be posted with a Notice sign as described in Section 4.7, and as detailed in Section 4.7.3.3.

4.3.9.2 Warning Signs – Purpose (Class 3R, Class 3B, or Class 4). The purpose of a laser area warning sign is to convey a rapid visual hazard-alerting message that:

(1) Warns of the presence of a laser hazard in the area

(2) Indicates specific policy in effect relative to laser controls

(3) Indicates the severity of the hazard (e.g., class of laser, NHZ extent, etc.)

(4) Instructs appropriate action(s) to take to reduce the hazard (eyewear requirements, etc.)

The laser warning signs shall utilize warning statements as defined in Section 5 of ANSI Z535.2-1998 (or latest revision thereof), Standard for Environmental and Facility Safety Signs, where the signal words have the following meanings:

"DANGER" indicates an imminently hazardous situation which, if not avoided, will result in death or serious injury. This signal word is to be limited to the most extreme conditions.

"CAUTION" indicates a potentially hazardous situation which, if not avoided, may result in minor or moderate injury. It may also be used to alert against unsafe practices.

"NOTICE" is used to indicate a statement of facility policy as the message relates directly or indirectly to the safety of personnel or the protection of property. This signal word shall not be associated directly with a hazard or hazardous situation and must not be used in place of "DANGER" or "CAUTION".

The laser area warning signs shall be designed as detailed in Section 4.7 and are to be posted as detailed in Sections 4.3.10.1, 4.3.10.2 and 4.3.11.1 and summarized in Table 11.

4.3.9.3 Warning Signs for Non-Beam Hazards. Warning signs for non-beam hazards (e.g., LGACs, electrical, compressed gases) as detailed in Section 7, shall be posted when the hazards are possible as specified in the current revision of ANSI 535.2 (see Multiple Hazard Labeling Requirements) and/or other standards applicable to the specific hazard(s) (see Section 10).

4.3.9.4 Activation Warning Systems (Class 3B or Class 4). An activation warning system should be used with Class 3B, and shall be used with Class 4 lasers or laser systems during activation or startup.

4.3.9.4.1 Audible Warning Devices (Class 3B and Class 4). For single-pulse lasers or laser systems, an audible system may commence operation when the laser power supply is charged for operation, for example, during the charging of capacitor banks.

Note that distinctive and clearly identifiable sounds which arise from auxiliary equipment (such as a vacuum pump or fan) and which are uniquely associated with the emission of laser energy are also acceptable as audible warnings.

4.3.9.4.2 Visible Warning Devices (Class 3B and Class 4). One form of visible warning device is a single red light or lighted laser warning sign that flashes when the laser is operating and is readably visible through laser protective eyewear and also viewable within the area. The light can be electrically interfaced and controlled by the laser power supply so that the light is on and flashing only when the laser is operating.

Another possible configuration can be a warning light assembly that may be interfaced to the laser controller to indicate conditions of enabled laser (high voltage on), laser on (beam on), and area clear (no high voltage or beam on). *(Note: Only a green light shall be used to indicate a safe condition.)* In this case, the green light will indicate when the laser is not operational (high voltage off) *and* by an additional (yellow) light when the laser is powered up (high voltage applied, but no laser emission) *and* by an additional (flashing optional) red light that activates when the laser is operating.

Note: The LSO shall consider alternative control measures for the hearing and visually impaired.

4.3.10 Indoor Laser Controlled Area (Class 3B or Class 4). A laser hazard analysis shall be effected by the LSO. If the analysis determines that the classification associated with the maximum level of accessible radiation is Class 3B or Class 4, a laser controlled area shall be established and adequate control measures instituted (see Section 4.3.10.1 or 4.3.10.2).

Note: The requirements for nonenclosed lasers or laser systems involving the general public are detailed in Section 4.5.1.

4.3.10.1 Class 3B Indoor Laser Controlled Area (Class 3B). The Class 3B laser controlled area shall:

(1) Be controlled to permit lasers and laser systems to be operated only by personnel who have been trained in laser safety and in the operation of the laser or laser system. (see Section 5.5).

(2) Be posted with the appropriate warning sign(s) (see Section 4.7), except as detailed in Section 4.5.1.10. An appropriate warning sign shall be posted at the entryway(s) and, if deemed necessary by the LSO, should be posted within the laser-controlled area.

(3) Be operated in a manner such that the path is well defined

(4) Be well defined and controlled if the laser beam must extend outdoors and projects into a controlled airspace, particularly under adverse atmospheric conditions, e.g., rain, fog, snow, etc. (see Section 4.3.11.1 or 4.3.11.2).

In addition to the above, a Class 3B controlled area should:

(5) Be under the direct supervision of an individual knowledgeable in laser safety

(6) Be located so that access to the area by spectators is limited and requires approval, except as detailed in Section 4.5

(7) Have any potentially hazardous beam terminated in a beamstop of an appropriate material

(8) Have only diffusely reflecting materials in or near the beam path, where feasible

(9) Provide personnel within the laser-controlled area with the appropriate eye protection as specified in Section 4.6

(10) Have the laser secured such that the exposed beam path is above or below eye level of a person in any standing or seated position, except as required for medical use

(11) Have all windows, doorways, open portals, etc. from an indoor facility either covered or restricted in such a manner as to reduce the transmitted laser radiation to levels at or below the applicable ocular MPE

(12) Require storage or disabling (for example, removal of the key) of the laser or laser system when not in use to prevent unauthorized use

4.3.10.2 Class 4 Laser Controlled Area (Class 4). All Class 4 area or entryway safety controls shall be designed to allow both rapid egress by laser personnel at all times and admittance to the laser controlled area under emergency conditions.

All personnel who require entry into a laser controlled area shall be appropriately trained, provided with appropriate protective equipment, and shall follow all applicable administrative and procedural controls (see Section 5). For requirements for spectators in a laser controlled area see Section 4.4.6.

4.3.10.2.1 Emergency Conditions. For emergency conditions there shall be a clearly marked "Emergency Stop" or other appropriately marked device appropriate for the intended purpose (remote controlled connector or equivalent device) available for deactivating the laser or reducing the output to levels at or below the applicable MPE.

4.3.10.2.2 Entryway Controls. The Class 4 laser controlled area shall be designed to fulfill the items of Section 4.3.10.1 and in addition shall incorporate one of the following alternatives:

(1) Non-defeatable (non-override) Area or Entryway Safety Controls.

Non-defeatable safety latches, entryway or area interlocks (e.g., electrical switches, pressure sensitive floor mats, infrared, or sonic detectors) shall be used to deactivate the laser or reduce the output to levels at or below the applicable MPE in the event of unexpected entry into the laser controlled area (see Figure 2a).

(2) Defeatable Area or Entryway Safety Controls.

Defeatable safety latches, entryway, or area interlocks shall be used if non-defeatable area/entryway safety controls limit the intended use of the laser or laser system. For example, during normal usage requiring operation without interruption (e.g., long term testing, medical procedures, surgery), if it is clearly evident that there is no laser radiation hazard at the point of entry, override of the safety controls shall be permitted to allow access to authorized personnel provided that they have been adequately trained and provided with adequate personal protective equipment (see Figure 2a).

(3) Procedural Area or Entryway Safety Controls.

Where safety latches or interlocks are not feasible or are inappropriate, for example during medical procedures, surgery, etc., the following shall apply (see Figure 2b):

(a) All authorized personnel shall be adequately trained and adequate personal protective equipment shall be provided upon entry.

(b) A door, blocking barrier, screen, curtains, etc. shall be used to block, screen, or attenuate the laser radiation at the entryway. The level of laser radiation at the exterior of these devices shall not exceed the applicable MPE, nor shall personnel experience any exposure above the MPE immediately upon entry.

(c) At the entryway there shall be an activation warning system indicating that the laser is energized and operating at Class 4 levels (see 4.3.9.4).

4.3.11 Outdoor Control Measures (All Classes).

4.3.11.1 General. All Class 3B and 4 lasers or laser systems used outdoors shall meet the following requirements:

(1) The LSO shall effect an analysis to establish the NHZ if not provided as part of the documentation furnished by the manufacturer.

(2) If visible lasers are used at night, the LSO shall effect an analysis to determine if the laser beams will visually interfere with critical tasks. For operation of visible lasers at night near airports, refer to FAA Order 7400.2 (or latest revision thereof) and ANSI Z136.6-2005 (or latest revision thereof).

(3) The NHZ shall be clearly posted with laser warning signs and demarcated and identified as the laser hazard area (see Section 4.3.9.2). For conditions of navigable airspace see Section 4.3.11.2.

(4) All personnel authorized to enter the NHZ shall be appropriately trained (see Section 5.2).

(5) Only personnel who have been authorized shall operate a laser or laser system.

(6) Appropriate combinations of physical barriers, screening, and personal protective equipment shall be provided and used by those personnel authorized within the NHZ (see Section 4.6).

(7) Appropriate administrative controls shall be used if personnel are permitted within the NHZ (see Section 4.4).

(8) Directing the laser beam toward automobiles, aircraft, or other manned structures or vehicles shall be prohibited unless adequate training and protective equipment is provided and used by all affected personnel, or as authorized by the LSO and permitted by FAA Order 7400.2 (latest revision). In such authorized cases, it is essential that adequate training and protective equipment are provided and used by all personnel within these areas.

(9) The exposed laser beam path shall not be maintained at or near personnel eye level without specific authorization of the LSO.

(10) The beam path shall be confined and terminated wherever possible (see Section 4.3.8).

(11) When the laser is not being used, it shall be disabled in a manner that prevents unauthorized use (see Section 4.3.4).

(12) The operation of Class 4 lasers or laser systems during rain, snowfall, fog, or dusty atmosphere may produce hazardous scattering near the beam. In such conditions, the LSO shall evaluate the need for, and specify the use of, appropriate personal protective equipment.

4.3.11.2 Use of Lasers in Navigable Airspace (All Classes). The Federal Aviation Administration (FAA) is responsible for regulating the use and efficient utilization of navigable airspace to ensure the safety of aircraft and the protection of people and property on the ground. Laser experiments or programs that will involve the use of lasers or laser systems in navigable airspace should be coordinated with the FAA (Washington, DC 20590, or any FAA regional office) and U.S. Space Command (please consult with the current ANSI Z136.6) in the planning stages to ensure proper control of any attendant hazard to airborne personnel or equipment. Also refer to FAA Order 7400.2 (or latest revision thereof) and ANSI Z136.6-2005 (or latest revision thereof). Laser light show demonstrations that use Class 3B or Class 4 laser systems to create visible open beams shall coordinate with the FDA prior to use (See 4.5.1).

4.3.12 Temporary Laser Controlled Area (All Classes). In those conditions where removal of panels or protective housings, overriding of protective housing interlocks, or entry into the NHZ becomes necessary (such as for service), and the accessible laser radiation exceeds the applicable MPE, a temporary laser controlled area shall be devised for the laser or laser system.

Such an area, which by its nature will not have the built-in protective features as defined for a laser controlled area, shall provide all safety requirements for all personnel, both within and outside the area.

A Notice sign (see Section 4.7.3.3) shall be posted outside the temporary laser controlled area to warn of the potential hazard.

4.3.13 Controlled Operation (Class 4). Whenever appropriate and possible, Class 4 lasers or laser systems should be controlled and monitored at a position as distant as possible from the emission portal of the laser or laser system.

4.3.14 Equipment Labels (All Classes)

Note: Labeling of laser equipment in accordance with the Federal Laser Product Performance Standard (FLPPS) or the IEC 60825-1 standard (or latest revision thereof) may be used to satisfy the equipment labeling requirements in this standard.

4.3.14.1 Warning Logotype Label for Equipment (All Classes Except Class 1). All lasers or laser systems (except Class 1) shall have appropriate warning labels (see Section 4.7.5) with the laser sunburst logotype symbol and the appropriate cautionary statement. The label shall be affixed to a conspicuous place on the laser housing or control panel. Such labels should be placed on both the housing and the control panel if these are separated by more than 2 meters.

4.3.14.2 Protective Housing Equipment Label (All Classes). An advisory protective housing label that indicates the relative hazard of laser radiation contained within the housing shall be placed on all removable protective housings which have no safety interlock and which can be removed or displaced during operation, maintenance, or service, and thereby allow access to laser radiation in excess of the applicable MPE. The laser sunburst logotype symbol is not required on such advisory labels. See Section 4.7.5 (1)(a-e) for suggested wording.

4.3.14.3 Long Distance Beam Conduit Label (All Classes Except Class 1). The LSO shall effect posting advisory protective housing labeling on long distance (>3 meters) beam conduits that contain beams operating above Class 1 levels. Such labeling shall be placed on the outside of the conduit at appropriate intervals (approximately 3 meters), to provide warning of the relative hazards of laser radiation contained within the conduit. The laser sunburst logotype symbol is not required on such advisory protective housing labels. See Section 4.7.5 (1)(a-e) for suggested wording.

Note: This does not apply to optical fiber cable used for telecommunications, i.e., optical fiber communications systems (OFCS). See ANSI Z136.2-1997 (or latest revision thereof) or IEC 60825-2 (or latest revision thereof) for OFCS labeling requirements.

4.4 Administrative and Procedural Controls

Administrative and procedural controls are methods or instructions which specify rules, or work practices, or both, which implement or supplement engineering controls and which may specify the use of personal protective equipment. Unless otherwise specified, administrative and procedural controls shall apply only to Class 3B and Class 4 lasers or laser systems.

The use of administrative and procedural controls are summarized in Table 10.

4.4.1 Standard Operating Procedures (Class 3B or Class 4). The LSO should require and approve written standard operating, maintenance and service procedures (SOPs) for Class 3B lasers or laser systems. The LSO shall require and approve written SOPs for Class 4 lasers or laser systems. These written SOPs shall be maintained with the laser equipment for reference by the operator, and maintenance or service personnel (see Section 4.4.5).

4.4.2 Output Emission Limitations (Class 3R, Class 3B, or Class 4). If, in the opinion of the LSO, excessive power or radiant energy is accessible during operation or maintenance of a Class 3R, 3B, or Class 4 laser or laser system, the LSO shall take such action as required to reduce the levels of accessible power or radiant energy to that which is commensurate with the required application.

4.4.3 Education and Training (All Classes except Class 1). Education and training shall be provided for operators, maintenance and service personnel for Class 3B or Class 4 lasers or laser systems. Education and training should be provided for operators, maintenance and service personnel for Class 1M, Class 2, Class 2M and Class 3R lasers or laser systems and Class 1 lasers or laser systems containing embedded Class 3B or Class 4 lasers. The level of training shall be commensurate with the level of potential hazard (see Section 5 and Appendix D).

4.4.4 Authorized Personnel (Class 3B or 4 or Embedded Class 3B or 4). Class 3B or Class 4 lasers or laser systems shall be operated, maintained, or serviced only by authorized personnel. Lasers or laser systems with enclosed Class 3B or Class 4 lasers shall be maintained or serviced only by authorized personnel if such procedures would permit access to levels which exceed the Class 3R AEL.

4.4.5 Alignment Procedures (All Classes except Class 1). Laser incident reports have repeatedly shown that an ocular hazard may exist during beam alignment procedures.

Alignment of Class 2, 3R, 3B, or Class 4 laser optical systems (mirrors, lenses, beam deflectors, etc.) shall be performed in such a manner that the primary beam, or a specular or diffuse reflection of a beam, does not expose the eye to a level above the applicable MPE (see Section 4.6.2.5.2(3)).

There are many instances, such as during service, when a temporary beam attenuator placed over the beam aperture can reduce the level of accessible laser radiation to levels at or below the applicable MPE.

Written standard operating procedures (SOPs) outlining alignment methods should be approved for Class 3B and shall be approved for Class 4 lasers or laser systems. SOPs shall also be applicable for all classes of lasers or laser systems which contain embedded Class 3B or Class 4 lasers under conditions which would allow access during alignment procedures.

The use of lower power (Class 1, Class 2 or Class 3R) visible lasers for path simulation of higher power lasers is recommended for alignment of higher power Class 3B or Class 4 visible or invisible lasers and laser systems.

4.4.5.1 Alignment Procedures for Class 3B and Class 4 Lasers

Alignments should be done only by those who have received laser safety training. In addition, the following actions should be taken:

(1) Exclude unnecessary personnel from the laser area during alignment.

(2) Whenever possible, use low-power visible lasers for path simulation of higher-power visible or invisible lasers.

(3) Wear protective eyewear and clothing to the extent practicable.

(4) When aligning invisible (and in some cases visible) laser beams, use beam display devices such as image converter viewers or phosphor cards to locate beams.

(5) Perform alignment tasks, that use high-power lasers, at the lowest possible power level.

(6) Use a shutter or beam block to block high-power beams at their source except when actually needed during the alignment process.

(7) Use a laser-rated beam block to terminate high-power beams down range of the optics being aligned.

(8) Use beam blocks and/or laser protective barriers in conditions where alignment beams could stray into areas with uninvolved personnel.

(9) Place beam blocks behind optics (e.g., turning mirrors) to terminate beams that might miss mirrors during alignment.

(10) Locate and block all stray reflections before proceeding to the next optical component or section.

(11) Be sure all beams and reflections are properly terminated before high-power operation.

(12) Post appropriate area warning signs during alignment procedures where lasers are normally Class 1 (enclosed). See Section 4.3.12.

4.4.6 Spectators (Class 3B or Class 4). Spectators should not be permitted within a laser controlled area (see Sections 4.3.10 and 4.3.11) which contains a Class 3B laser or laser system and spectators shall not be permitted within a laser controlled area which contains a Class 4 laser or laser system unless:

(1) Appropriate approval from the supervisor has been obtained;

(2) The degree of hazard and avoidance procedure has been explained; and

(3) Appropriate protective measures are taken.

Laser demonstrations involving the general public shall be governed by the requirements of Section 4.5.1.

4.4.7 Service Personnel (All Classes). Personnel who require access to Class 3B or Class 4 lasers or laser systems enclosed within a protective housing or protected area enclosure shall comply with the appropriate control measures of the enclosed or embedded laser or laser system. The LSO shall confirm that service personnel have the education and safety training commensurate with the class of the laser or laser system contained within the protective housing.

4.5 Special Considerations.

4.5.1 Laser Demonstrations Involving the General Public.

4.5.1.1 General. Except as noted below, only Class 1 lasers or laser systems shall be used for general public demonstration, display, or entertainment in unsupervised areas without additional requirements. The use of Class 3B or 4 lasers in an artistic, demonstration or entertainment application will typically require a laser light show variance. This variance is issued by the U.S. Department of Health and Human Services, Food and Drug Administration, Center for Devices and Radiological Health. For further information, please reference Code of Federal Regulations – Performance Standard for Laser Products, 21 CFR Part 1010.10 and 1040.11(c) and the regulations addressing variance from performance standards, 21 CFR Part 1010.4. Note that the CDRH has established a form for applying for a variance for Class IIIb or IV laser light shows and displays. More information is available at the CDRH Internet site: http://www.fda.gov/cdrh/comp/rad_ nonion_products.html.

The following special control measures shall be employed for those situations where lasers or laser systems are used for demonstration, artistic display, entertainment, or other related uses where the intended viewing group is the general public.

Such demonstrations can be, but are not limited to, trade show demonstrations, artistic light performances, planetarium laser shows, discotheque lighting, stage lighting effects, and similar special lighting effects that use lasers or laser systems emitting in the visible wavelength range (0.4 to 0.7 μm).

For outdoor artistic laser operations, ANSI Z136.6-2005 (or latest revision thereof) and FAA Order 7400.2 (or latest revision thereof) should be consulted.

The applicable MPE may be determined by using the classification duration defined as the total combined operational time of the laser during the performance or demonstration within any single period of 3×10^4 seconds.

4.5.1.2 Operational Requirements - General. The use of Class 3B or Class 4 lasers or laser systems shall be permitted only when the LSO has assured that appropriate controls are incorporated which provide for adequate protection to the general public, and under the following conditions:

(1) When the laser operation is under the control of an experienced, trained operator as specified in Section 4.5.1.7

(2) When the laser is operated in an unsupervised laser installation provided that a designated person, present at all times at the show or display, is responsible for the immediate termination of the laser beam(s) in the event of equipment malfunction, audience unruliness, or other unsafe conditions. For training of operators see Section 5.

(3) When all federal, state, and local requirements for a safe operation have been met prior to the operation of the laser or laser system

(4) When pre-show alignment and verification have been completed

4.5.1.3 Invisible Laser Emission Limitations. The general public shall not be exposed nor have access to laser radiation emission at wavelengths outside the visible range (0.4 to

0.7 μm) at levels exceeding the applicable MPEs under any reasonably foreseeable conditions of operation.

4.5.1.4 Operators and Performers. All operators, performers, and employees shall be able to perform their required functions without the need for exposure to laser radiation levels in excess of the applicable MPE.

4.5.1.5 Scanning Devices. Scanning devices, including rotating mirrored balls, shall incorporate a means to prevent laser emission if scan failure or other failure resulting in a change in either scan velocity or amplitude would result in failure to fulfill the criteria given in Sections 4.5.1.3 and 4.5.1.4.

4.5.1.6 Unsupervised Installations - Distance Requirements. If a laser demonstration using a Class 3B or Class 4 laser does not operate at all times under the direct supervision or control of an experienced, trained operator, the laser radiation levels to which access can be gained shall be limited by barriers, windows, or other means so as not to exceed the limits of the applicable MPE. This limitation applies at any point less than 6 m above any surface upon which a person in the general public is permitted to stand and to any point less than 2.5 m in lateral separation from any position where a person in the general public is permitted to be present during a performance or display (see Figure 2c).

4.5.1.7 Supervised Laser Installations. Laser demonstrations which do not meet the criteria stated in Section 4.5.1.6 (applicable to Class 3B and Class 4) shall be operated at all times under the direct supervision or control of an experienced, trained operator who shall maintain constant surveillance of the laser display and terminate the laser emission in the event of equipment malfunction, audience unruliness, or other unsafe conditions.

The operator shall have visual access to the entire area of concern. If obstacles or size preclude visual access by the operator, then multiple observers shall be used, with a communication link to the operator. In such supervised installations accessible laser radiation shall be limited by barriers, windows, or other means so as to not exceed the applicable MPE at any point unless the following requirements are met:

(1) The accessible laser radiation is maintained a minimum distance of 3.0 m above any surface upon which the general public would be able to stand during a performance (see Figure 2d).

(2) The accessible laser radiation is maintained a minimum distance of 2.5 m in lateral separation from any position where the general public is permitted to be present during the performance or demonstration (see Figure 2e).

As a general practice, the largest practical vertical and lateral separation distances should be employed wherever possible. However, if specific physical limitations of the space in which the lasers are to be used preclude compliance with the required minimum separations specified in (1) and (2), shorter separation distances may be utilized, provided that the LSO assures that alternative measures are established which assure an equivalent degree of protection to the general public.

4.5.1.8 Beam Termination Requirements. All laser demonstration systems (applicable to Class 3B and Class 4) shall be provided with a readily accessible means to effect immediate termination of the laser radiation. If the demonstration does not require continuous supervision or operator control during its operation, there must be a designated person at all times at the show or display who is responsible for the immediate termination of the laser radiation in the event of equipment malfunction, audience unruliness, or other unsafe conditions.

4.5.1.9 Maximum Power Limitations. The maximum output power of the laser shall be limited to the level required to produce the desired and intended effect within the limitations outlined in Sections 4.5.1.1 through 4.5.1.8.

4.5.1.10 Posting of Warning Signs and Logos. If the laser installation fulfills all requirements as detailed in Sections 4.5.1.1 through 4.5.1.9 - or as alternatively provided by the LSO (see, for example, Section 4.5.1.7) - then posting of area warning signs shall not be required.

4.5.1.11 Federal, State, or Local Requirements. The laser operator or LSO responsible for producing the laser demonstration shall ensure that all applicable federal, state, or local requirements are satisfied.

4.5.2 Laser Optical Fiber Transmission Systems (All Classes). Laser transmission systems which employ optical cables shall be considered enclosed systems with the optical cable forming part of the enclosure. If disconnection of a connector results in accessible radiation being reduced to below the applicable MPE by engineering controls, then connection or disconnection may take place in an uncontrolled area and no other control measures are required. When the system provides access to laser radiation above the applicable MPE via a connector, the conditions given in Section 4.5.2.1 or 4.5.2.2 shall apply.

Note: The requirements and nomenclature for optical fiber systems used for telecommunications (OFCS) may differ from those pertaining to laser optical fiber transmission systems used for other purposes, e.g., optical power delivery. See ANSI Z136.2-1997 (or latest revision thereof) and IEC 60825-2 (latest revision) for requirements specific to optical fiber systems used for telecommunications.

4.5.2.1 Connection or disconnection during operation shall take place in an appropriate laser controlled area, in accordance with the requirements of Section 4.3.12, if the MPE is exceeded.

4.5.2.2 Connection or disconnection during maintenance, modification, or service shall take place in a temporary laser controlled area, in accordance with Section 4.3.12, if the MPE is exceeded. When the connection or disconnection is made by means of a connector, other than one within a secured enclosure, such a connector shall be disconnected only by the use of a tool.

Optical fibers or optical fiber cables attached to Class 3B or Class 4 lasers or laser systems shall not be disconnected prior to termination of transmission of the beam into the fiber. In this case, if laser radiation above the applicable MPE can be made accessible by disconnection of a connector, the connector shall bear a label or tag bearing the words "Hazardous Laser Radiation when Disconnected."

It is recommended that appropriate procedures be instituted to prevent inadvertent personnel exposure from an unterminated or severed fiber, such as lockout/tagout requirements at the laser source.

When the connection or disconnection is made within a secured enclosure, no tool for connector disconnection shall be required, but a warning sign appropriate to the class of laser or laser system shall be visible when the enclosure is open.

4.5.3 Laser Robotic Installations (Class 3B and Class 4). In many industrial applications Class 3B and Class 4 lasers and laser systems are used in conjunction with robots. In these situations, the robot working envelope (typically 3-6 meters) should also include the NHZ associated with the laser. In all cases where the beam is focused by a lens associated with the robotic device, appropriate laser-robotic safeguards can be assured if:

(1) The design or control measures in combination provide for a positive beam termination during operation.

(2) The beam geometry is limited to only the necessary work task.

(3) All workers are located at a distance greater than or equal to the lens-on-laser NHZ value for the laser robotic system.

In many instances, including those created by hardware failure and software errors, the laser beam from robotic delivery systems can be incident on the target surface at angles that could lead to potential scattering geometries that are very complex and require extensive evaluation. Measurements are often required to confirm the NHZ boundaries.

4.6 Protective Equipment.

4.6.1 General. Enclosure of the laser equipment or beam path is the preferred method of control, since the enclosure will isolate or minimize the hazard.

When other control measures do not provide adequate means to prevent access to direct or reflected beams at levels above the MPE, it may be necessary to use personal protective equipment such as protection in the form of goggles or spectacles, barriers, windows, clothing and gloves, and other devices that have been specifically selected for suitable protection against laser radiation.

It should be noted that personal protective equipment may have serious limitations when used as the only control measure with higher-power Class 4 lasers or laser systems; the protective equipment may not adequately reduce or eliminate the hazard, and may be damaged by the incident laser radiation.

4.6.2 Protective Eyewear (Class 3B or Class 4).

4.6.2.1 Eye Protection (Class 3B or Class 4). Eye protection devices which are specifically designed for protection against radiation from Class 3B lasers or laser systems should be administratively required within the NHZ and their use enforced when engineering or other procedural and administrative controls are inadequate to eliminate potential exposure in excess of the applicable MPE.

Eye protection devices which are specifically designed for protection against radiation from Class 4 lasers or laser systems shall be administratively required and their use enforced when engineering or other procedural and administrative controls are inadequate to eliminate potential exposure in excess of the applicable MPE.

Laser protective eyewear is usually not required for Class 2 or Class 3R lasers or laser systems except in conditions where intentional long-term (> 0.25 s) direct viewing is required.

Laser protective eyewear may include goggles, face shields, spectacles, or prescription eyewear using special filter materials or reflective coatings (or a combination of both) to reduce the potential ocular exposure below the applicable MPE.

Laser protective eyewear shall be specifically selected to withstand either direct or diffusely scattered beams depending upon the anticipated circumstances of exposure. In this case, the protective filter shall exhibit a damage threshold for a specified exposure time, typically 10 seconds (see Appendix C). The eyewear shall be used in a manner so that the damage threshold is not exceeded in the "worst case" exposure scenario. Important in the selection of laser protective eyewear is the factor of flammability (see ANSI Z87.1-2003, American National Standard for Occupational and Educational Personal Eye and Face Protection Devices, or the latest revision thereof).

Recent studies have indicated that existing laser eye protective filters (plastic, glass, interference, or hybrid filters) often exhibit non-linear effects such as saturable absorption when exposed to ultrashort (e.g., femtosecond) pulse durations. Laser users should request test data from laser eyewear manufacturers.

4.6.2.2 UV Laser Protection. Particular care shall be taken when using UV lasers or laser systems. Thus, in addition to other laser controls which apply to all laser systems, the following requirements shall also apply. Exposure to UV radiation shall be minimized by using beam shields and clothing which attenuate the radiation to levels below the applicable MPE for the specific UV wavelengths.

Hazardous byproducts: Special attention shall be given to the possibility of producing undesirable reactions in the presence of UV radiation. For example, formation of skin sensitizing agents, ozone, LGACs, etc. (see Section 7.4). Personal Protective Equipment (PPE), shall be used when working with open beam Class 3B or Class 4 UV lasers. This shall include both eye and skin protection.

4.6.2.3 Eyewear for Protection Against Other Agents. Physical and chemical hazards to the eye can be reduced by the use of face shields, goggles, and similar protective devices. Consult American National Standard for Occupational and Educational Personal Eye and Face Protection, ANSI Z87.1-2003 (or latest revision thereof).

4.6.2.4 Factors in Selecting Appropriate Eyewear. The following factors shall be considered in selecting the appropriate laser protective eyewear to be used:

(1) Laser power and/or pulse energy

(2) Wavelength(s) of laser output

(3) Potential for multi-wavelength operation

(4) Radiant exposure or irradiance levels for which protection (worst case) is required

(5) Exposure time criteria (see Section 4.6.2.5.2)

(6) Maximum permissible exposure (MPE) (see Section 8)

(7) Optical density requirement of eyewear filters at laser output wavelength(s) (see Table 2)

(8) Angular dependence of protection afforded

(9) Visible light transmission requirement and assessment of the effect of the eyewear on the ability to perform tasks while wearing the eyewear

(10) Need for side-shield protection and maximum peripheral vision requirement; side shields shall be considered and should be incorporated where appropriate

(11) Radiant exposure or irradiance and the corresponding time factors at which laser safety filter characteristics change occurs, including transient bleaching especially for ultrashort pulse lengths

(12) Need for prescription glasses

(13) Comfort and fit

(14) Degradation of filter media, such as photobleaching

(15) Strength of materials (resistance to mechanical trauma and shock) (see ANSI Z87.1-2003, or latest revision thereof, for appropriate criteria)

(16) Capability of the front surface to produce a hazardous specular reflection

(17) Requirement for anti-fogging design or coatings

4.6.2.5 Optical Density.

4.6.2.5.1 Specification of Optical Density, D_λ. The optical density (attenuation), D_λ, of laser protective eyewear at a specific wavelength shall be specified. Many lasers radiate at more than one wavelength; thus eyewear designed to have an adequate D_λ for a particular wavelength could have a completely inadequate D_λ at another wavelength radiated by the same laser. This problem may become particularly serious with lasers that are tunable over broad wavelength bands. In such cases, alternative methods of eye protection, such as indirect viewing, may be more appropriate (e.g., image converters, closed circuit TV).

If the potential eye exposure level or value is given by H_p, the optical density, D_λ, required of protective eyewear to reduce this exposure to the MPE is given by

$$D_\lambda = \log_{10} (H_p / \text{MPE}) = -\log_{10} \tau_\lambda$$

where H_p is expressed in the same units as the appropriate MPE and τ_λ is the transmittance of the filter at the specific wavelength (see Section 8).

Note: When the laser beam is smaller than the limiting aperture (D_f), the value of H_p is determined by averaging the beam energy over the limiting aperture (7 mm for the 0.4 to 1.4 μm region). This is necessary since the MPE has been established (normalized) relative to the limiting aperture area. Use of the beam diameter (a) to evaluate H_p for cases where $a < D_f$ will result in excessively large D_λ specifications.

Table 4 provides values for optical density for given values of H_p/MPE. If the beam size is larger than the size of the protective eyewear, it should be noted that optical densities greater than 3 or 4 (depending upon exposure time) could reduce eye exposure below the ocular

MPE but leave the unprotected skin surrounding the eyewear exposed to values in excess of the skin MPE as specified in section 8.4.

The optical density of the protective material shall be determined for all anticipated viewing angles and wavelengths.

4.6.2.5.2 Optical Density Time Basis Criteria. The duration of intended use of the laser or laser system shall be used as the time factor upon which the MPE computation is based when computing the optical density of a filter material (see Tables 2 and 4). The following are recommendations that are applicable in determining the time factor criteria:

(1) **Aversion Response Criteria to Visible Lasers (0.4-0.7 μm) (Class 3B or Class 4).** When long-term intrabeam exposure to visible lasers is not intended, the applicable MPE used to establish the optical density requirement for eye protection should be based on an exposure time of 0.25 second (see Section 8.2 and Table 4). This time factor is based upon the human aversion time for a bright light stimulus. Thus, this becomes the "first line of defense" for unexpected exposure to some lasers (see Section 8.2.2).

(2) **Near infrared Criteria (Class 3B or Class 4).** When long-term exposure to point source, near infrared (0.7-1.4 μm) lasers is not intended, the applicable MPE used to establish the optical density requirement for eye protection should be based on a 10 second exposure (see Section 8.2.2). This represents a realistic "worst case" time period because natural eye motions dominate for periods longer than 10 s.

(3) **Diffuse Viewing Criteria (Class 3B or Class 4).** When viewing an extended source or the diffuse reflection of the beam from a Class 3B or Class 4 laser or laser system where intermediate viewing time is intended, e.g., optical alignment procedures, the applicable MPE should be based upon the maximum viewing time which may be required during any given 8 hour period.

When long-term exposure to visible (0.4-0.7 μm) CW lasers is not specifically intended, the applicable MPE used to establish the optical density requirement for eye protection may be based on a 600-second exposure. This represents a typical "worst case" time period during tasks such as alignment and is applicable for most alignment procedures when viewing a diffusely reflecting target. In some situations where prolonged staring is anticipated, such as during surgical laser usage, even longer times should be considered, based upon actual conditions of use.

Note that if the extended source criteria (see Section 8.1) are not applicable due to a small beam size, then the exposure at the cornea from a diffuse reflector may be estimated using the inverse square law relationship, and the point source MPE criteria shall apply. In that case,

$$E = \rho\, \Phi \cos \theta_v / (\pi\, r_1^2)$$

where E is the irradiance produced at a distance r_1 (cm) from a diffuse surface, when the surface is irradiated by a laser with output Φ (watts), and where ρ is the reflection coefficient of the surface, and θ_v is the viewing angle relative to the normal to the surface.

If the angular source size exceeds α_{min} at the distance r_1, then the extended source criteria apply (see Section 8.1).

(4) **Daily Occupational Exposure Criteria (Class 3B or Class 4).** The time period of 30,000 seconds represents a full one-day (8-hour) occupational exposure and is determined from the approximate number of seconds in an 8 hour period.

The exposure duration is equal to the maximum time of anticipated direct exposure, which in a 24 hour period will not exceed 30,000 seconds except for ultraviolet wavelengths where additivity may occur (see Section 8.2.3.1).

When long-term exposure to any laser is possible, the applicable MPE used to establish the optical density requirement for eye protection shall be based on a 30,000 second exposure.

4.6.2.5.3 Optical Density for Non-Laser Emissions. Eye protection shall be provided for the ultraviolet and blue-green spectral region (0.18 to 0.55 μm) for laser welding processes. On the basis of currently available data, a minimum optical density, D_λ, of 2.0-3.0 (neutral density) or welding shade 6 (see American National Standard for Occupational and Educational Personal Eye and Face Protection, ANSI Z87.1-2003, or the latest revision thereof) is recommended for emission in the ultraviolet and blue-green spectral regions. The optical density values given above would apply for the laser induced plasma, such as that associated with typical laser welding systems. Greater optical densities are required for higher power laser welding systems.

The plasma emission optical density specified does not replace the optical density requirements for laser emission as specified in Section 4.6.2.5.1. See Section 7.2.2 for optical radiation hazards.

The luminous transmission of the protective filter that is needed to accomplish the task should be considered to allow adequate visibility without reducing the optical density (D_λ) necessary for laser protection.

4.6.2.6 Visible Transmission. Adequate optical density, D_λ, at the laser wavelength of interest shall be weighed with the need for adequate visible transmission.

4.6.2.7 Identification of Eyewear. All laser protective eyewear shall be clearly labeled with the optical density and wavelength for which protection is afforded (see Section 4.6.2.5). Color coding or other distinctive identification of laser protective eyewear is recommended in multi-laser environments.

4.6.2.8 Cleaning and Inspection. Periodic cleaning and inspection shall be made of protective eyewear to ensure the maintenance of satisfactory condition. The frequency of the safety inspection should be once per year, or as determined by the LSO. This shall include:

(1) Periodic cleaning of laser eyewear. Care should be observed when cleaning lenses of protective eyewear to avoid damage to the absorbing and reflecting surfaces. In some uses (e.g., surgery) eyewear may require cleaning (and sterilization) after each use. Consult eyewear manufacturers for instructions for proper cleaning methods.

(2) Inspection of the attenuation material for pitting, crazing, cracking, discoloration, etc.

(3) Inspection of the frame for mechanical integrity.

(4) Inspection for light leaks and coating damage.

Eyewear in suspicious condition should be tested for acceptability or discarded.

4.6.2.9 Purchasing Information for Protective Eyewear. Purchasers of laser safety protective eyewear should require that the following information accompanies each item:

(1) Wavelength(s) and corresponding optical density for which protection is afforded;

(2) Pertinent data such as damage threshold for laser safety purposes (see Appendix C for reference material); and

(3) Manufacturers' recommendations on shelf life, storage conditions, cleaning and use.

4.6.3 Facility Window Protection (Class 3B or Class 4). Facility windows (exterior or interior) that are located within the NHZ of a Class 3B or Class 4 laser or laser system shall be provided with an appropriate absorbing filter, scattering filter, blocking barrier, or screen which reduces any transmitted laser radiation to levels below the applicable MPE.

Such laser windows shall be specifically selected to withstand direct and diffusely scattered beams. In this case, the window barrier shall exhibit a damage threshold for beam penetration for a specified exposure time commensurate with the total hazard evaluation for the facility and specific application (see Appendix C).

Important in the selection of the window are the factors of flammability and decomposition products of the window material. It is essential that the window not support combustion or release toxic airborne contaminants following a laser exposure.

4.6.4 Laser Protective Barriers and Curtains (Class 3B or Class 4). A blocking barrier, screen, or curtain which can block or filter the laser beam at the entryway should be used inside the controlled area to prevent the laser light from exiting the area at levels above the applicable MPE. In some cases, where the barrier does not extend completely to the ceiling or to the floor, the LSO shall conduct an NHZ analysis to assure safety is afforded to all workers outside the barrier protected area.

Laser barriers shall be specifically selected to withstand direct and diffusely scattered beams. The barrier shall exhibit a damage threshold for beam penetration for a specified exposure time commensurate with the total hazard evaluation for the facility and specific application (see Appendix C).

Important in the selection of the barrier are the factors of flammability and decomposition products of the barrier material. It is essential that the barrier not support combustion or release toxic fumes following a laser exposure.

4.6.5 Labeling of Protective Equipment (Class 3B or Class 4). All protective equipment shall be permanently labeled as specified below:

4.6.5.1 Labeling of Laser Protective Eyewear. All laser protective eyewear shall be labeled with the optical density and wavelength(s) for which protection is afforded (see Section 4.6.2.4). Color coding or other distinctive identification of laser protective eyewear is also suggested when rapid eyewear identification is needed in multi-laser environments (e.g., surgery, research labs).

4.6.5.2 Labeling of Laser Protective Windows. All laser protective windows, sold other than as an integral part of a product, shall be labeled with the optical density and wavelength(s) for which protection is afforded (see Section 4.6.2.4). Such windows should also be labeled with the exposure time for which the limit applies and the conditions under which protection is afforded.

4.6.5.3 Labeling of Collecting Optics Filters. All permanently mounted collecting optics housings containing laser protective filters sold other than as an integral part of a product shall be labeled with the optical density and wavelength(s) for which protection is afforded (see Section 4.6.2.5). All collecting optics filter housings should also be labeled with the threshold limit (TL) and exposure time for which the limit applies and the conditions under which protection is afforded.

4.6.5.4 Labeling of Laser Protective Barriers. All laser protective barriers sold other than as an integral part of a product shall be labeled with the barrier exposure time for which the limit applies and the beam exposure conditions under which protection is afforded (see Appendix C2.4).

4.6.5.5 Labeling of Laser Protective Viewports and Films. All laser protective viewports and films sold other than as an integral part of a product should be labeled with the optical density and the spectral region for which protection is afforded (see Appendix C2.3). This information shall be provided by the manufacturer.

4.6.6 Skin Protection (Class 3B or Class 4). In some laser applications, such as use of excimer lasers operating in the ultraviolet, the use of a skin cover shall be employed if chronic (repeated) exposures are anticipated at exposure levels at or near the applicable MPEs for skin.

Skin protection can best be achieved through engineering controls. If the potential exists for a damaging skin exposure, particularly for ultraviolet lasers (0.295-0.400 μm) and/or laser welding/cutting application, then skin-covers and / or "sun screen" creams are recommended. Most gloves will provide some protection against laser radiation. Tightly woven fabrics and opaque gloves provide the best protection. In some cases a laboratory jacket or coat may fulfill the requirement. For Class 4 lasers, consideration shall be given to flame-retardant materials.

For wavelengths greater than 1.4 μm, "large-area" exposures can cause heat loading — causing skin dryness and with excessive exposure, may lead to heat stress (see Section 8.4.2). In these cases, personnel exposures shall be minimized.

Chronic exposure may have long term adverse health effects which are not fully understood at this time.

4.6.7 Other Personal Protective Equipment. Respirators, additional local exhaust ventilation, fire extinguishers, and hearing protection may be required whenever engineering controls cannot provide protection from a harmful ancillary environment (see Section 7).

4.7 Area Warning Signs and Equipment Labels.

4.7.1 Design of Signs. Sign dimensions, letter size and color, etc., shall be in accordance with American National Standard Specification for Accident Prevention Signs, ANSI Z535 series. Figures 1a and 1b show sample signs for Class 2, Class 2M, Class 3R, Class 3B, and Class 4 lasers or laser systems.

4.7.2 Symbols. Two similar laser symbol designs are accepted for laser signs and labels.

4.7.2.1 Laser Symbol Design. There are two possible designs that can be used:

4.7.2.1.1 ANSI Z535 Design. The laser hazard symbol shall be a sunburst pattern consisting of two sets of radial spokes of different lengths and one long spoke, radiating from a common center. This is as specified in the ANSI Z535 series of the National Standard Specification for Accident Prevention Signs. The wording can be used for area warning signs only, or alternatively as specified in Section 4.7.3.

4.7.2.1.2 IEC 60825-1 Design. The laser hazard symbol shall be composed of an equilateral triangle surrounding a sunburst pattern consisting of two sets of radial spokes of different lengths and one spoke, radiating from a common center (see Figure 1c). This is as specified in IEC 60825-1:2001 (or latest revision thereof).

4.7.2.2 Safety Alert Symbol. A symbol which indicates a potential personal safety hazard. It is composed of an equilateral triangle surrounding an exclamation mark and conforms to ANSI Z535.3-1998 (or latest revision thereof), Criteria for Safety Symbols. The symbol is to be located to the left of the signal word on the "Danger" or "Caution" signs. It is not used on the "Notice" signs.

4.7.3 Signal-Words Laser Warning Signs—Purpose (Class 3R, Class 3B, or Class 4). The purpose of a laser area warning sign is to convey a rapid visual hazard-alerting message that:

(1) Warns of the presence of a laser hazard in the area

(2) Indicates specific policy in effect relative to laser controls

(3) Indicates the severity of the hazard (e.g., class of laser, NHZ extent, etc.)

(4) Instructs appropriate action(s) to take to avoid the hazard (eyewear requirements, etc.)

The laser warning signs shall utilize warning statements as defined in Section 5 of ANSI Z535.2-1998 (or latest revision thereof), where the signal words have the following meanings:

"DANGER" indicates an imminently hazardous situation which, if not avoided, will result in death or serious injury. This signal word is to be limited to the most extreme conditions.

"CAUTION" indicates a potentially hazardous situation which, if not avoided, may result in minor or moderate injury. It may also be used to alert against unsafe practices.

"NOTICE" is used to indicate a statement of facility policy as the message relates directly or indirectly to the safety of personnel or the protection of property. This signal word shall not be associated directly with a hazard or hazardous situation and must not be used in place of "DANGER" or "CAUTION."

The laser area warning signs shall be designed as detailed in Section 4.7 and are to be posted as detailed in Sections 4.3.10.1, 4.3.10.2 and 4.3.11.1, and summarized in Table 11.

The following signal words are used with the ANSI Z535 design laser signs and labels:

4.7.3.1 Danger. The signal word "Danger" shall be used with all signs and labels associated with all lasers and laser systems that exceed the applicable MPE for irradiance, including all Class 3R, Class 3B, and Class 4 lasers and laser systems (see Figure 1b). The OD of protective eyewear and wavelength shall be shown on the sign for a location requiring the use of eyewear.

4.7.3.2 Caution. The signal word "Caution" shall be used with all signs and labels associated with Class 2 and Class 2M lasers and laser systems, which do not exceed the applicable MPE for irradiance (see Figure 1a).

4.7.3.3 Notice. The signal word "Notice" shall be used on signs posted outside a temporary laser controlled area (see Sections 4.3.12 and 4.3.9.2), for example, during periods of service (see Figure 1d).

Note: when a temporary laser controlled area is created, the area outside the temporary area remains Class 1, while the area within is either Class 3B or Class 4 and the appropriate danger warning is also required within the temporary laser controlled area (see Figure 1b and Section 4.3.12).

4.7.4 Pertinent Sign Information. Sign information and warnings shall conform to the following specifications.

4.7.4.1 The appropriate signal word (Danger, Caution, or Notice) shall be located in the upper panel.

4.7.4.2 Adequate space shall be available on all signs to allow for the inclusion of pertinent information. Such information may be included during the printing of the sign or may be handwritten in a legible manner, and shall include the following:

(1) At position 1 above the tail of the sunburst, special precautionary instructions or protective action that may be applicable. For example:

- (a) Laser Protective Eyewear Required
- (b) Invisible Laser Radiation
- (c) Knock Before Entering
- (d) Do Not Enter When Light is On
- (e) Restricted Area

Note: The class-based warning descriptions given in Section 4.7.5 (1) (a-e) can alternatively be used in position 1.

(2) At position 2 below the tail of the sunburst, the type of laser (Nd:YAG, Helium-Neon, etc.), or the emitted wavelength, pulse duration (if appropriate), and maximum output; and

(3) At position 3, the class of the laser or laser system.

Note: The word "Radiation" on signs and labels may be replaced by the word "Light" for lasers operating in the visible range at wavelengths greater than 0.4 μm and equal to or less than 0.7 μm. For lasers operating outside of this visible range the word "Invisible" shall be placed prior to the words "Laser Radiation."

4.7.4.3 Location of Signs. All signs shall be conspicuously displayed in locations where they best will serve to warn onlookers (see Sections 4.3.9, 4.3.10.1, 4.3.10.2, 4.3.11, and 4.3.12).

4.7.5 Pertinent Equipment Label Information. Equipment labels shall conform to the following specifications:

(1) At position 1 above the tail of the sunburst, special precautionary instructions or protective actions required by the reader such as:

(a) For Class 2 lasers and laser systems, "Laser Radiation - Do Not Stare into Beam"

(b) For Class 2M and 3R lasers and laser systems where the accessible irradiance does not exceed the applicable MPE based upon a 0.25 s exposure for wavelengths between 0.4 and 0.7 μm (see Section 3.3.3.1), "Laser Radiation – Do Not Stare into Beam or View Directly with Optical Instruments"

(c) For all other Class 3R lasers and laser systems, "Laser Radiation – Avoid Direct Eye Exposure"

(d) For all Class 3B lasers and laser systems, "Laser Radiation – Avoid Direct Exposure to Beam"

(e) For Class 4 lasers and laser systems, "Laser Radiation – Avoid Eye or Skin Exposure to Direct or Scattered Radiation"

Note: Labeling of laser equipment in accordance with the Federal Laser Product Performance Standard (FLPPS) or the IEC 60825-1 standard (or latest revision thereof) may be used to satisfy the labeling requirements in this standard.

(2) At position 2 below the tail of the sunburst, type of laser (Nd:YAG, Helium-Neon, etc.), or the emitted wavelength, pulse duration (if appropriate), and maximum output; and

(3) At position 3, the class of the laser or laser system.

4.7.5.1 Location of Equipment Labels. All equipment warning labels shall be conspicuously displayed in locations on the equipment where they best will serve to warn onlookers (see Section 4.3.14).

4.7.6. Existing Signs and Labels. Signs and labels prepared in accordance with previous revisions of this standard are considered to fulfill the requirement of the standard.

5. Education and Training

5.1 General.

Training shall be provided to each LSO and employee routinely working with or potentially exposed to Class 3B or Class 4 laser radiation. Training should be provided to employees working with or potentially exposed to Class 1M, Class 2, Class 2M or Class 3R laser radiation (see Appendix D). The level of training shall be commensurate with the degree of potential laser hazards, both from the laser radiation and non-beam hazards. The course topics selected from Appendix D, and the depth and skill level of content, shall largely be determined based on the results from a complete hazard evaluation as detailed in Section 3.

The employer should address the recommendations in Appendix D when determining the requirements for a laser safety training program. The laser safety program includes provisions for training the Laser Safety Officer (LSO) and users.

5.2 Refresher Training.

The employer shall address the needs for maintaining the appropriate level of laser safety proficiency through the use of periodic training.

The implementation and frequency of refresher training shall be considered on the basis of the total hazard evaluation criteria presented in Section 3 of this standard. The evaluation of personnel working with lasers and the amount of time they spend working with lasers are equally important considerations as the potential hazards from a laser. Occasional work with lasers may be a stronger justification for refresher or more frequent laser safety training than working daily with lasers, because the user's degree of familiarity is usually less with occasional work with lasers or laser systems. The level of education of the user is another major point for consideration.

Refresher training may be an abbreviated version of the original training, or it may simply be a generic overview of laser safety. Whatever form refresher training takes, the end result should be that the users have the necessary laser safety awareness and knowledge to continue to work safely with their lasers.

5.3 Trainer Qualifications.

Education and training programs shall be conducted by individuals with training skills adequate and appropriate to the subject matter being taught. For example, this would include, but not be limited to: knowledge of lasers, laser safety concepts, and laser safety standards.

Note: Experience has shown that the important factors are experience with lasers, good presentation skills, and a thorough knowledge of the applicable standards.

5.4 LSO Training.

Management (employer) shall provide for LSO training on the potential hazards (including bioeffects), control measures, applicable standards, medical surveillance (if applicable) and any other pertinent information pertaining to laser safety and applicable standards, or provide to the LSO adequate consultative services. The training shall be commensurate to at least the highest class of laser under the jurisdiction of the LSO. The training shall also include consideration for the evaluation and control of any non-beam hazards associated with the lasers and the laser systems under the jurisdiction of the LSO.

5.5 User Training.

Laser safety training shall be provided to the users of Class 3B or Class 4 lasers and laser systems. Laser safety training should be provided to users of Class 1M, Class 2, Class 2M and Class 3R lasers. Laser safety training shall include warnings against the misuse of lasers.

Users shall include operators, technicians, engineers, maintenance and service personnel, and any other persons working with or potentially exposed to laser radiation in excess of Class 1. The training shall ensure that the users are knowledgeable of the potential hazards and the control measures for laser equipment they may have occasion to use. All training shall be commensurate with the greatest potential for hazards associated with each laser operation, and shall be consistent with the results of the completed hazard evaluation as performed in accordance with Section 3 of this standard, which considers the laser, the environment, and the personnel.

Where appropriate, training shall include cardiopulmonary resuscitation (CPR) and safety procedures for applicable non-beam hazards associated with laser systems in use.

6. Medical Examinations

6.1 Examinations Following a Suspected or Actual Laser-Induced Injury.

Medical examinations shall be performed as soon as practical (usually within 48 hours) when a suspected injury or adverse effect from a laser exposure occurs. In addition to the acute symptoms, consideration shall be given to the exposure wavelength, emission characteristics and exposure situation to assure appropriate medical referral. See Appendix E for recommended examination protocol commensurate with the observed symptoms and laser system. For injury to the eye from lasers operating in the retinal hazard region, examinations shall be performed by an ophthalmologist.

6.2 Medical Surveillance.

The rationale for medical surveillance requirements for personnel working in a laser environment and specific information of value to examining or attending physicians are included in Appendix E. Medical surveillance should be limited to those who are clearly known to be at risk from particular kinds of laser radiation. Medical laser surveillance is not recommended for personnel using Class 1, Class 1M, Class 2, Class 2M or Class 3R lasers and laser systems as defined in Section 3.3, and should be required for Class 3B and Class 4 lasers and laser systems. Some employers may wish to provide their employees with additional examinations for medical-legal reasons, to conform to established principles of what constitutes a thorough ophthalmologic or dermatologic examination, or as part of a planned epidemiologic study. Further information is provided in Appendix E.

6.2.1 Personnel Categories. Each employee's category shall be determined by the LSO in charge of the installation involved. The individuals who should be under laser medical surveillance are defined in Sections 6.2.2 and 6.2.3.

6.2.2 Incidental Personnel. Incidental personnel are those whose work makes it possible (but unlikely) that they will be exposed to laser energy sufficient to damage their eyes or skin, e.g., custodial, military personnel on maneuvers, clerical, and supervisory personnel not working directly with laser devices.

6.2.3 Laser Personnel. Laser personnel are those who work routinely in laser environments. These individuals are ordinarily fully protected by engineering controls or administrative procedures, or both.

6.3 General Procedures.

6.3.1 Incidental personnel should have an eye examination for visual acuity (see Appendix E for further details).

6.3.2 Laser personnel should be subject to the following baseline eye examination:

Ocular history (see Appendix E3.2.1). If the ocular history shows no problems and visual acuity (see Appendix E3.2.2) is found to be 20/20 (6/6 in each eye for far and near) with corrections (whether worn or not), and Amsler Grid Test (see Appendix E3.2.3) and Color Vision (see Appendix E3.2.4) responses are normal, no further examination is required. Laser workers with medical conditions noted in Appendix E3.2.1 should be evaluated carefully with respect to the potential for chronic exposure to laser radiation. Any deviations from acceptable performance will require an identification of the underlying pathology either by a funduscopic examination (see Appendix E3.2.5), or other tests as determined appropriate by the responsible medical or optometric examiner.

6.4 Frequency of Medical Examinations.

For both incidental and laser personnel, required examinations should be performed prior to participation in laser work. Following any suspected laser injury, the pertinent required examinations will be repeated, in addition to whatever other examinations may be desired by the attending physician. Periodic examinations are not required.

7. Non-Beam Hazards

7.1 General.

It is important to address hazards associated with the use of lasers not related to exposure of the eye and skin to the laser beam. Non-beam hazards are a class of hazards that do not result from direct human exposure to a laser beam.

Non-beam hazards include physical, chemical, and biological agents. Non-beam hazards may occur when a material is exposed to a laser beam (e.g., fire or airborne contaminants); when materials used to generate the beam (e.g., flow-through gases, dyes and solvents) are released into the atmosphere; or when individuals contact system components (e.g., shock or electrocution).

In some cases, these hazards can be life threatening (e.g., electrocution). As a result, the hazards discussed in this section require use of control measures different from those discussed in Section 4. Also, all written SOPs shall address non-beam hazards as well as beam hazards.

Because of the diversity of non-beam hazards, the LSO may employ safety and/or industrial hygiene personnel to effect evaluations. Appendix F provides additional background material and references on non-beam hazards to assist the LSO in recognizing potential hazards.

7.2 Physical Agents.

7.2.1 Electrical Hazards. Electrical equipment in general presents three potential hazards: shock, resistive heating, and ignition of flammable materials.

7.2.1.1 Shock. The use of lasers or laser systems can present an electric shock hazard. This may occur from contact with energized electrical conductors contained in device control systems, power supplies, and other devices that operate at potentials of 50 volts and above. These exposures can occur during laser set up or installation, maintenance, modification, and service, where equipment protective covers are often removed to allow access to active components as required for those activities. Those exposed can be equipment installers, users, technicians, and uninformed members of the public, such as passers by.

The effect upon those who accidentally come into contact with energized conductors at or above 50 volts can range from a minor "tingle," to startle reaction, to serious personal injury, or death. Current pathways depend on complex parameters, so electric shock occurrence and outcome are difficult to predict. Electric shock is a very serious opportunistic hazard, and loss of life has occurred during electrical servicing and testing of laser equipment incorporating high-voltage power supplies.

Protection against accidental contact with energized conductors by means of a barrier system is the primary methodology to prevent electric shock accidents with laser equipment. Hazard warnings and safety instructions extend the safety system to embody exposures caused by conditions of use, maintenance, and service, and provide protection against the hazards of possible equipment misuse. It is recommended that electrical surge protection be provided to minimize transients, spikes, harmonics, outage, and electromagnetic interference (EMI).

7.2.1.2 Resistive Heating. Heating of a conductor due to electric current flow increases with the conductor's resistance. Unchecked and increasing resistive heating can produce excessive heat build up and potentially damage/corrode system components. While laser system designers generally provide sufficient cooling for routine operations, it is important that this equipment be regularly checked for excessive resistive heating symptoms such as component warping, discoloration, or corrosion, and repaired as needed.

7.2.1.3 Electric Spark Ignition of Flammable Materials. Equipment malfunctions can lead to electrical fires. In addition, electrical sparks can serve as an ignition source in the presence of a flammable vapor.

7.2.1.4 Electrical Hazard Control Measures. Additional electrical safety requirements are imposed upon laser devices, systems, and those who work with them, by the United States Department of Labor, Occupational Safety and Health Administration (OSHA), the National

Electrical Code (NFPA 70), and related state and local laws and regulations. These requirements govern equipment connection to the electrical utilization system, electrical protection parameters, and specific safety training. These requirements must be observed with all laser installations. In addition, it is recommended that fire extinguishers designed for electrical fires be used with laser systems. A "Panic Button" as described in Section 4 can also serve to eliminate or minimize electrical hazards in an emergency if the button cuts power to the system.

The following potential electrical problems have frequently been identified during laser facility audits:

(1) Uncovered and improperly insulated electrical terminals

(2) Hidden "power-up" warning lights

(3) Lack of personnel trained in current cardiopulmonary resuscitation practices, or lack of refresher training (see Section 5.2)

(4) "Buddy system" or equivalent safety measure not being practiced during maintenance and service

(5) Failure to properly discharge and ground capacitors

(6) Non earth-grounded or improperly grounded laser equipment

(7) Non-adherence to the OSHA lock-out standard (29 CFR 1910.147)

(8) Excessive wires and cables on floor that create fall or slip hazards

7.2.2 Collateral and Plasma Radiation. Collateral radiation is radiation other than that associated with the primary laser beam and is produced by system components such as power supplies, discharge lamps and plasma tubes. Such radiation may take the form of x-radiation, UV, visible, IR, microwave and radio-frequency (RF) radiation.

Plasma radiation is generated when an energetic laser beam interacts with matter, typically metals. This occurs when high power pulsed laser beams (peak irradiance of the order of 10^{12} $W{\cdot}cm^{-2}$) are focused on a target.

7.2.2.1 Collateral Radiation.

7.2.2.1.1 Radiation. X-radiation may be generated by electronic components of the laser system, e.g., high-voltage vacuum tubes (usually greater than 15 kV) and from laser-metal induced plasmas. The characteristics and intensity of x-radiation emanating from laser power supplies and components therein should be investigated. Additional radiation such as neutrons and high energy X-rays can be emitted by targets exposed to high irradiance beam interactions. All generated radiation (intentional or not) should be controlled in accordance with the provisions listed in applicable federal, state, or local codes and regulations.

7.2.2.1.2 Ultraviolet (UV) and Visible Radiation. Collateral UV emitted from laser discharge tubes and pump lamps shall be suitably shielded so that personnel exposures are maintained within exposure limits specified by the ACGIH (see latest version of Threshold Limit Values for Chemical Substances and Physical Agents and Biological Exposure Indices). UV radiation may cause photodermatitis or photokeritits. Photosensitizing agents from industrial chemicals or medications can make an individual more susceptible to those effects. See Appendix E for representative list of such agents. The presence of UV radiation at short wavelengths may produce ozone that will need to be exhausted.

7.2.2.1.3 Electric, Magnetic and Electromagnetic Fields. Power supplies and other electrical equipment associated with some lasers are capable of generating intense power frequency electric and magnetic fields (50 or 60 Hz and harmonics). MPEs for exposure to such fields at frequencies below 3 kHz are found in the latest version of the IEEE Standard for Safety Levels with Respect to Human Exposure to Electromagnetic Fields, 0 to 3 kHz (C95.6-2002). Some lasers contain radio frequency (RF) excited components, e.g., plasma tubes and Q-switches. MPEs for RF exposure are found in the latest version of the IEEE Standard for Safety Levels with Respect to Human Exposure to Radio Frequency Electromagnetic Fields, 3 kHz to 300 GHz (C95.1-2005); guidance for an RF safety program can be found in the IEEE Recommended Practice for Radio Frequency Safety Programs (C95.7-2005); appropriate RF warning signs and labels can be found in IEEE Standard for Radio-Frequency Energy and Current-Flow Symbols (C95.2-1999) (or latest revisions thereof).

7.2.2.2 Plasma Radiation. Plasma emissions created during laser-material interaction processes may contain sufficient UV and blue light (0.18 to 0.55 μm) to raise concern about long-term ocular viewing without protection. Studies have shown that the integrated blue-light irradiance levels are much higher for CO_2 than for Nd:YAG lasers. Also, welding events yield higher plume radiation levels than cutting events (see references in Appendix F).

7.2.3 Fire Hazards. Class 4 laser beams represent a fire hazard. Enclosure of Class 4 laser beams can result in potential fire hazards if enclosure materials are likely to be exposed to irradiances exceeding 10 $W{\cdot}cm^{-2}$ or beam powers exceeding 0.5 W. *(Note: The National Fire Protection Agency (NFPA) states that for CW lasers 0.5 $W{\cdot}cm^{-2}$ is a possible ignition hazard.)* Under some situations where flammable compounds or substances exist, it is possible that fires can be initiated by Class 3B lasers. The LSO should encourage the use of flame retardant materials wherever applicable with all laser applications.

Opaque laser barriers, e.g., curtains, can be used to block the laser beam from exiting the work area during certain operations (see Section 4.6). While these barriers can be designed to offer a range of protection, they normally cannot withstand high irradiance levels for more than a few seconds without some damage, e.g., production of smoke, open fire, or penetration. Users of commercially available laser barriers should obtain appropriate fire prevention information from the manufacturer. Users can also refer to NFPA Code #115 for further information on controlling laser induced fires.

Operators of Class 4 lasers should be aware of the ability of unprotected wire insulation and plastic tubing to catch on fire from intense reflected or scattered beams, particularly from lasers operating at invisible wavelengths.

7.2.4 Explosion Hazards. High-pressure arc lamps, filament lamps, and capacitor banks in laser equipment shall be enclosed in housings which can withstand the maximum explosive pressure resulting from component disintegration. The laser target and elements of the optical train which may shatter during laser operation shall also be enclosed or equivalently protected to prevent injury to operators and observers. Explosive reactions of chemical laser reactants or other laser gases may be a concern in some cases.

There have been several reports of explosions caused by the ignition of dust that has collected in ventilation systems serving laser processes. The potential for such can be greatly minimized by good maintenance practice.

7.2.5 Mechanical Hazards Associated with Robotics. In many industrial applications lasers are employed in conjunction with robots. Robots can punch holes in protective housing, damage the beam delivery system, and cause a laser beam to be aimed at operators or enclosures. In addition to such hazards, the mechanical safety of the robot installation must be carefully considered.

A number of accidents have occurred where a worker has been pinned between a robot and a confining object ("pinch effect"). The LSO should ensure that control measures to prevent these types of accidents are in place. These control measures may include the use of surface interlock mats, interlocked light curtains, or non-rigid walls and barriers. The installation should conform to recommendations contained in the latest version of ANSI/RIA R15.06 Standard for Industrial Robots and Robot Systems-Safety Requirements (or latest revision thereof).

7.2.6 Noise. Noise levels from certain lasers, such as pulsed excimers, and their work environment, may be of such intensity that noise control may be necessary. Consult the US Department of Labor, Occupational Safety and Health Administration Regulations and the ACGIH TLVs.

7.3 Chemical Agents.

These include laser generated airborne contaminants, compressed gases, dyes and solvents, and assist gases.

7.3.1 Laser generated Air Contaminants (LGAC). Air contaminants may be generated when certain Class 3B and Class 4 laser beams interact with matter. The quantity, composition, and chemical complexity of the LGAC depend greatly upon target material, cover gas, and the beam irradiance. The LSO shall ensure that industrial hygiene aspects of exposure to LGAC are addressed and that appropriate control measures are effected.

While it is difficult to predict what LGAC may be released in any given interaction situation, it is known that contaminants, including a wide variety of new compounds, can be produced with many types of lasers. When the target irradiance reaches a given threshold, approximately 10^7 $W \cdot cm^{-2}$ (see Table F1(a) in Appendix F), target materials including plastics, composites, metals, and tissues may liberate carcinogenic, toxic and noxious airborne contaminants. The amount of the LGAC may be greater for lasers that have most of their energy absorbed at the surface of the material.

Such compounds may be gaseous or particulate and can, under certain conditions, pose occupational concern (see Appendix F for a compilation of some LGAC).

Special optical materials used for far infrared windows and lenses have been the source of potentially hazardous levels of airborne contaminants. For example, calcium telluride and zinc telluride will burn in the presence of oxygen when beam irradiance limits are exceeded. Exposure to cadmium oxide, tellurium, and tellurium hexafluoride should also be controlled.

The LSO shall ensure that appropriate industrial hygiene characterizations of exposure to LGAC are effected in accordance with applicable federal, state, and local requirements. Exposure criteria are included in 29 CFR 1910 Subpart Z and The Threshold Limit Values for Chemical Substances and Physical Agents and Biological Exposure Indices (or latest version thereof) by the ACGIH. The LSO should refer to any Material Safety Data Sheet (MSDS) from the manufacturer of the laser system, laser machine or target material. This may provide some useful information, but many MSDS contain little information on the biological effects of decomposition products and/or LGAC. After characterization of the contaminant, it may be necessary for the LSO to effect appropriate control methods

7.3.2 Compressed Gases. Presently many hazardous gases are used in lasers and laser applications including chlorine, fluorine, hydrogen chloride, and hydrogen fluoride. All compressed gases having a hazardous material information system (HMIS) health, flammability, or reactivity rating of 3 or 4 shall be contained in an approved and appropriately exhausted gas cabinet that is alarmed with sensors to indicate potential leakage conditions. Standard operating procedures shall be developed for safely handling compressed gases. Some safety problems that occur with compressed gases are:

(1) Working with a free-standing cylinder not isolated from personnel

(2) Failure to protect open cylinders (regulator disconnected) from atmosphere and contaminants

(3) No remote shutoff valve or provisions for purging gas before disconnect or reconnect

(4) Labeled hazardous gas cylinders not maintained in appropriate exhausted enclosures

(5) Gases of different categories (toxic, corrosive, flammable, oxidizer, inert, high pressure, and cryogenic) not stored separately in accordance with OSHA and Compressed Gas Association requirements

7.3.3 Laser Dyes and Solvents. Laser dyes are complex fluorescent organic compounds which, when in solution with certain solvents, form a lasing medium for dye lasers. Certain dyes are highly toxic or carcinogenic. Since these dyes frequently need to be changed, special care must be taken when handling them to prepare solutions from them, and operating dye lasers. An MSDS for dye compounds shall be available to all appropriate workers.

The use of dimethylsulfoxide (DMSO) as a solvent for cyanine dyes in dye lasers should be discontinued if possible. DMSO aids in the transport of dyes through the skin and into the blood stream. If another solvent cannot be found, low permeability gloves should be worn by personnel any time a situation arises where contact with the solvent may occur.

Dye lasers containing at least 100 milliliters of flammable liquids shall be in conformance with the provisions of the NFPA (NFPA 30 and 45), and the NEC (Article 500 - Hazardous (classified) Locations). Laser dyes shall be prepared in a laboratory fume hood. Dye pumps and reservoirs should be placed in secondary containment vessels to minimize leakage and spills in conformance with NFPA 115.

7.3.4 Assist Gases. These gases may be used to produce an inert atmosphere, to remove material from the beam-interaction site, and to minimize deposition on components (e.g., mirrors or lenses). Assist gases have been shown to appear in types of LGAC and the spectral distribution of plasma radiation.

7.3.5 Control Measures. In general there are three major control measures available to reduce the concentration of chemical agents to acceptable levels. They are exhaust ventilation, respiratory protection, and isolation of the process. The priority of control requires that engineering controls be used as the primary control measure, with respiratory protection (and other forms of PPE) used as supplementary controls.

7.3.5.1 Exhaust Ventilation. Recirculation of LGAC should be avoided wherever possible. Exhaust ventilation shall be used to ensure that all personnel exposures to hazardous concentrations of LGAC are maintained at or below the allowable levels specified by OSHA, NIOSH, ACGIH, or other applicable authorities.

Whenever possible, enclosing hoods should be used to control LGAC. Enclosing hoods afford better control with lower air volumes than exterior hoods, are less susceptible to drafts, and may provide protection from reflected and scattered radiation.

Exhaust ventilation systems (including hoods, ducts, air cleaners, and fans) should be designed in accordance with recommendations in the latest revision of Industrial Ventilation (ACGIH) and Fundamentals Governing the Design and Operation of Local Exhaust Systems, ANSI Z9.2 (or latest revision thereof).

7.3.5.2 Respiratory Protection. Respiratory protection may be used to control brief exposures, or as an interim control measure until other engineering or administrative controls are implemented. If respiratory protection is utilized, the program shall comply with the provisions specified by the US Department of Labor, Occupational Safety and Health Administration (29 CFR 1910.134) (or latest revision thereof).

7.3.6 Process Isolation. The laser process may be isolated by physical barriers, master-slave manipulators, or remote control apparatus. Process isolation should be used with laser welding or cutting of targets such as plastics, biological material, coated metals, and composite substrates. In addition, during biomedical applications the work area and personal protective equipment shall be disinfected or sterilized immediately after use.

7.3.7 Sensors and Alarms. Sensors shall be installed in hazardous gas cabinets and other locations as appropriate, including exhaust ventilation ducts. Exhaust ductwork should be of rigid construction, especially for hazardous gases.

Sensors and associated alarm systems should be used for toxic and corrosive chemical agents such as halogen gases. Sensors should always be able to detect the hazardous gas in a mixture of emitted gases, i.e., fluorine versus hydrogen fluoride. Gas detection systems must be properly shielded to minimize susceptibility to electromagnetic interference (EMI).

7.4 Biological Agents.

These include LGAC and infectious materials. LGAC may be generated when high power laser beams interact with tissue. Infectious materials, such as bacteria and viral organisms, may survive beam irradiation and become airborne. For more information, see Appendix F and ANSI Z136.3-2005 (or latest revision thereof).

7.5 Human Factors.

7.5.1 Ergonomics. The LSO shall be aware of hazards created by neglecting ergonomic principles in laser system designs, such as poor workstation layout, worker-machine interface, manual handling techniques, and area illumination. Painful arm, hand, and wrist injuries (e.g., carpal tunnel syndrome) may result from repetitive motions occurring during the use of some laser products.

Recently, ergo-ophthalmological issues such as glare, startle reactions, afterimages and temporary flash blindness have been reported in the laser environment as distractions that lead to other primary or secondary effects of a more serious biological nature. The LSO should be aware that these types of ergo-ophthalmologic issues may create visual distractions in the workplace. While these types of low-level acute distractions can occur and need to be noted, they are not presently considered in this standard.

7.5.2 Limited Work Space. There is limited work space or area in many laser system installations. Such limited work space can present a problem while working near or around mechanical (e.g., robotics; see Section 7.2.5) or high voltage equipment (see the National Electric Code, Section 110-16). There must be sufficient room for personnel to turn around and maneuver freely (see OSHA 29 CFR 1910). This issue is further compounded when more than one type of laser is being operated at the same time. Audits have also shown that the presence of wires and cables on the floor of limited work areas can and do create trip and slip hazards. Whenever lasers or laser systems are used in limited work space, local exhaust, mechanical ventilation and respiratory protection shall be used if LGACs are present.

7.5.3 Work Patterns. Swing and third shift work patterns have been shown to affect worker alertness, as well as extended or excessive work hours, and hence safety compliance.

7.5.4 Laser and Laser Waste Disposal.

7.5.4.1 Laser Disposal. There are three basic ways to dispose of lasers that are no longer being used. The first method is to give/donate the laser to an organization that can use it. Such organizations might be schools, industrial companies, hospitals, etc. The donor should assure that the equipment being given complies with all applicable product safety standards, such as the FLPPS, and is provided with adequate safety instructions for operations and maintenance. The donor should ensure that the laser will be used by individuals who are trained in laser safety. Another approach would be to return the laser to the manufacturer for credit onto a new laser if applicable.

The second method is to eliminate the possibility of activating the laser by removing all means by which it can be electrically activated. Once this has happened the laser could then be disposed.

The third method would be to destroy the laser. The last two methods could have some land fill restrictions due to the possibility of hazardous materials being found inside the laser components, such as mercury switches, oils, and other chemicals.

7.5.4.2 Laser Waste Disposal. Proper waste disposal of contaminated laser-related material, such as flue and smoke filters, organic dyes, and solvent solutions shall be handled in conformance with appropriate federal, state, and local guidelines.

7.5.5 Chillers. Lasers can produce as much as 2-1000 watts of heat for every watt of optical power generated. In order to control this heat, laser manufacturers design laser systems to be conductivity-cooled, air-cooled, or cooled with a closed loop chiller. A chiller is a system designed to remove a certain heat load at a given temperature. It is recommended that users consult the manufacturer to obtain information on cooling approaches before activating the laser. If cooled water is used to aid in reducing heat loads, it may be useful to filter the incoming water to ensure that minerals and particulate matter are removed to minimize damage to equipment.

8. Criteria for Exposures of Eye and Skin

Maximum permissible exposures (MPEs) are below known hazardous levels. Appendix G provides reference material on biological effects. Exposure to levels at the MPE may be uncomfortable to view or feel upon the skin. Thus, it is good practice to maintain exposure levels sufficiently below the MPE to avoid discomfort. Distractions from the laser beam, such as flashblindness, glare, and startle, which can create secondary hazards, have become an increasing concern. These low-level effects are not covered in this standard, but are covered for nighttime use in FAA Order 7400.2 (or latest revision thereof) and in the ANSI Z136.6-2005 Standard for the Safe Use of Lasers Outdoors (or latest revision thereof).

The MPEs are expressed (normalized) relative to the limiting aperture area and, therefore, a limiting aperture or cone angle shall be used for measurements or calculations with all MPEs. The limiting aperture is the maximum circular area over which irradiance and radiant exposure can be averaged. (See Sections 3 and 9 for selection and application of the appropriate aperture or cone angle. See Section 8.2.3 for repeated exposures.)

The irradiance values for the MPEs in Tables 5a and 5b can be obtained by dividing the radiant exposure by the exposure duration, *t*, in seconds. Values for the radiant exposure can be obtained by multiplying the irradiance by the exposure duration, *t*, in seconds. For photochemical effects, the MPEs are provided in Table 5b as radiance or integrated radiance. See Section 9.1, Tables 8a and 8b, Appendix B7.2 and Figure B10 for limiting apertures and cone angles.

8.1 Ocular Exposures From Point Sources and Extended Sources.

For the purpose of this standard, within the retinal hazard region (0.4 to 1.4 μm) sources are considered either point or extended. Point sources subtend a visual angle less than or equal to α_{min} (1.5 mrad). Viewing a laser from within a collimated beam produces a small (20-30 μm) or nearly diffraction limited retinal image, which will be nearly a "point source." Point source MPEs are listed in Table 5a. These MPEs in the wavelength range of 0.4 μm to 0.6 μm are based on both thermal and photochemical effects to the retina. The computed time, T_1, separates which effect is dominant for a particular wavelength. Extended sources subtend an angle greater than α_{min}. The MPEs for extended sources are listed in Table 5b. Instead of using a computed time, T_1 as in Table 5a, both the thermal and photochemical MPEs in the wavelength range of 0.4 μm to 0.6 μm must be computed to determine which produces the lower MPE. For thermal effects the extended source correction factor C_E is used to modify the point source MPEs for exposures less than or equal to 10 s. (See Section 2 and Table 6 for definition of C_E). For photochemical effects C_E does not apply and the MPE is provided in Table 5b as radiance or integrated radiance averaged over a limiting cone angle γ. See Section 9.2.1.1, Appendix B7.2 and Figure B10.

Non-uniform sources such as laser arrays, multiple diode lasers, or non-uniform diffuse reflections require special considerations if the source subtends an angle greater than α_{min}. For non-circular sources, the effective diameter is determined as the arithmetic mean of the two dimensions (average dimension). When computing this average value, dimensions less than α_{min} are set equal to α_{min}, and values greater than α_{max} are set equal to α_{max}. For circular sources, the angular subtense is based on an effective Gaussian image at $1/e$ of peak irradiance points. In addition, laser energy not contained within a cone defined by α_{max}, centered on the source of laser emission, is not considered as contributing to the retinal exposure. (The MPE for sources larger than α_{max} are based on retinal irradiance or retinal radiant exposure.)

Each independent subsource of the extended source shall be considered as a separate source and the results compared with the MPE based on the source size of the separate source. Then the entire source (or any combination of subsources) shall be considered as a single source and the MPE shall be based on the size of the combination of subsources. Combinations of sources whose centers are separated by an angle greater than α_{max} (100 mrad) are considered independent.

Note: The angular subtense is not the divergence of the source. It is the apparent visual angle as calculated from the source size and distance from the eye. The limiting angular subtense, α_{min}, is that apparent visual angle which divides point source viewing from extended source viewing (see Appendix B3.5).

8.2 MPE for Ocular Exposures.

The single-pulse or single-exposure MPEs for ocular exposures are given in Tables 5a and 5b. In order to apply these MPE values, the information in the remainder of this Section is required (see Section 8.3 for special qualifications of use; see also Figures 3, 4, 5, and 9).

When a laser emits radiation at several widely different wavelengths or where pulses are superimposed on a CW background, the calculation of the MPE is complex. The effects of simultaneous exposure to pulsed and CW laser radiation can act synergistically. Caution should be used in these exposure situations until more data are available.

8.2.1 Wavelength. The wavelength (λ) must be specified to establish which spectral region is applicable. The MPEs in Tables 5a and 5b are arranged in broad wavelength regions expressed in micrometers (µm). For multiple wavelength laser emissions, the MPE must first be determined for each wavelength separately. Exposures from several wavelengths in the same time domain are additive on a proportional basis of spectral effectiveness with due allowance for all correction factors. In the ultraviolet region, special considerations may apply for multiple exposures (see Section 8.2.3.1).

8.2.2 Exposure Duration. For single-pulse lasers, the exposure duration is equal to the pulse duration t, defined at its half-power points.

When laser pulses are superimposed on a CW background, both thermal and photochemical exposure limits must be calculated separately and the exposure within any exposure duration T must not exceed the MPE for time T (see Appendix B3.3, Examples 10-16).

For non-visible wavelengths ($\lambda < 0.4$ μm and $\lambda > 0.7$ μm), the CW exposure duration is the maximum time of anticipated direct exposure, T_{max}. For the hazard evaluation of retinal exposures in the near infrared (0.7 – 1.4 μm) a T_{max} of 10 s (T_2 for extended sources) provides an adequate hazard criterion for either incidental viewing or purposeful staring conditions. In this case, eye movements provide a natural exposure limitation, eliminating the need for calculations based on exposure durations greater than 10 s, except for unusual viewing conditions. In special applications, such as health care or experimental conditions, longer exposure durations may be appropriate (see Section 8.3).

The MPEs for single-pulse exposures between 10^{-13} and 10^{-9} seconds, at 0.4 μm - 1.4 μm are listed in Tables 5a and 5b. Exposure limits for pulse durations less than 100 fs are not provided for the retinal hazard region (0.4 μm $< \lambda <$ 1.4 μm) and for all pulse durations less than 1 ns outside this spectral region because of a lack of biological data. For pulse durations less than 100 fs in the retinal hazard region (0.4 μm $< \lambda <$ 1.4 μm), it is recommended that the peak irradiance be limited to the MPEs applicable to 100 fs pulses. For pulse durations less than 1 ns outside of the retinal hazard region ($\lambda < 0.4$ μm and $\lambda > 1.4$ μm) it is recommended that the peak irradiance be limited to the MPEs applicable to 1 ns pulses.

For a CW or multiple-pulsed visible (0.4 – 0.7 μm) laser, the exposure duration is the maximum time of anticipated exposure, T_{max}. If purposeful staring into the beam is not intended or anticipated, the aversion response time, 0.25 s, may be used.

Note: For a CW laser under these conditions the MPE can be rounded to 2.6 mW·cm^{-2}.

8.2.3 Repeated Exposures. For repetitive-pulse lasers, no single pulse in the train can exceed the single-pulse MPE. The radiant exposure from a modulated output or from a group of pulses of duration T shall not exceed the MPE applicable to a single unmodulated exposure of time T. The total exposure duration T_{max} of the train of pulses is determined in the same manner as for CW laser exposures.

Rule 1: Single-Pulse MPE. The exposure from any single pulse in a train of pulses shall not exceed the MPE for a single pulse of that pulse duration. (Rule 1 protects against thermal injury from any single pulse having greater than average energy.)

Rule 2: Average Power MPE for Thermal and Photochemical Hazards. The exposure from any group of pulses (or sub-group of pulses in a train) delivered in time T shall not exceed the MPE for time T. That is, the total radiant exposure of all pulses within any part of the train shall not exceed the MPE for the duration of that part. Depending upon the complexity of the pulse train, the calculation of several potential MPEs (for different pulse groupings) may be required. The calculation of Rule 2 usually provides a lower MPE for lasers with a high duty cycle than by applying Rule 3 below. (Rule 2 protects against cumulative injury from photochemical damage mechanisms and also against heat buildup from average power for thermal injury.)

Rule 3: Multiple-pulse MPE for Thermal Hazards. The exposure for any single pulse ($t < 0.25$ sec) or group of pulses ($T < 0.25$ sec) (each separated by at least t_{min}) shall not exceed the single-pulse MPE (for $t \geq t_{min}$) multiplied by a multiple-pulse correction factor C_P.

The multiple-pulse correction factor C_P is $n^{-0.25}$, where n is the number of pulses (see Figure 13 for a graphical representation of $n^{-0.25}$). Rule 3 applies only to MPEs for thermal injury, where all pulses delivered in less than t_{min} are treated as a single pulse. (Rule 3 protects against sub-threshold pulse-cumulative thermal injury.) For individual pulses or groups of pulses, either delivered within a time frame less than t_{min}, or when the inter-pulse spacing between pulses or pulse groups is less than t_{min}, these pulse structures are treated as a single pulse in applying this rule. When all separations between pulses are less than t_{min} during the exposure duration, T_{max}, no C_P is necessary since the exposure is treated as CW for this rule.

Note: For repetition rates which are so high that multiple pulses occur in a time frame less than t_{min}, pulse energies delivered within those time frames are summed directly. It is assumed that the energy within t_{min} acts as if it were delivered in a single pulse.

The methods of applying the three rules for determining the MPEs for repetitive laser exposures for specific spectral bands and determination of t_{min} are given in 8.2.3.1 to 8.2.3.3. See 8.2.3.3 for proper apertures to use with each rule.

8.2.3.1 Repeated Exposures, Ultraviolet (0.180 to 0.400 µm) – Special Considerations. Photochemical effects generally are dominant in this spectral region, but dual limits do exist. The Rules from 8.2.3 are used to find those limits. Rules 1 and 2 apply to both limits, but Rule 3 applies only to the thermal limit (i.e., the MPE expressed as $0.56\ t^{\ 0.25}$), where t_{min} is 1 ns. Repeated exposures are additive over a 24-hour duration regardless of the repetition rate for the wavelength range of 0.180 to 0.400 µm, if the MPE is to protect against photochemical effects (i.e., those MPEs expressed as a constant radiant exposure for up to 30,000 s). Additionally, for the wavelength range of 0.280 to 0.400 µm, the applicable MPE for any 24-hour period is reduced by a factor of 2.5 times, if exposures on succeeding days are expected to approach that MPE.

8.2.3.2 Repeated Exposures, Visible (0.4 to 0.7 µm) and Infrared (0.7 to 1.4 µm). Dual limits apply in the short-wavelength part of the spectral region and the values from 8.2.3 are used for the calculations. For repeated exposures, the MPE per pulse is the lowest of the three calculated results using Rules 1, 2, and 3. For wavelengths between 0.4 to 1.05 µm, the value of t_{min} is 18 µs; whereas between 1.05 and 1.4 µm, t_{min} is 50 µs. The MPE to protect against photochemically induced retinal injury applies only to the visible part of the spectrum between 0.4 and 0.6 µm, and for exposure durations greater than 0.7 s. The exposure dose is linearly additive up to T_{max}. The MPE is also limited by the radiance of the source and can be expressed as 100 C_B $J{\cdot}cm^{-2}{\cdot}sr^{-1}$. For exposure durations of 0.7 s or less, the MPE computed by Rule 2 will result in a radiance less than this value. In all cases, the maximum duration to apply in determining "n" for Rule 3 from the duration of the pulse train T shall be T_2 seconds.

Note: In this spectral region (0.4 to 1.4 µm), the dividing line between Rules 2 and 3 is the critical frequency. For a short, unintentional exposure (0.25 to 10 s) to nanosecond (or longer) pulses, the critical frequency is 55 kHz for wavelengths between 0.4 and 1.05 µm, and 20 kHz for wavelengths between 1.05 and 1.4 µm. For longer exposure durations (0.4 to 0.7 µm) when the product of n and the pulse duration exceeds 10 s, Rule 2 often produces the lower limit, mainly due to photochemical interaction.

8.2.3.3 Repeated Exposures, Infrared (1.4 µm to 1 mm). Only thermal effects occur in this spectral region. The lower MPE calculated from Rules 2 and 3 from Section 8.2.3

determines the actual MPE. The critical frequency is much lower for these middle and far infrared wavelengths, and is often just a few hertz or less. Since different limiting and measurement apertures apply for pulsed versus CW exposures, the aperture for Rule 1 is determined from the duration of a single pulse. For Rule 2, the potential exposure for all exposure durations, T, less than or equal to T_{max} is compared with the MPE for T with the corresponding limiting aperture determined from T. For Rule 3, the aperture is determined from the duration of a single pulse ($\leq$ 0.25 s). The energy from a group of pulses with an inter-pulse spacing of t_{min} or less is considered a single pulse for Rule 3.

Note: For lasers with wavelengths greater than 1.5 μm but less than 1.8 μm, the single-pulse MPE [Rule 1] is the same as the CW MPE [Rule 2] for a 10 s exposure. Therefore, t_{min} is 10 s for such lasers; the MPE for each pulse in a train of pulses is simply the single-pulse MPE divided by the number of pulses in the train. For lasers with wavelengths greater than 2.6 μm, t_{min} is only 100 ns. For other infrared wavelengths, t_{min} is 1 ms.

8.3 Special Qualifications for Ocular Exposures.

Lower exposure MPEs are required for visible lasers (0.4 to 0.7 μm) when the eye is immobilized or has a large pupil such as in health care with ophthalmic instruments or in research situations. Lower MPEs are needed in order to protect against injury to the eye by visible light exposure (0.4 to 0.7 μm), while the normal protective mechanisms such as eye movement and pupil constriction have been prevented by drugs or other means.

When the exposure time exceeds 0.1 s and pupil constriction is inhibited by drugs or other means, the ocular MPEs shall be reduced as follows:

(1) To protect against photochemically induced retinal injury, the integrated radiance of the source must be below 20 C_B $J \cdot cm^{-2} \cdot sr^{-1}$ averaged over a cone angle of γ. This integrated radiance limit corresponds to a retinal radiant exposure limit of 2.7 C_B $J \cdot cm^{-2}$, ignoring intraocular transmission losses.

(2) To protect against thermally induced retinal injury for both point source viewing and viewing of extended sources, the MPE for exposures between 0.07 s and 0.7 s should remain that which is applicable for a 0.07 s exposure. For exposure durations longer than 0.7 s, the MPE should be reduced by a factor of 5.4 for wavelengths between 0.4 and 0.6 μm, and by a factor of $10^{7.4(0.700-\lambda)}$ for wavelengths between 0.6 and 0.7 μm.

When the eye is immobilized or otherwise constrained so that the image on the retina is stabilized, both the point source viewing and the extended source exposure are limited to 20 C_B $J \cdot cm^{-2} \cdot sr^{-1}$ averaged over 1.5 mrad.

8.4 MPE for Skin Exposure to a Laser Beam.

MPEs for skin exposure to a laser beam are given in Table 7. These levels are for worst-case conditions and are based on the best available information.

8.4.1 MPE for Skin, Repeated Exposures. For repetitive-pulse lasers the MPEs for skin exposure are applied as follows: Exposure of the skin shall not exceed the MPE based upon a single-pulse exposure, and the average irradiance of the pulse train shall not exceed the MPE applicable for the total pulse train, duration T. Rule 3 does not apply to skin exposure.

8.4.2 Large Area Exposures (Wavelengths Greater than 1.4 μm). For beam cross-sectional areas between 100 cm^2 and 1000 cm^2, the MPE for exposure durations exceeding 10 s is 10,000/A_s mW·cm^{-2}, where A_s is the area of the exposed skin in cm^2. For exposed skin areas exceeding 1000 cm^2, the MPE is 10 mW·cm^{-2}.

9. Measurements

9.1 General.

Measurements are appropriate under the following circumstances: when the laser or laser system has not been classified by the manufacturer in accordance with the FLPPS or IEC 60825-1 (or latest revision thereof); when alterations to a system may have changed its classification, or when the borders of a NHZ cannot be determined from an analysis of the beam parameters. Measurements should not be necessary when the laser or laser system has been classified by the manufacturer in accordance with the FLPPS or IEC 60825-1 (or latest revision thereof).

When comparing measured results to the MPE or AEL, the combined uncertainty due to all sources of inaccuracy shall not exceed ± 20%, or, if this is not possible, the best that the state of the art reasonably will permit. It is important to recognize that measurements improperly performed may be worse than no measurements, since they may imply a safe condition that does not actually exist. Guidance on laser measurements can be found in the ANSI Recommended Practice for Laser Safety Measurements and Hazard Evaluation, Z136.4-2005 (or latest revision thereof).

If measurements are performed, the accuracy of the instrumentation should be traceable to national standards, either directly to the National Institute of Standards and Technology (NIST) or to other transfer standards traceable to NIST. NIST establishes and maintains national measurement standards for characterizing laser radiation.

Measurements should be attempted only by personnel trained or experienced in laser technology and radiometry. Routine survey measurements of lasers or laser systems are neither required nor advisable when the laser classifications are known and the appropriate control measures implemented.

If a laser or laser system is used outdoors over long ranges, where the uncertainties of propagation influence exposures, or where the beam divergence is uncertain, measurements at specific locations may be useful.

Measurements shall be made with the laser adjusted to produce the most hazardous exposure conditions for the intended use.

9.2 Point Source and Extended Source Measurements.

If measurements or calculations are required, distinction shall first be made between point source viewing and extended source viewing in the 0.4 to 1.4 μm wavelength region. For the purpose of this standard, an extended source subtends an angle at the observer's eye greater than the angular subtense, α_{min}, (1.5 mrad), across the largest angular dimension of the source as viewed by the observer. A field of view of 100 mrad (α_{max}) is sufficient to evaluate retinal hazards since the MPE is related to retinal irradiance or radiant exposure for images larger than α_{max}. For photochemical MPEs and AELs over the wavelength range from 0.4 μm to 0.6 μm, the specified field of view γ shall be used for averaging radiance.

9.2.1 Measurements Relating to MPE and AEL. For comparing laser beam characteristics to the MPE, that radiant energy or power which can be collected in a circular limiting aperture having a diameter as given in Tables 8a and 8b shall be used for comparison with the MPE at any location where exposure can occur. For laser classification, beam measurements shall be made at the point of greatest hazard but no closer than those distances given in Table 9 from the point of closest access.

9.2.1.1 Radiant Energy or Power. For classification, the radiant energy or power which can be collected in circular measurement apertures located at the distances given in Table 9 (Condition 1 and Condition 2) shall be used for comparison with the AEL to determine the appropriate hazard class.

9.2.2 Irradiance or Radiant Exposure.

9.2.2.1 Limiting Aperture. The limiting aperture diameters specified in Tables 8a and 8b are intended for averaging exposures. Apertures with diameters smaller than those specified may be used for measurements, but may produce conservative results. If measurements with a smaller diameter aperture than specified in Table 8a indicate a moderate hazard, then the averaging aperture specified in Table 8a shall be used to determine if the exposure is actually above or below the MPE.

The sensitivity per unit area shall be sufficiently uniform, when mapped with a 1 mm diameter beam, to ensure the required accuracy of measurement.

No correction for beam size or homogeneity is necessary in cases where the entire beam enters the effective limiting aperture. For larger beams, the measurement shall be made in the area of the beam that gives the maximum reading.

For distinguishing between Class 3B and Class 4 pulsed lasers, the maximum radiant power or energy which is transmitted through the measurement apertures listed in Table 9 shall be used.

9.2.2.2 Field of View (0.18 to 0.40 μm and 1.4 μm to 1 mm Wavelengths). In measuring the irradiance or radiant exposure from ultraviolet and far infrared diffuse sources, care shall be taken to make sure that the field of view of the instrument is adequate to ensure the required accuracy of measurement.

9.3 Instruments.

Many optical power, energy, pulse shape, and PRF measuring devices available commercially can be used to determine classification and compliance with this standard. Instruments shall be calibrated sufficiently well to permit overall measurement accuracies of ± 20% wherever possible.

Measurements with instruments having smaller effective limiting apertures than those in Table 9 are permitted provided the appropriate correction factors are applied to ensure the required accuracy of measurement.

10. Revision of Standards Referred to in this Document

10.1 ANSI Standards.

When any of the following American National Standards referred to in this document is revised, the latest revision approved by the American National Standards Institute, Inc., shall apply:

American National Standard Compressed Gas Cylinder Value Outlet and Inlet Connections, ANSI/CGA V-1.

American National Standard National Electrical Code, ANSI/NFPA 70.

American National Standard Safety Standard for Radio Receivers, Audio Systems, and Accessories, ANSI/UL 1270.

American National Standard General Safety Standard for Installations Using Non-Medical X-Ray and Sealed Gamma-Ray Sources, Energies up to 10 MeV, ANSI/N43.3.

American National Standard Specifications for Accident Prevention Signs, ANSI Z535.1.

American National Standard Criteria for Safety Symbols, ANSI Z535.2-1998.

American National Specification for Accident Prevention Signs, ANSI Z535.3-1998.

American National Standard for Occupational and Educational Personal Eye and Face Protection, ANSI Z87.1-2003.

American National Standard for Industrial Robots and Robot Systems-Safety Requirements, ANSI/RIA R15.06.

American National Standard Fundamentals Governing the Design and Operation of Local Exhaust Systems, ANSI Z9.2.

10.2 Other Standards and Codes.

ACGIH: Industrial Ventilation: A Manual of Recommended Practice (latest revision thereof).

ACGIH: Threshold Limit Values for Chemical Substances and Physical Agents and Biological Exposure Indices (latest revision thereof).

FDA/CDRH Laser Products – Conformance with IEC 60825-1, Am. 2 and IEC 60601-2-22; Final Guidance for Industry and FDA (Laser Notice No. 50).

FDA/CDRH Federal Laser Product Performance Standard (FLPPS), 21CFR Part 1040.

IEC 60825-1, Ed 1.2: 2001-08 Safety of Laser Products – Part 1: Equipment Classification, Requirements, and User's Guide.

IEEE Standard for Safety Levels with Respect to Human Exposure to Radio Frequency Electromagnetic Fields, 3 kHz to 300 GHz, C95.1-2005.

IEEE Standard for Radio-Frequency Energy and Current-Flow Symbols, C95.2-1999

IEEE Standard for Safety Levels with Respect to Human Exposure to Electromagnetic Fields, 0 to 3 kHz, IEEE C95.6-2002.

IEEE Recommended Practice for Radio Frequency Safety Programs, 3 kHz to 300 GHz, C95.7-2005

National Fire Protection Association: NFPA 30, Flammable and Combustible Liquids; NFPA 45, Fire Protection for Laboratories Using Chemicals; NFPA 115, Laser Fire Protection.

NEC, Section 110-16, Work Space About Electric Equipment (600 Volts Nominal or Less).

NEC: National Electrical Code, Article 500, Hazardous (Classified) Locations.

OSHA: Occupational Safety and Health Standards for General Industry, 29 CFR 1910:

1910.95	Occupational Noise Exposure
1910.169,170,171	Compressed Gas and Compressed Air Equipment
1910.134	Respiratory Protection
1910.147	The Control of Hazardous Energy (lockout/tagout)
1910.309-330	Electrical Safety Related Work Practices
Subpart Z	Toxic and Hazardous Substance

Table 2. Recommended Limiting Exposure Durations for CW and Repetitive-Pulse MPE Calculations*

Wavelength Range	Diffuse (seconds)	Intrabeam (seconds)
UV 0.18 to 0.4 μm	30,000	30,000
Visible 0.4 to 0.7 μm	600	0.25**
NIR 0.7 to 1.4 μm	600	10
FIR 1.4 μm to 1 mm	10	10

* For single pulse lasers (PRF < 1 Hz) use actual laser pulse duration.

** For unintended or accidental viewing only. For other conditions, use the time of *intended* viewing.

Table 3. Diffusely Reflected Beam Energy in Joules that does not Exceed the MPE

Pulsed Lasers (1 ns to 50 μs Pulse Duration: Wavelengths Between 0.400 to 1.400 μm).[†]

Beam Diameter (cm)	Viewing Distance, r_1 (cm) 20	100	1000
0.1	$0.002 \times C_A$	$0.016 \times C_A$	$1.6 \times C_A$
0.2	$0.004 \times C_A$	$0.021 \times C_A$	$1.6 \times C_A$
0.3	$0.006 \times C_A$	$0.032 \times C_A$	$1.6 \times C_A$
0.4	$0.008 \times C_A$	$0.042 \times C_A$	$1.6 \times C_A$
0.5	$0.011 \times C_A$	$0.053 \times C_A$	$1.6 \times C_A$
0.6	$0.013 \times C_A$	$0.063 \times C_A$	$1.6 \times C_A$
0.7	$0.015 \times C_A$	$0.074 \times C_A$	$1.6 \times C_A$
0.8	$0.017 \times C_A$	$0.084 \times C_A$	$1.6 \times C_A$
0.9	$0.020 \times C_A$	$0.095 \times C_A$	$1.6 \times C_A$
1.0	$0.022 \times C_A$	$0.11 \times C_A$	$1.6 \times C_A$
1.5	$0.034 \times C_A$	$0.16 \times C_A$	$1.6 \times C_A$
2.0	$0.046 \times C_A$	$0.21 \times C_A$	$2.1 \times C_A$
2.5	$0.074 \times C_A$	$0.27 \times C_A$	$2.6 \times C_A$
3.0	$0.11 \times C_A$	$0.32 \times C_A$	$3.2 \times C_A$
3.5	$0.15 \times C_A$	$0.38 \times C_A$	$3.7 \times C_A$
4.0	$0.20 \times C_A$	$0.44 \times C_A$	$4.2 \times C_A$
4.5	$0.26 \times C_A$	$0.49 \times C_A$	$4.7 \times C_A$
5.0	$0.33 \times C_A$	$0.55 \times C_A$	$5.3 \times C_A$
6.0	$0.50 \times C_A$	$0.68 \times C_A$	$6.3 \times C_A$
7.0	$0.7 \times C_A$	$0.79 \times C_A$	$7.4 \times C_A$
8.0	$0.9 \times C_A$	$0.91 \times C_A$	$8.4 \times C_A$
9.0	$1.3 \times C_A$	$1.0 \times C_A$	$9.5 \times C_A$
10.0	$1.6 \times C_A$	$1.2 \times C_A$	$11.0 \times C_A$

[†] The table shows the values for pulsed lasers with 1 ns to 18 μs pulse durations for the wavelength region 0.400 to 1.050 μm and 1 ns to 50 μs for the wavelength region 1.050 to 1.400 μm.

Note 1: The diffuse reflection values Q are based on the MPE values in Tables 5a and 5b and are calculated from the general equation

$$Q = \frac{\pi(\text{MPE})(r_1 + D_\rho / 2)^2}{\rho_\lambda \cos\theta_v}$$

which is valid for all exposure durations where the MPE in Tables 5a and 5b is expressed in J•cm^{-2}, including those for 100 fs to 1 ns. D_ρ is the diameter of the laser beam at the reflection site, θ_v is the viewing angle, ρ_λ is the spectral reflectance as a function of wavelength (where this is not known, the value 1 is used), and r_l is the viewing distance. In calculating the above values, the following was assumed: $\theta_v = 90°$; $\rho_\lambda = 1$; and n = 1 (that is, these values are for the single-pulse case). The MPE values substituted into the above equation must include the correction factors C_A, C_C, C_E, and C_P where appropriate, and for wavelengths between 0.4 and 0.55 μm, the MPE is the lower value of the thermal and photochemical MPE computations (see Tables 5 and 6 and Section 8.2.3.2).

Note 2: In the wavelength region 1.050 to 1.400 μm, the tabular values above are to be multiplied by the term 2 × C_C (see Table 6).

Note 3: For targets of known reflectance, the above values may be divided by the reflectance of the target.

Table 4. Simplified Method for Selecting Laser Eye Protection for Point Source Viewing (Wavelengths Between 0.400 and 1.400 μm)†

Q-Switched Laser (10^{-9} - 10^{-2} s)		Non-Q-Switched Lasers (0.4×10^{-3} - 10^{-2} s)		Continuous-Wave Lasers Momentary (0.25 - 10 s)		Continuous-Wave Lasers Long-Term Staring (< 1 hr)		Attenuation	
Maximum Output Energy (J)	Max Beam Radiant Exposure ($J \cdot cm^{-2}$)	Max Laser Output Energy (J)	Max Beam Radiant Exposure ($J \cdot cm^{-2}$)	Max Power Output (W)	Max Beam Irradiance ($W \cdot cm^{-2}$)	Max Power Output (W)	Max Beam Irradiance ($W \cdot cm^{-2}$)	Attenuation Factor	OD
10	20	100	200	10^5 *	2×10^5 *	100 *	200 *	10^8	8
1	2	10	20	10^4 *	2×10^4 *	10 *	20 *	10^7	7
10^{-1}	2×10^{-1}	1	2	10^3 *	2×10^3 *	1	2	10^6	6
10^{-2}	2×10^{-2}	10^{-1}	2×10^{-1}	100 *	200 *	10^{-1}	2×10^{-1}	10^5	5
10^{-3}	2×10^{-3}	10^{-2}	2×10^{-2}	10	20	10^{-2}	2×10^{-2}	10^4	4
10^{-4}	2×10^{-4}	10^{-3}	2×10^{-3}	1	2	10^{-3}	2×10^{-3}	10^3	3
10^{-5}	2×10^{-5}	10^{-4}	2×10^{-4}	10^{-1}	2×10^{-1}	10^{-4}	2×10^{-4}	10^2	2
10^{-6}	2×10^{-6}	10^{-5}	2×10^{-5}	10^{-2}	2×10^{-2}	10^{-5}	2×10^{-5}	10	1

† Use of this table may result in optical densities (OD) greater than necessary. See Section 4.6.2 for other wavelengths.

* Not recommended as a control procedure at these levels. These levels of power could damage or destroy the attenuating material used in the eye protection. The skin also needs protection at these levels.

Table 5a. Maximum Permissible Exposure (MPE) for Point Source Ocular Exposure to a Laser Beam †

Wavelength (μm)	Exposure Duration, t (s)	MPE ($J \cdot cm^{-2}$)	MPE ($W \cdot cm^{-2}$)	Notes
Ultraviolet				In the Dual Limit Wavelength Region (0.180 to 0.400 μm), the lower MPE considering photochemical and thermal effects must be chosen.
Dual Limits for λ between 0.180 and 0.400 μm				
Thermal				
0.180 to 0.400	10^{-9} to 10	$0.56\ t^{0.25}$		
Photochemical				
0.180 to 0.302	10^{-9} to 3×10^{4}	3×10^{-3}		See Tables 8a and 8b for limiting aperture and Table 9 for measurement aperture.
0.302 to 0.315	10^{-9} to 3×10^{4}	$10^{200(\lambda-0.295)} \times 10^{-4}$		
0.315 to 0.400	10 to 3×10^{4}	1.0		
Visible				
0.400 to 0.700	10^{-13} to 10^{-11}	1.5×10^{-8}		In the Wavelength Region (0.400 to 0.500 μm), T_1 determines whether the photochemical or thermal MPE is lower.
0.400 to 0.700	10^{-11} to 10^{-9}	$2.7\ t^{0.75}$		
0.400 to 0.700	10^{-9} to 18×10^{-6}	5.0×10^{-7}		
0.400 to 0.700	18×10^{-6} to 10	$1.8\ t^{0.75} \times 10^{-3}$		
0.500 to 0.700	10 to 3×10^{4}		1×10^{-3}	
Thermal				For extended sources in the retinal hazard region (0.400 to 1.4 μm), see Table 5b.
0.450 to 0.500	10 to T_1		1×10^{-3}	
Photochemical				
0.400 to 0.450	10 to 100	1×10^{-2}		See Table 6 and Figures 8 and 9 for correction factors C_A, C_B, C_C, C_P, C_E, and times T_1 and T_2.
0.450 to 0.500	T_1 to 100	$C_B \times 10^{-2}$		
0.400 to 0.500	100 to 3×10^{4}		$C_B \times 10^{-4}$	
Near Infrared				
0.700 to 1.050	10^{-13} to 10^{-11}	$1.5\ C_A \times 10^{-8}$		For repeated (pulsed) exposures, see Section 8.2.3. A correction factor, C_P applies to thermal limits, but not to photochemical limits.
0.700 to 1.050	10^{-11} to 10^{-9}	$2.7\ C_A\ t^{0.75}$		
0.700 to 1.050	10^{-9} to 18×10^{-6}	$5.0\ C_A \times 10^{-7}$		
0.700 to 1.050	18×10^{-6} to 10	$1.8\ C_A\ t^{0.75} \times 10^{-3}$		
0.700 to 1.050	10 to 3×10^{4}		$C_A \times 10^{-3}$	
1.050 to 1.400	10^{-13} to 10^{-11}	$1.5\ C_C \times 10^{-7}$		The wavelength region λ_1 to λ_2 means $\lambda_1 \leq \lambda < \lambda_2$, e.g., 0.180 to 0.302 μm means $0.180 \leq \lambda < 0.302$ μm.
1.050 to 1.400	10^{-11} to 10^{-9}	$27.0\ C_C\ t^{0.75}$		
1.050 to 1.400	10^{-9} to 50×10^{-6}	$5.0\ C_C \times 10^{-6}$		
1.050 to 1.400	50×10^{-6} to 10	$9.0\ C_C\ t^{0.75} \times 10^{-3}$		
1.050 to 1.400	10 to 3×10^{4}		$5.0\ C_C \times 10^{-3}$	
Far Infrared				
1.400 to 1.500	10^{-9} to 10^{-3}	0.1		Note: The MPEs must be in the same units.
1.400 to 1.500	10^{-3} to 10	$0.56\ t^{0.25}$		
1.400 to 1.500	10 to 3×10^{4}		0.1	
1.500 to 1.800	10^{-9} to 10	1.0		
1.500 to 1.800	10 to 3×10^{4}		0.1	
1.800 to 2.600	10^{-9} to 10^{-3}	0.1		
1.800 to 2.600	10^{-3} to 10	$0.56\ t^{0.25}$		
1.800 to 2.600	10 to 3×10^{4}		0.1	
2.600 to 1000	10^{-9} to 10^{-7}	1×10^{-2}		
2.600 to 1000	10^{-7} to 10	$0.56\ t^{0.25}$		
2.600 to 1000	10 to 3×10^{4}		0.1	

Table 5b. Maximum Permissible Exposure (MPE) for Extended Source Ocular Exposure[†]

Wavelength (μm)	Exposure Duration, t (s)	MPE ($J \cdot cm^{-2}$) except as noted	MPE ($W \cdot cm^{-2}$) except as noted	Notes
Visible				
0.400 to 0.700	10^{-13} to 10^{-11}	$1.5\ C_E \times 10^{-8}$		(See Tables 8a and 9 for limiting apertures)
0.400 to 0.700	10^{-11} to 10^{-9}	$2.7\ C_E\ t^{0.75}$		
0.400 to 0.700	10^{-9} to 18×10^{-6}	$5.0\ C_E \times 10^{-7}$		
0.400 to 0.700	18×10^{-6} to 0.7	$1.8\ C_E\ t^{0.75} \times 10^{-3}$		
Dual Limits for λ between 0.400 and 0.600 μm visible laser exposure for $t > 0.7$ s				
Photochemical				
For $\alpha \le 11$mrad, the MPE is expressed as irradiance and radiant exposure*				
0.400 to 0.600	0.7 to 100	$C_B \times 10^{-2}$		(See Tables 8a and 9 for limiting apertures)
0.400 to 0.600	100 to 3×10^4		$C_B \times 10^{-4}$	
For $\alpha > 11$mrad, the MPE is expressed as radiance and integrated radiance*				
0.400 to 0.600	0.7 to 1×10^4	$100\ C_B\ J \cdot cm^{-2} \cdot sr^{-1}$		(See Table 8a for limiting cone angle γ)
0.400 to 0.600	1×10^4 to 3×10^4		$C_B \times 10^{-2}\ W \cdot cm^{-2} \cdot sr^{-1}$	
	and			
Thermal				
0.400 to 0.700	0.7 to T_2	$1.8\ C_E\ t^{0.75} \times 10^{-3}$		
0.400 to 0.700	T_2 to 3×10^4		$1.8\ C_E\ T_2^{-0.25} \times 10^{-3}$	
Near Infrared				
0.700 to 1.050	10^{-13} to 10^{-11}	$1.5\ C_A\ C_E \times 10^{-8}$		(See Tables 8a and 9 for limiting apertures)
0.700 to 1.050	10^{-11} to 10^{-9}	$2.7\ C_A\ C_E\ t^{0.75}$		
0.700 to 1.050	10^{-9} to 18×10^{-6}	$5.0\ C_A\ C_E \times 10^{-7}$		
0.700 to 1.050	18×10^{-6} to T_2	$1.8\ C_A\ C_E\ t^{0.75} \times 10^{-3}$		
0.700 to 1.050	T_2 to 3×10^4		$1.8\ C_A\ C_E\ T_2^{-0.25} \times 10^{-3}$	
1.050 to 1.400	10^{-13} to 10^{-11}	$1.5\ C_C\ C_E \times 10^{-7}$		
1.050 to 1.400	10^{-11} to 10^{-9}	$27.0\ C_C\ C_E\ t^{0.75}$		
1.050 to 1.400	10^{-9} to 50×10^{-6}	$5.0\ C_C\ C_E \times 10^{-6}$		
1.050 to 1.400	50×10^{-6} to T_2	$9.0\ C_C\ C_E\ t^{0.75} \times 10^{-3}$		
1.050 to 1.400	T_2 to 3×10^4		$9.0\ C_C\ C_E\ T_2^{-0.25} \times 10^{-3}$	

[†] See Table 6 and Figures 8, 9 and 13 for correction factors C_A, C_B, C_C, C_E, C_P, and times T_1 and T_2.

* For sources subtending an angle greater than 11 mrad, the limit may also be expressed as an integrated radiance $L_p = 100\ C_B\ J \cdot cm^{-2} \cdot sr^{-1}$ for $0.7\ s \le t < 10^4$ s and $L_e = C_B \times 10^{-2}\ W \cdot cm^{-2} \cdot sr^{-1}$ for $t \ge 10^4$ s as measured through a limiting cone angle γ. These correspond to values of $J \cdot cm^{-2}$ for $10\ s \le t < 100$ s and $W \cdot cm^{-2}$ for $t \ge 100$ s as measured through a limiting cone angle γ.

$\gamma = 11$ mrad for $0.7\ s \le t < 100$ s,
$\gamma = 1.1 \times t^{0.5}$ mrad for $100\ s \le t < 10^4$ s
$\gamma = 110$ mrad for $10^4\ s \le t < 3 \times 10^4$ s

See Figure 3 for γ and Appendix B7.2 for examples.

Note 1: For repeated (pulsed) exposures, see Section 8.2.3.
Note 2: The wavelength region λ_1 to λ_2 means $\lambda_1 \le \lambda < \lambda_2$, e.g., 1.180 to 1.302 μm means $1.180 \le \lambda < 1.302\ \mu m$.
Note 3: Dual Limit Application: In the Dual Limit wavelength region (0.400 to 0.600 μm), the exposure limit is the lower value of the determined photochemical and thermal exposure limit.
Note 4: The MPEs must be in the same units.

Table 6. Parameters and Correction Factors

Parameters/ Correction Factors	Wavelength (μm)	Figure with Graphical Representation
$C_A = 1.0$	0.400 to 0.700	8a
$C_A = 10^{2(\lambda-0.700)}$	0.700 to 1.050	8a
$C_A = 5.0$	1.050 to 1.400	8a
$C_B = 1.0$	0.400 to 0.450	8c
$C_B = 10^{20(\lambda-0.450)}$	0.450 to 0.600	8c
$C_C = 1.0$	1.050 to 1.150	8b
$C_C = 10^{18(\lambda-1.150)}$	1.150 to 1.200	8b
$C_C = 8$	1.200 to 1.400	8b
$C_E = 1.0 \quad \alpha < \alpha_{min}$*	0.400 to 1.400	—
$C_E = \alpha / \alpha_{min} \quad \alpha_{min} \le \alpha \le \alpha_{max}$*	0.400 to 1.400	—
$C_E = \alpha^2 / (\alpha_{max}\, \alpha_{min}) \quad \alpha > \alpha_{max}$*	0.400 to 1.400	—
$C_P = n^{-0.25}$ **	0.180 to 1000	13
$T_1 = 10 \times 10^{20(\lambda-0.450)}$ ***	0.450 to 0.500	9a
$T_2 = 10 \times 10^{(\alpha-1.5)/98.5}$ ****	0.400 to 1.400	9b

* For wavelengths between 0.400 and 1.400 μm: $\alpha_{min} = 1.5$ mrad, and $\alpha_{max} = 100$ mrad

** See 8.2.3 for discussion of C_P and 8.2.3.2 for discussion of pulse repetition frequencies below 55 kHz (0.4 to 1.05 μm) and below 20 kHz (1.05 to 1.4 μm).

*** $T_1 = 10$ s for $\lambda = 0.450$ μm, and $T_1 = 100$ s for $\lambda = 0.500$ μm.

**** $T_2 = 10$ s for $\alpha < 1.5$ mrad, and $T_2 = 100$ s for $\alpha > 100$ mrad.

Note 1: Wavelengths must be expressed in micrometers and angles in milliradians for calculations.

Note 2: The wavelength region λ_1 to λ_2 means $\lambda_1 \le \lambda < \lambda_2$, e.g., 0.550 to 0.700 μm means $0.550 \le \lambda < 0.700$ μm.

Table 7. Maximum Permissible Exposure (MPE) for Skin Exposure to a Laser Beam

Wavelength (μm)	Exposure Duration, t (s)	MPE (J·cm^{-2}) except as noted	MPE (W·cm^{-2}) except as noted	Notes
Ultraviolet				
	Dual Limits for λ between 0.180 to 0.400 μm			In the Dual Limit Wavelength Region (0.180 to 0.400 μm), the lower MPE considering photochemical and thermal effects must be chosen.
Thermal				
0.180 to 0.400	10^{-9} to 10	$0.56\ t^{0.25}$		
Photochemical				
0.180 to 0.302	10^{-9} to 3×10^4	3×10^{-3}		
0.302 to 0.315	10^{-9} to 3×10^4	$10^{200(\lambda-0.295)} \times 10^{-4}$		3.5 mm limiting aperture applies for all wavelengths and exposure durations (see Table 8a).
0.315 to 0.400	10 to 10^3	1.0		
0.315 to 0.400	10^3 to 3×10^4		1×10^{-3}	
Visible and Near Infrared				The wavelength region λ_1 to λ_2 means $\lambda_1 \le \lambda < \lambda_2$, e.g., 0.180 to 0.302 μm means $0.180 \le \lambda < 0.302$ μm.
0.400 to 1.400	10^{-9} to 10^{-7}	$2\ C_A \times 10^{-2}$		
0.400 to 1.400	10^{-7} to 10	$1.1\ C_A\ t^{0.25}$		
0.400 to 1.400	10 to 3×10^4		$0.2\ C_A$	
Far Infrared				
1.400 to 1.500	10^{-9} to 10^{-3}	0.1		The exposure duration t_1 to t_2 means $t_1 \le t < t_2$, e.g., 10 to 10^3 s means 10 s $\le t < 10^3$ s.
1.400 to 1.500	10^{-3} to 10	$0.56\ t^{0.25}$		
1.400 to 1.500	10 to 3×10^4		0.1	
1.500 to 1.800	10^{-9} to 10	1.0		
1.500 to 1.800	10 to 3×10^4		0.1	
1.800 to 2.600	10^{-9} to 10^{-3}	0.1		
1.800 to 2.600	10^{-3} to 10	$0.56\ t^{0.25}$		See Section 8.4.2 for large beam cross sections and Table 6 for correction factor C_A
1.800 to 2.600	10 to 3×10^4		0.1	
2.600 to 1000	10^{-9} to 10^{-7}	1×10^{-2}		
2.600 to 1000	10^{-7} to 10	$0.56\ t^{0.25}$		
2.600 to 1000	10 to 3×10^4		0.1	

Table 8a. Limiting Apertures (Irradiance and Radiant Exposure) and Limiting Cone Angles γ (Radiance and Integrated Radiance) for Hazard Evaluation

Spectral Region (μm)	Duration† (s)	Aperture Diameter (mm) Eye	Skin
0.180 to 0.400	10^{-9} to 0.3	1.0	3.5
	0.3 to 10*	$1.5\ t^{0.375}$	3.5
	10 to 3×10^4	3.5	3.5
0.400 to 1.400	10^{-13} to 3×10^4	7.0	3.5
1.400 to 10^2	10^{-9} to 0.3	1.0	3.5
	0.3 to 10*	$1.5\ t^{0.375}$	3.5
	10 to 3×10^4	3.5	3.5
10^2 to 10^3	10^{-9} to 3×10^4	11.0	11.0
		Limiting Cone Angle, γ (mrad)	
0.400 to 0.600	0.7 to 100	11	
	100 to 10^4	$1.1\ t^{0.5}$	
	10^4 to 3×10^4	110	

* Under normal conditions these exposure durations would not be used for hazard evaluation.

† For guidance on exposure durations less than 10^{-13} seconds, see 8.2.2.

Note: The wavelength region λ_1 to λ_2 means $\lambda_1 \le \lambda < \lambda_2$ μm, e.g., 0.315 to 0.400 μm means $0.315 \le \lambda < 0.400$ μm. Additionally, the exposure duration region t_1 to t_2 means $t_1 \le t < t_2$ s, e.g., 0.3 to 10 s means $0.3 \le t < 10$ s.

Table 8b. Limiting Apertures for AEL Determination

Spectral Region (μm)	Duration* (s)	Aperture Diameter (mm)	Area of Limiting Aperture (cm^2)
0.180 to 0.400	10^{-9} to 0.3	1.0	7.85×10^{-3}
	0.3 to 10	$1.5\ t^{0.375}$	$2.25 \times 10^{-2}\ t^{0.75}$
	10 to 3×10^4	3.5	9.6×10^{-2}
0.400 to 1.400	10^{-13} to 3×10^4	7.0	0.385
1.400 to 10^2	10^{-9} to 0.3	1.0	7.85×10^{-3}
	0.3 to 10	$1.5\ t^{0.375}$	$2.25 \times 10^{-2}\ t^{0.75}$
	10 to 3×10^4	3.5	9.6×10^{-2}
10^2 to 10^3	10^{-9} to 3×10^4	11.0	0.95

* Since different limiting and measurement apertures apply for pulsed versus CW exposures, the aperture for Rule 1 is determined from the duration of a single pulse. For Rule 2, the potential exposure for all exposure durations, *T*, less than or equal to T_{max} is compared with the MPE for *T* with the corresponding limiting aperture determined from *T*. For Rule 3, the aperture is determined from the duration of a single pulse, (≤ 0.25 s). The energy from pulses contained within exposure duration t_{min} is considered a single pulse for Rule 3. Information on these Rules is available in Section 8.2.3.

Note: The wavelength region λ_1 to λ_2 means $\lambda_1 \le \lambda < \lambda_2$ μm e.g., 0.315 to 0.400 μm means $0.315 \le \lambda < 0.400$ μm. Additionally, the exposure duration region t_1 to t_2 means $t_1 \le t < t_2$ s, e.g., 0.3 to 10 s means $0.3 \le t < 10$ s.

Table 9. Measurement Apertures for Laser Classification*

		Condition 1		Condition 2	
Spectral Region** (µm)	Exposure† Duration (s)	Aperture Diameter§ (mm)	Measurement Distance (cm)	Aperture Diameter (mm)	Measurement Distance# (cm)
	10^{-9} to 0.3			1.0	
0.180 to 0.302	0.3 to 10	N/A	N/A	$1.5t^{0.375}$	10
	10 to 3 × 10			3.5	
	10^{-9} to 0.3	7.0		1.0	
0.302 to 0.4	0.3 to 10	$11\,t^{0.375}$	200	$1.5t^{0.375}$	10
	10 to 3 × 10^4	25.0		3.5	
0.4 to 1.4	10^{-13} to 3 × 10^4	50.0	200	7.0	10
	10^{-9} to 0.3	7.0		1.0	
1.4 to 2.8	0.3 to 10	$11\,t^{0.375}$	200	$1.5t^{0.375}$	10
	10 to 3 × 10^4	25.0		3.5	
	10^{-9} to 0.3			1.0	
2.8 to 10^2	0.3 to 10	N/A	N/A	$1.5t^{0.375}$	10
	10 to 3 × 10^4			3.5	
10^2 to 10^3	10^{-9} to 3×10^4	N/A	N/A	11.0	10

* These apertures are used for the measurement of optical power or energy for the purpose of laser classification (see 3.3). The standardized measurement apertures and distances actually simulate many viewing conditions and do not necessarily refer only to viewing at those measurement distances. For high power scopes used for examining optical fiber communication systems (OFCS) fibers, the guidance provided in ANSI Z136.2 (1997) should be followed.

**Condition 1 in this standard does not apply for lasers having wavelengths exceeding 2.8 µm since most telescopic optics do not transmit beyond 2.8 µm; however, the IEC 60825-1 applies Condition 1 to lasers that have wavelengths up to 4.0 µm in consideration of special purpose telescopes that have transmission over an extended spectral range.

† For guidance on exposure durations less than 10^{-13} seconds see 8.2.2. Exposure durations between 0.3 s and 10 s would not normally be used for classification.

§Under use conditions, when the laser output is intended to be viewed with optics (excluding ordinary eyeglasses) or the Laser Safety Officer determines that there is a reasonable probability of accidental viewing with optics, the apertures listed in Tables 8a and 8b for hazard evaluation apply to the exit beam from the particular optical instrument being considered. For situations where the default conditions do not apply, refer to the hazard analysis techniques in the examples in B6.4.3 Appendix B.

#The default measurement distance for Condition 2 in the IEC 60825-1 is 7 cm.

Note: The wavelength region λ_1 to λ_2 means $\lambda_1 \le \lambda < \lambda_2$, e.g., 0.315 to 0.400 µm means $0.315 \le \lambda < 0.400$ µm.

Table 10. Control Measures for the Seven Laser Classes

Engineering Control Measures	Classification						
	1	1M	2	2M	3R	3B	4
Protective Housing (4.3.1)	X	X	X	X	X	X	X
Without Protective Housing (4.3.1.1)	LSO shall establish Alternative Controls						
Interlocks on Removable Protective Housings (4.3.2)	∇	∇	∇	∇	∇	X	X
Service Access Panel (4.3.3)	∇	∇	∇	∇	∇	X	X
Key Control (4.3.4)	—	—	—	—	—	•	X
Viewing Windows, Display Screens and Collecting Optics(4.3.5.1)	Assure viewing limited < MPE						
Collecting Optics (4.3.5.2)							
Fully Open Beam Path (4.3.6.1)	—	—	—	—	—	X NHZ	X NHZ
Limited Open Beam Path (4.3.6.2)	—	—	—	—	—	X NHZ	X NHZ
Enclosed Beam Path (4.3.6.3)	None is required if 4.3.1 and 4.3.2 fulfilled						
Remote Interlock Connector (4.3.7)	—	—	—	—	—	•	X
Beam Stop or Attenuator (4.3.8)	—	—	—	—	—	•	X
Activation Warning Systems (4.3.9.4)	—	—	—	—	—	•	X
Indoor Laser Controlled Area (4.3.10)	—	*	—	*	—	X NHZ	X NHZ
Class 3B Indoor Laser Controlled Area (4.3.10.1)	—	—	—	—	—	X	—
Class 4 Laser Controlled Area (4.3.10.2)	—	—	—	—	—	—	X
Outdoor Control Measures (4.3.11)	X	* NHZ	X NHZ	* NHZ	X NHZ	X NHZ	X NHZ
Laser in Navigable Airspace (4.3.11.2)	X	* NHZ	X NHZ	* NHZ	X NHZ	X NHZ	X NHZ
Temporary Laser Controlled Area (4.3.12)	∇ MPE	∇ MPE	∇ MPE	∇ MPE	∇ MPE	—	—
Controlled Operation (4.3.13)	—	—	—	—	—	—	•
Equipment Labels (4.3.14 and 4.7)	X	X	X	X	X	X	X
Laser Area Warning Signs and Activation Warnings (4.3.9)	—	—	—	—	•	X NHZ	X NHZ

LEGEND:
- X Shall
- • Should
- — No requirement
- ∇ Shall if enclosed Class 3B or Class 4
- MPE Shall if MPE is exceeded
- NHZ Nominal Hazard Zone analysis required
- * May apply with use of optical aids

Table 10. Control Measures for the Seven Laser Classes (cont.)

Administrative and Procedural Control Measures	Classification						
	1	1M	2	2M	3R	3B	4
Standard Operating Procedures (4.4.1)	—	—	—	—	—	•	X
Output Emission Limitations (4.4.2)	—	—	—	—	LSO Determination		
Education and Training (4.4.3)	—	•	•	•	•	X	X
Authorized Personnel (4.4.4)	—	*	—	*	—	X	X
Alignment Procedures (4.4.5)	∇	∇	∇	∇	∇	X	X
Protective Equipment (4.6)	—	*	—	*	—	•	X
Spectators (4.4.6)	—	*	—	*	—	•	X
Service Personnel (4.4.7)	∇	∇	∇	∇	∇	X	X
Demonstration with General Public (4.5.1)	—	*	X	*	X	X	X
Laser Optical Fiber Transmission Systems (4.5.2)	MPE	MPE	MPE	MPE	MPE	X	X
Laser Robotic Installations (4.5.3)	—	—	—	—	—	X NHZ	X NHZ
Protective Eyewear (4.6.2)	—	—	—	—	—	•	X
Window Protection (4.6.3)	—	—	—	—	—	X	X NHZ
Protective Barriers and Curtains (4.6.4)	—	—	—	—	—	•	•
Skin Protection (4.6.6)	—	—	—	—	—	X	X NHZ
Other Protective Equipment (4.6.7)	Use may be required						
Warning Signs and Labels (4.7) (Design Requirements)	—	—	•	•	•	X NHZ	X NHZ
Service Personnel (4.4.7)	LSO Determination						
Laser System Modifications (4.1.2)	LSO Determination						

LEGEND:

X	Shall
•	Should
—	No requirement
∇	Shall if enclosed Class 3B or Class 4
MPE	Shall if MPE is exceeded
NHZ	Nominal Hazard Zone analysis required
*	May apply with use of optical aids

Table 11a. Summary of Area Warning Signs

Clause	Title	Classification				Required Statement or Comment
		2	3R	3B	4	
3.5.1	Personnel	X	X	X	X	Some individuals may be unable to read or understand signs
4.3.9.1	Warning Sign Posting	-	X	X	X	Specifies which sign required Caution, Danger, Notice
4.3.9.2	Laser Warning Sign Purpose	-	X	X	X	States the four purposes of warning signs
4.3.9.3	Warning Sign Non-Beam Hazard	X	X	X	X	Must follow requirements of other appropriate documents
4.3.9.4.1	Audible Warning Devices	-	-	X	X	Audible warning should be required for Class 3B and shall for Class 4
4.3.9.4.2	Visible Warning Devices	-	-	X	X	Visible warning should be required for Class 3B and shall for Class 4
4.7.1	Design of Signs		X	X	X	Per ANSI Z535 requirements
4.7.2.1.1	Laser Symbol		X	X	X	Laser sun burst required on all signs per ANSI
4.7.2.1.2	International Laser Symbol					International symbol as specified in IEC 60825-1 is acceptable
4.7.2.2	Safety Alert Symbol		X	X	X	The alert symbol is required on all Caution & Danger Signs
4.7.3.1	Signal Word "Danger"		X	X	X	Specifies when to use "Danger" word and format
4.7.3.2	Signal Word "Caution"		X			Specifies when to use "Caution" word and format
4.7.3.3	Signal Word "Notice"		X	X	X	Specifies when to use "Notice" word and format
4.7.4	Pertinent Sign Information		X	X	X	Specifies the location of words on signs
4.7.4.3	Location of Signs		X	X	X	Specifies location of signs

Note: Signs and labels prepared in accordance with previous revisions of this standard are considered to fulfill the requirement of the standard.

Table 11b. Summary of Labeling Requirements

Clause	Title	Classification					Required Statement or Comment
		1	2	3R	3B	4	
3.5.1	Personnel	X	X	X	X	X	Some individuals may be unable to read or understand labels
4.3.14.1	Warning Label	-	X	X	X	X	Class label with symbols & specific words
4.3.14.2	Protective Housing	X	X	X	X	X	Specific word depending on internal laser (see Section 4.7.5 for suggested words)
4.3.14.3	Conduit Label		X	X	X	X	
4.3.3	Service Access Panel	X	X	X	X	X	Label required if removal permits access to laser
4.5.2	Optical Fiber Transmission			X	X	X	Words required if disconnect not in a laser controlled area
4.7.5	Equipment Label Information	X	X	X	X	X	Specifies specific wording by class

Note1: Labeling of laser equipment in accordance with the Federal Laser Product Performance Standard (FLPPS) or IEC 60825-1 (or latest revision thereof) may be used to satisfy the equipment labeling requirements in this standard.

Note 2: Signs and labels prepared in accordance with previous revisions of this standard are considered to fulfill the requirement of the standard.

Table 11c. Summary of Protective Equipment Labeling

Clause	Title	Summary
4.6.5.1	Protective Eyewear	OD and wavelength marking required
4.6.5.2	Protective Windows	OD, wavelength and exposure time marking required
4.6.5.3	Collecting Optics Filters	OD, wavelength and threshold limit marking required
4.6.5.4	Protective Barrier	Threshold limit and exposure time marking required, see Appendix C2.4.

Note 1: Signs and labels prepared in accordance with previous revisions of this standard are considered to fulfill the requirement of the standard.

Note 2: Marking is only required when windows, filters or barriers are not sold as an integral part of the product.

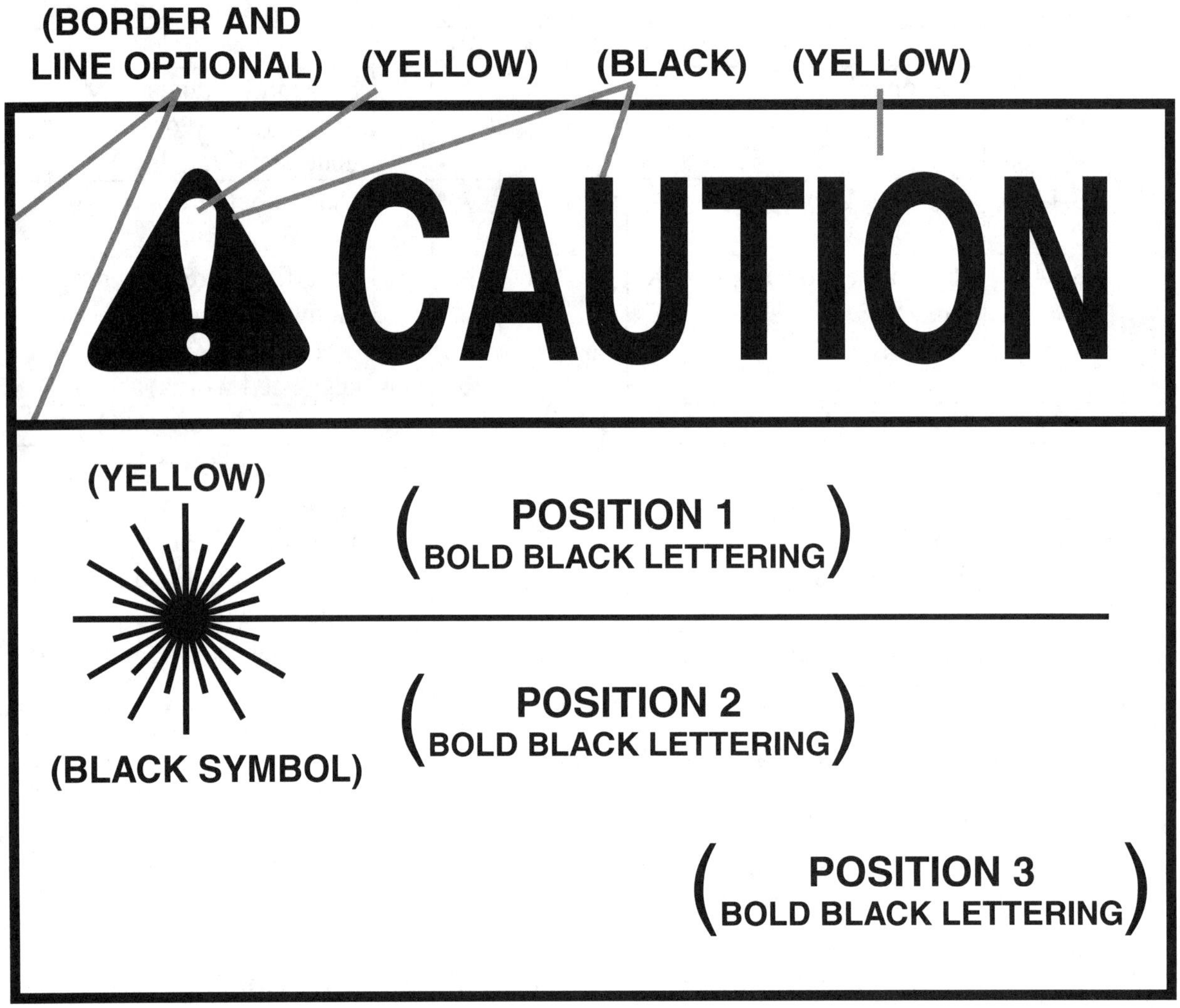

Figure 1a. Sample Warning Sign for Class 2 and Class 2M Lasers

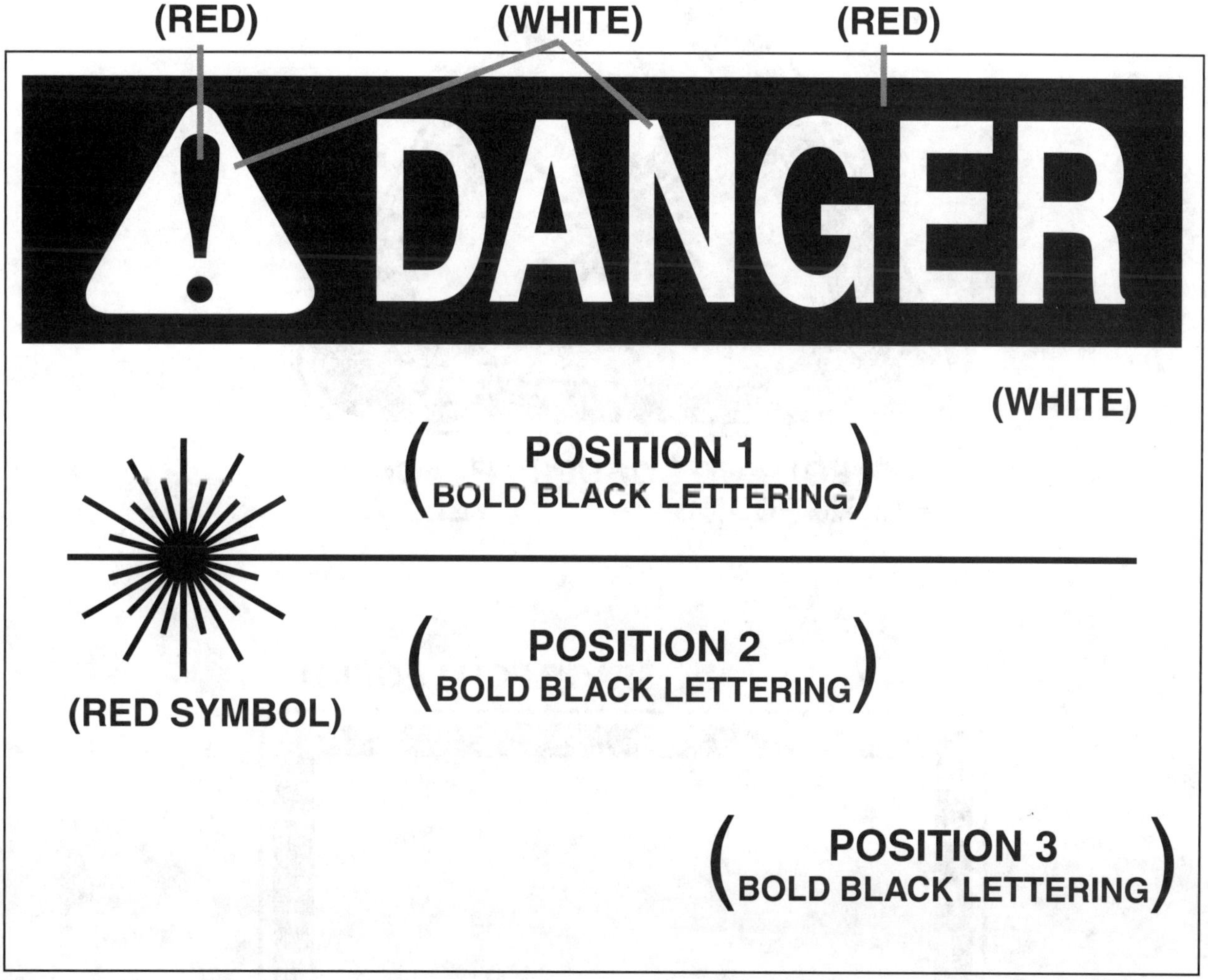

Figure 1b. Sample Warning Sign for Class 3R, Class 3B, and Class 4 Lasers

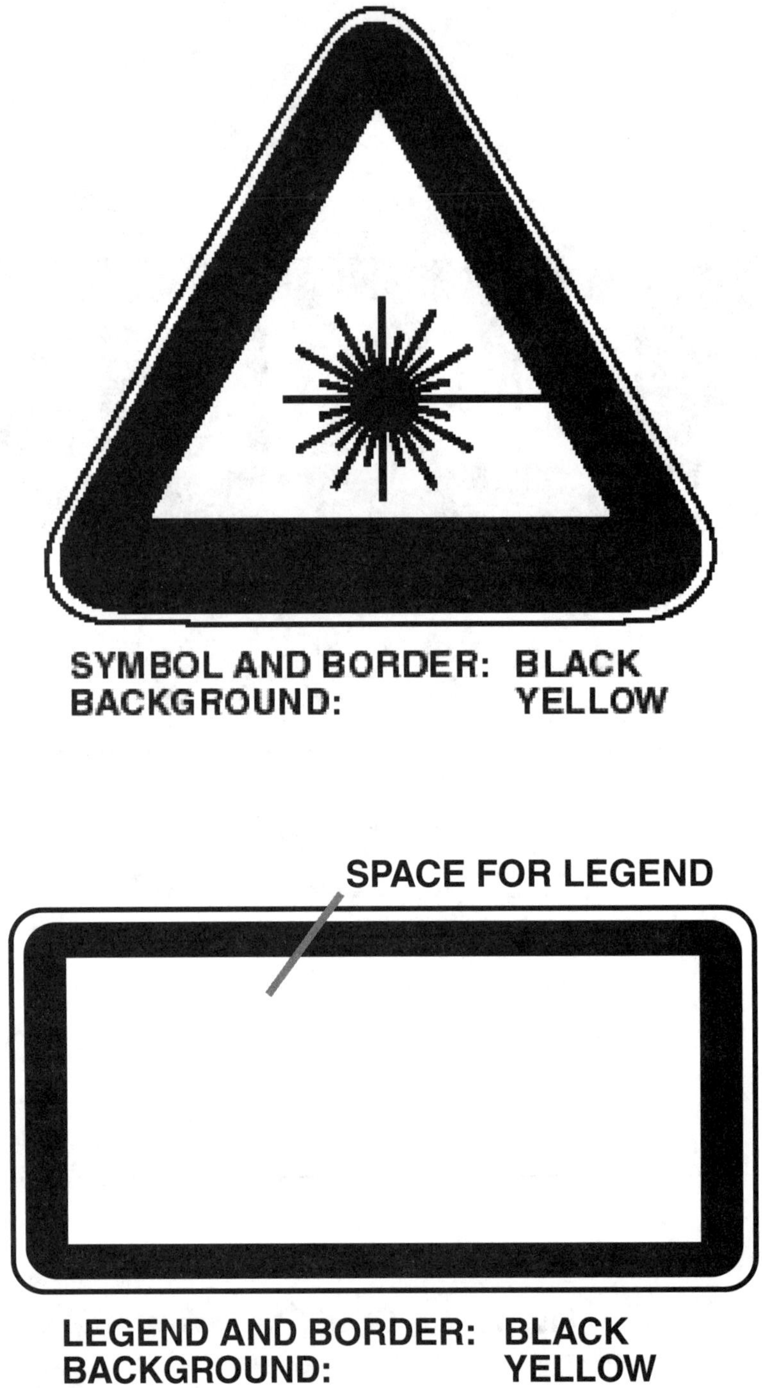

Figure 1c. IEC Warning Logo and Information Label

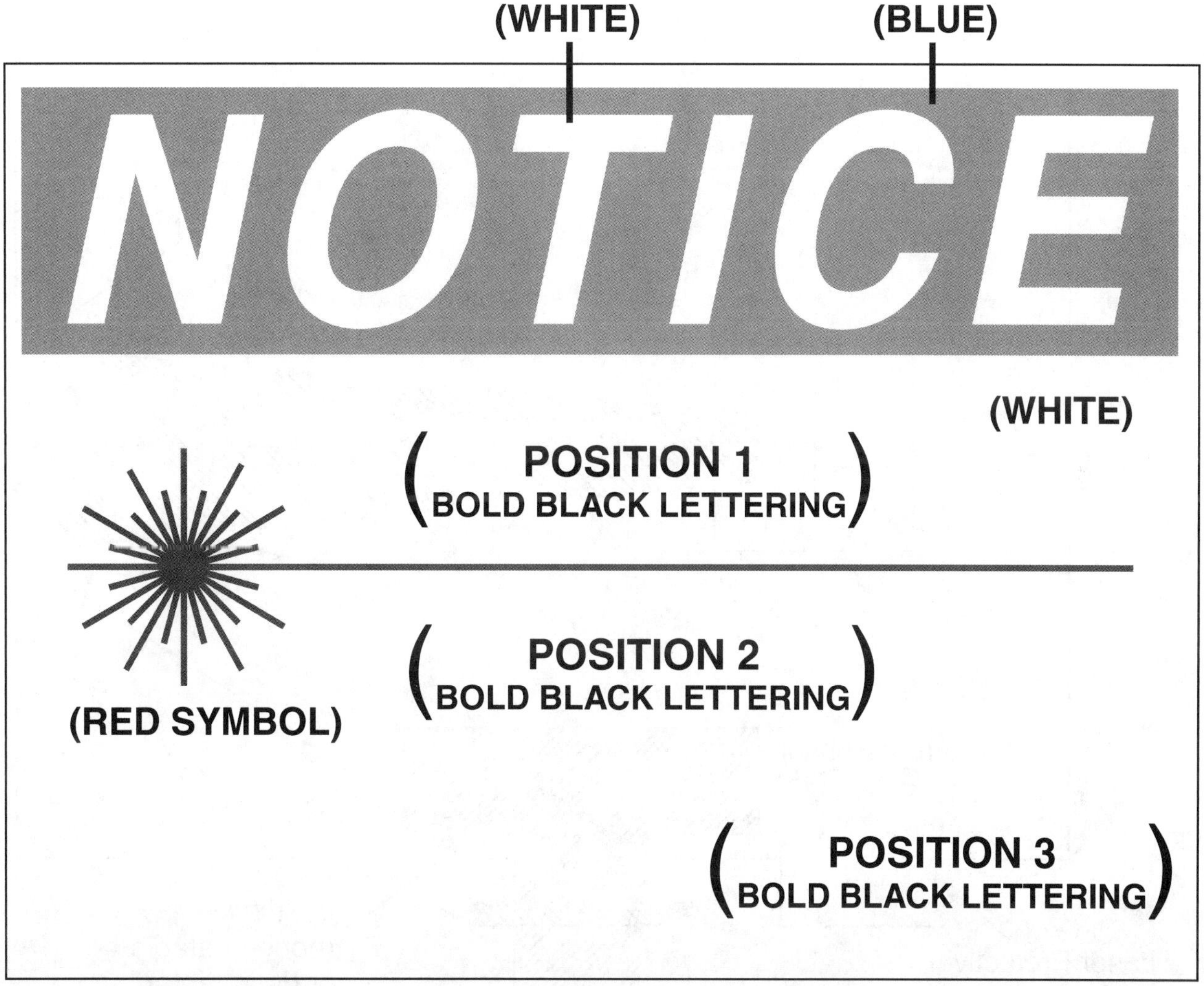

Figure 1d. Sample Warning Sign for Facility Policy, for example, Outside a Temporary Laser Controlled Area During Periods of Service

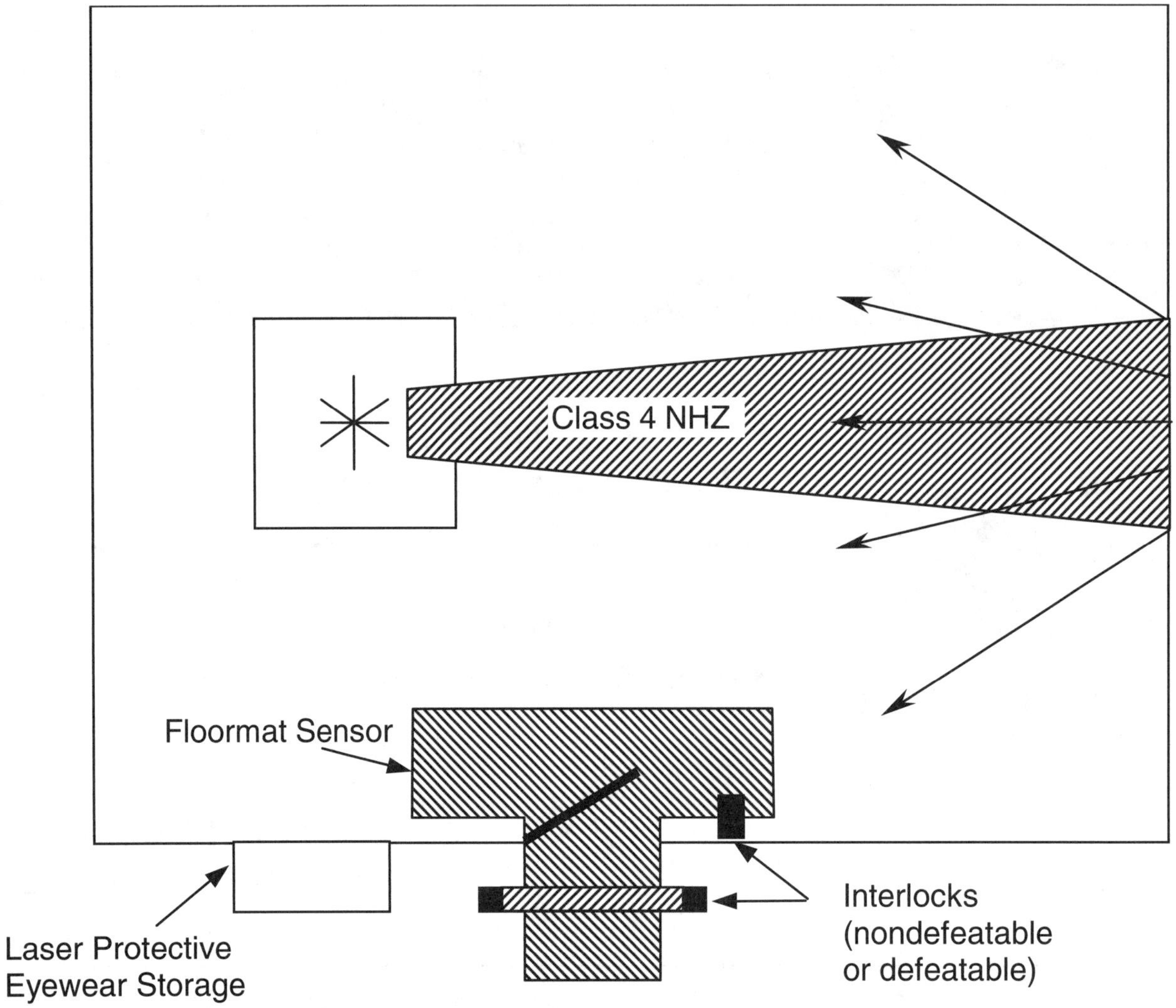

Figure 2a. Area/Entryway Safety Controls for Class 4 Lasers Utilizing Entryway Interlocks

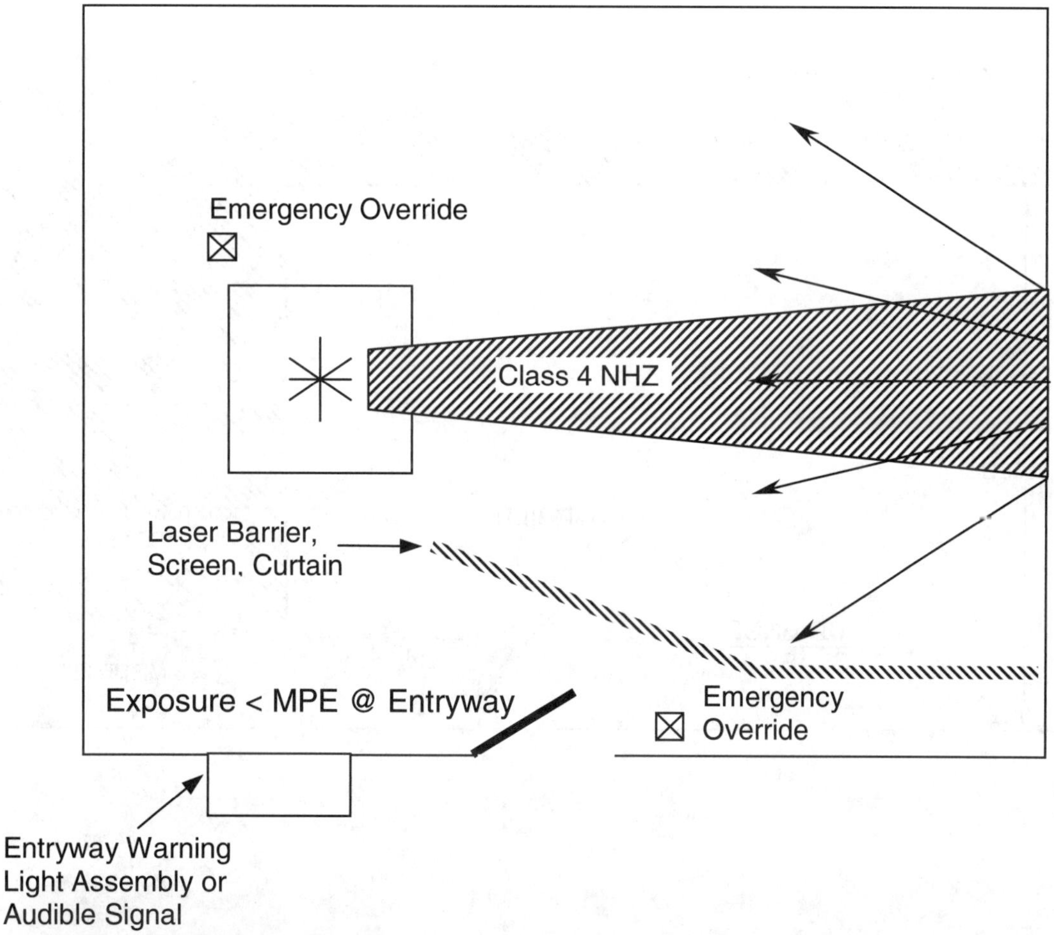

Figure 2b. Entryway Safety Controls for Class 4 Lasers without Entryway Interlocks

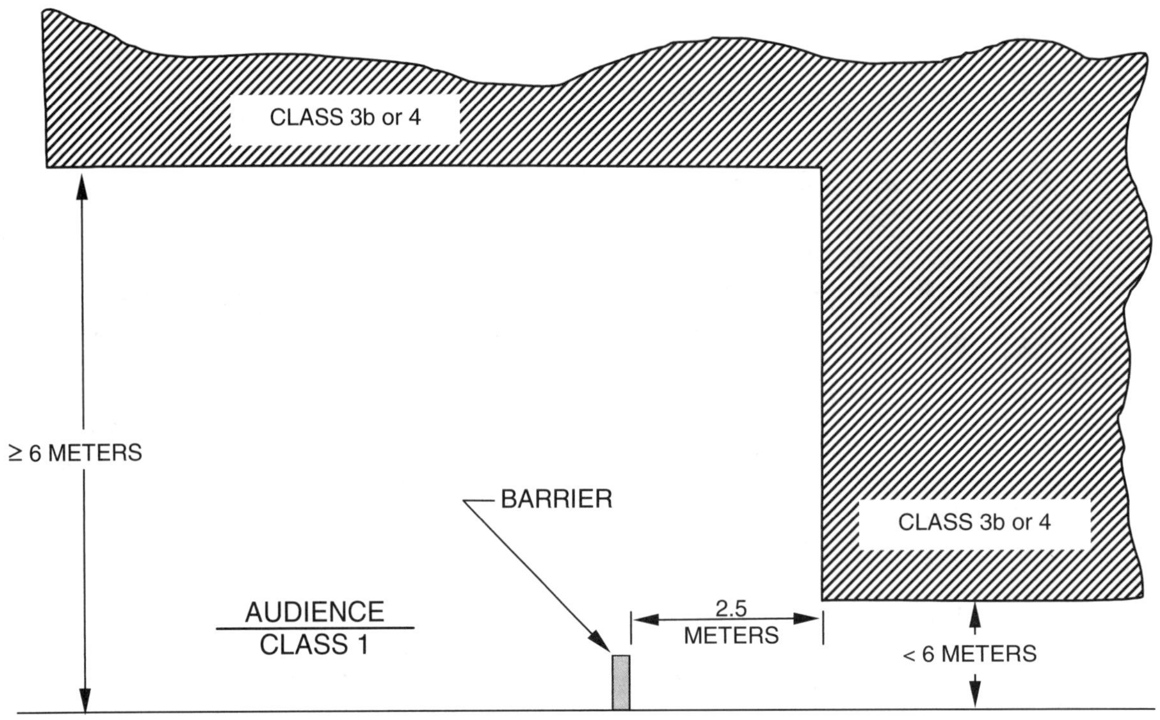

Figure 2c. Unsupervised Laser Installation for Demonstration Laser

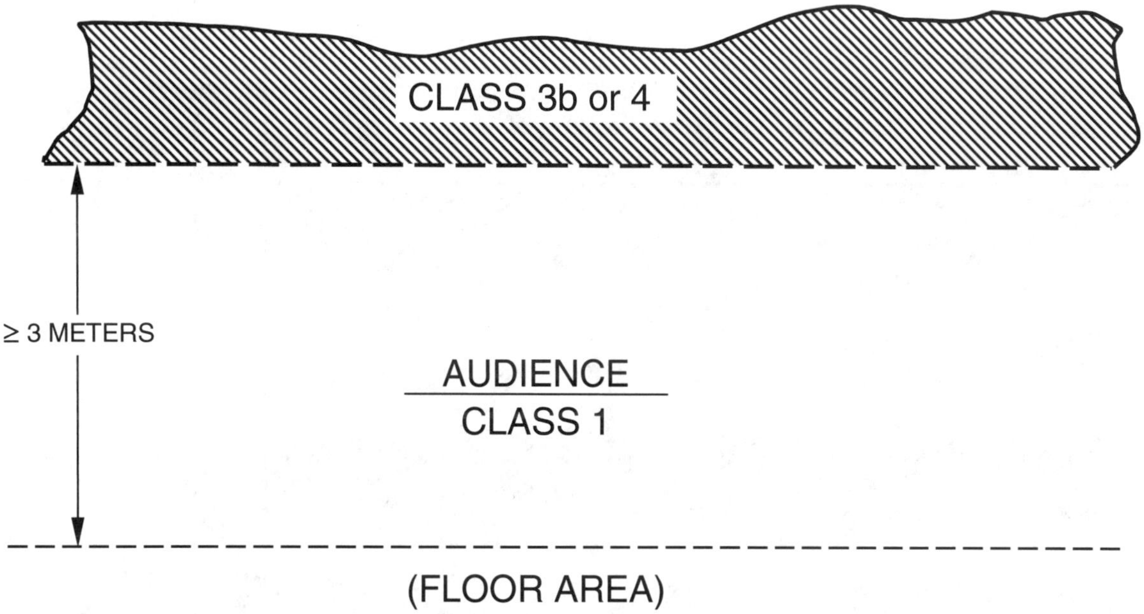

Figure 2d. Supervised Laser Installation for Demonstration Laser

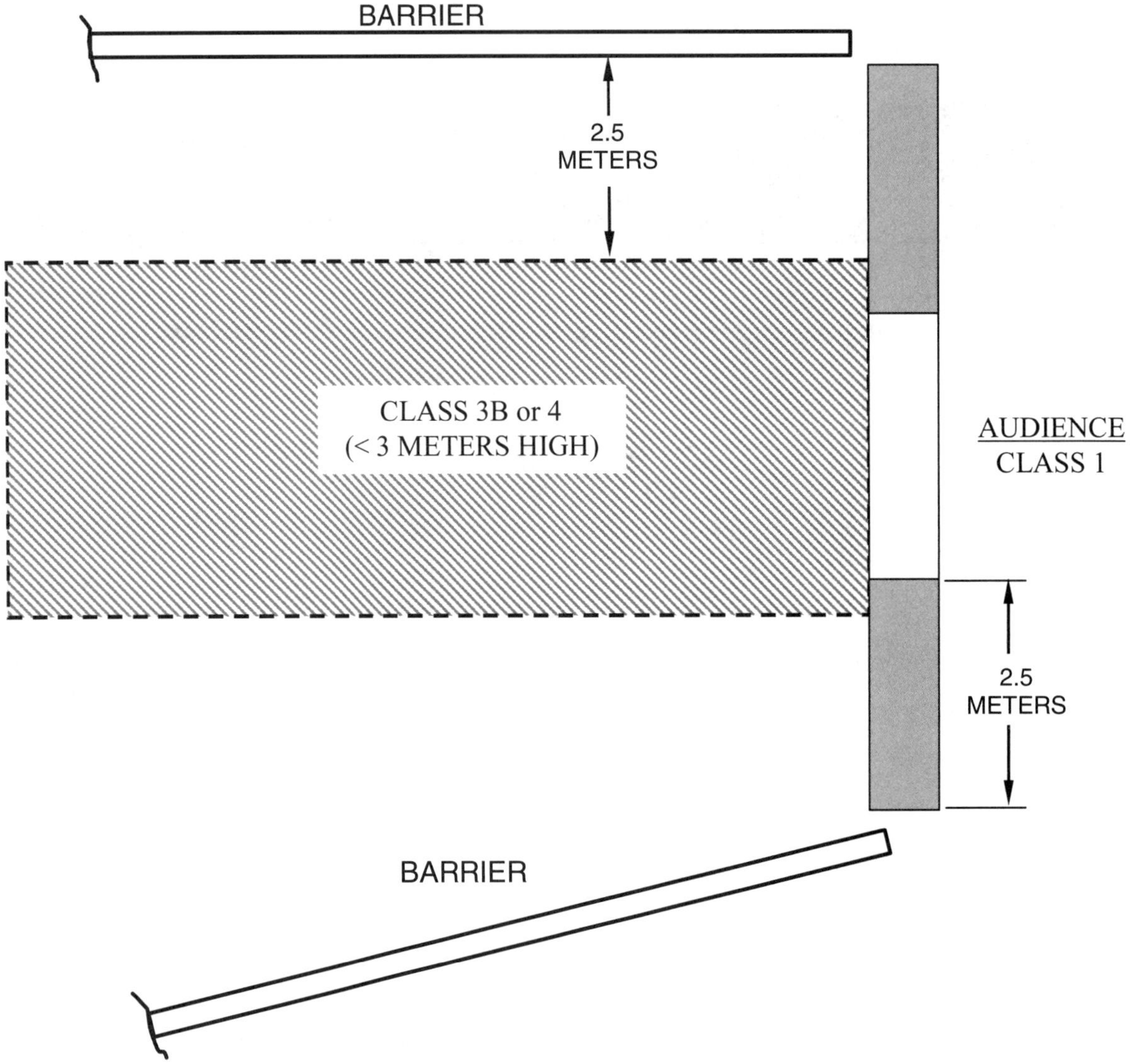

Figure 2e. Supervised Laser Installation for Demonstration Laser

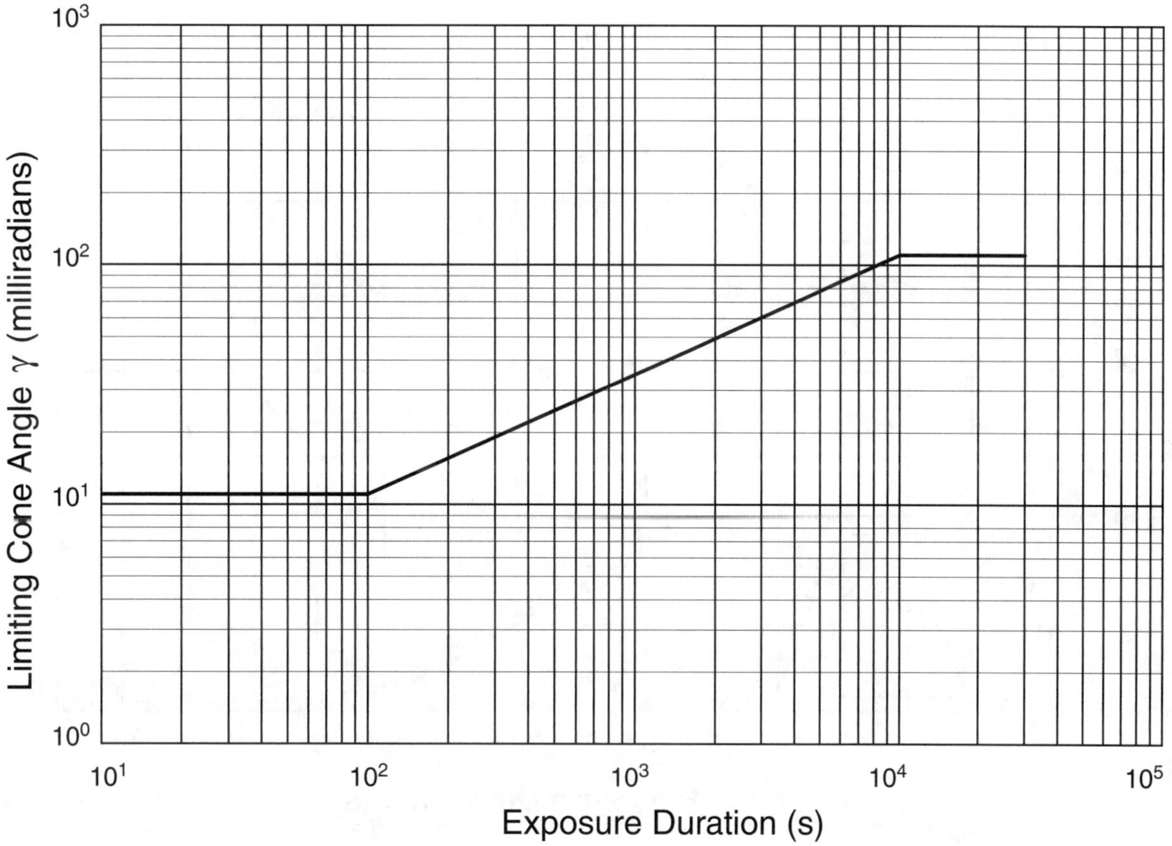

Figure 3. Limiting Cone Angle γ, Photochemical MPEs

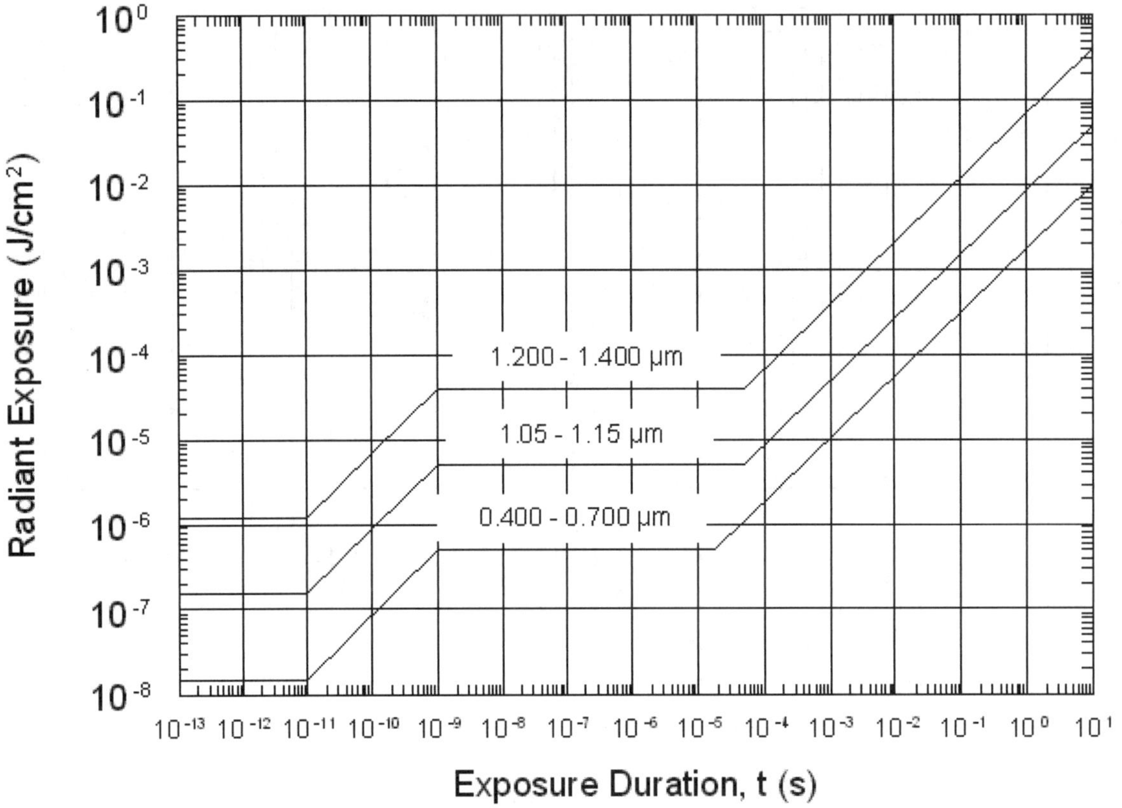

Figure 4. Point Source MPEs for Visible and Near Infrared Pulsed Sources (Wavelengths from 0.400 to 1.400 μm)

See Table 5a.

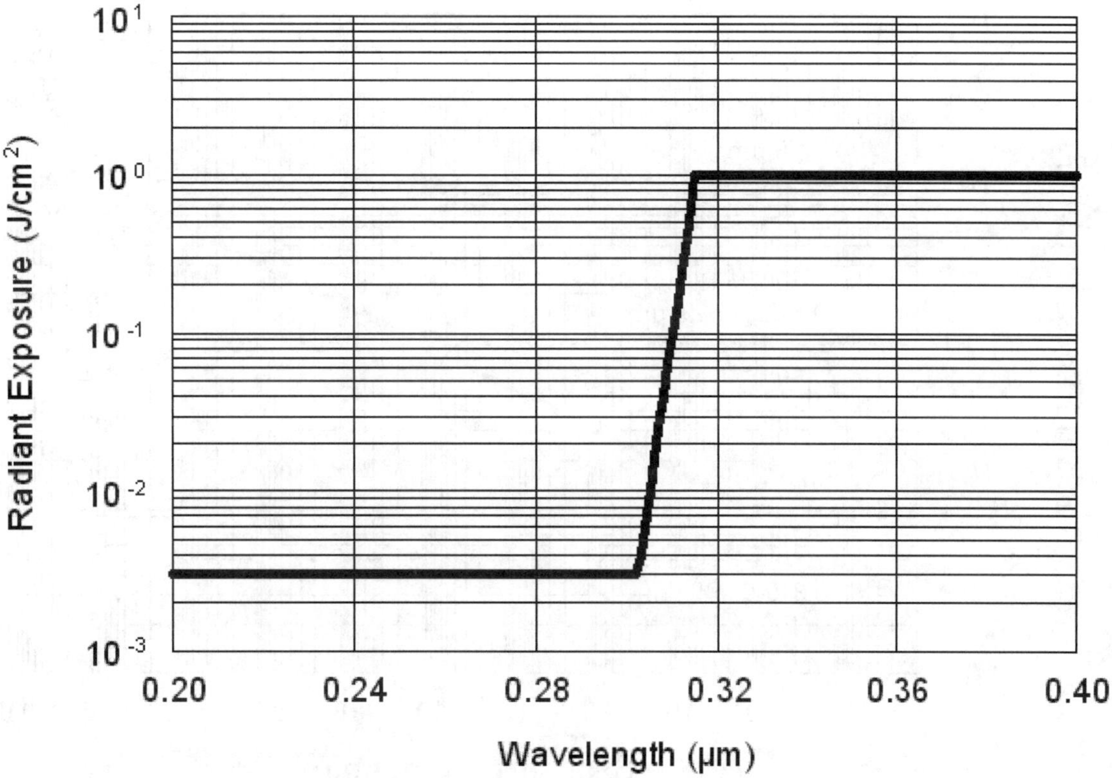

Figure 5. MPE for Ultraviolet Radiation (Small and Extended Sources) for Exposure Duration from 10^{-9} to 3×10^{4} s for Ocular Exposure and 10^{-9} to 10^{3} s for Skin Exposure*

* Unless 0.56 $t^{0.25}$ is exceeded (possible for exposure durations < 10 s at wavelengths from 0.305 to 0.315 µm).

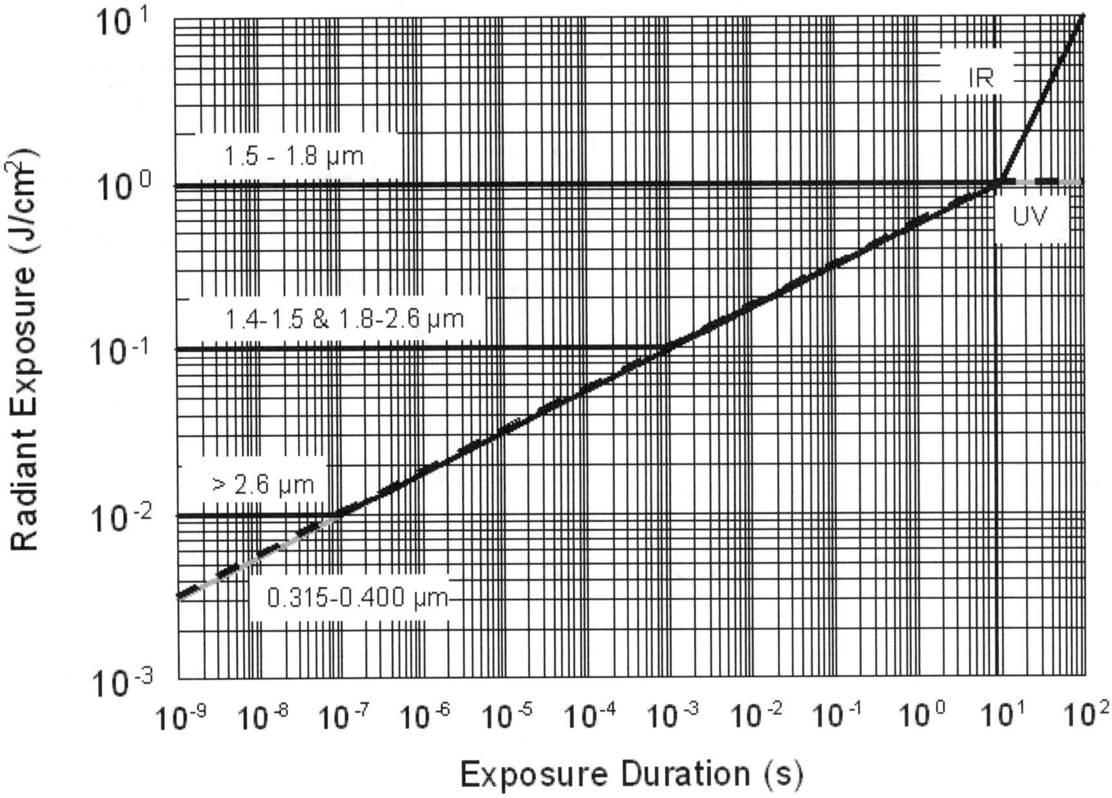

Figure 6. MPE for Ultraviolet (Wavelengths from 0.315 to 0.400 µm) and Infrared Radiation (Wavelengths from 1.400 µm to 1mm) for Single Pulses or Continuous Exposure (Small or Extended Sources)

See Figure 5 for Wavelengths less than 0.315 µm.

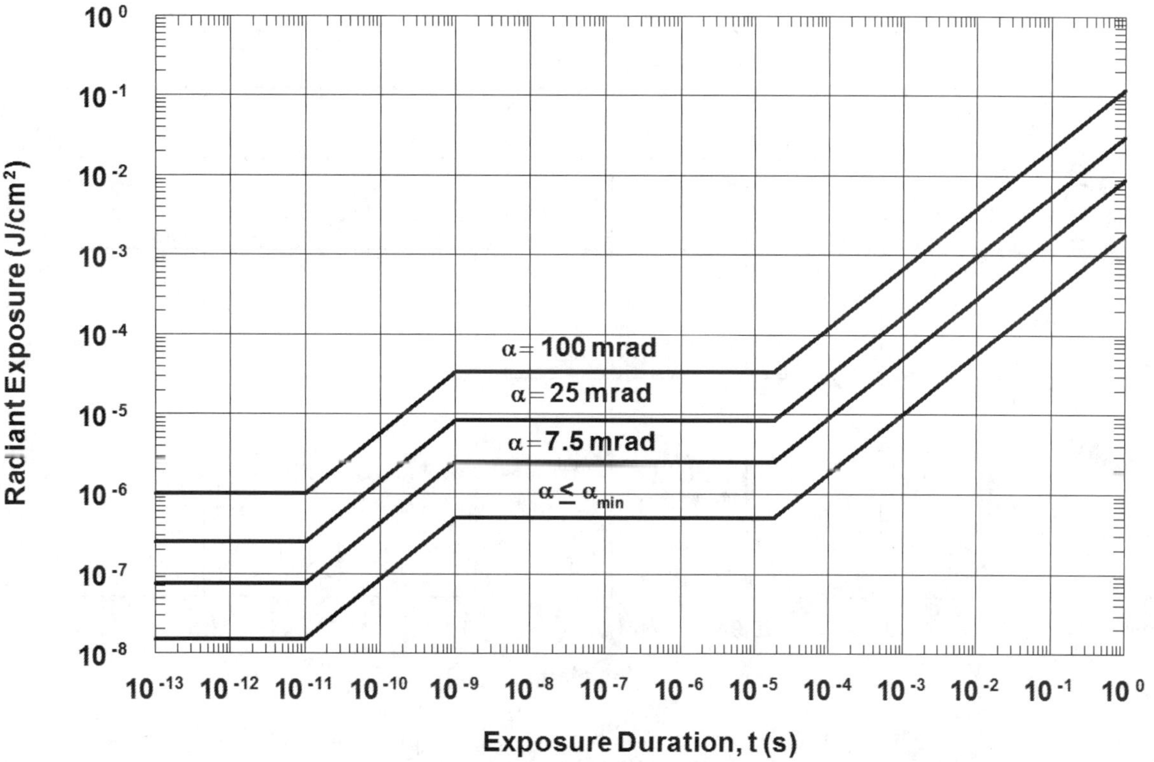

Figure 7. MPE for Ocular Exposure to Visible Laser Radiation (Wavelengths from 0.400 to 0.700 μm) for Single Pulses or Continuous Exposure (Small or Extended Sources)

See Tables 5a and 5b.

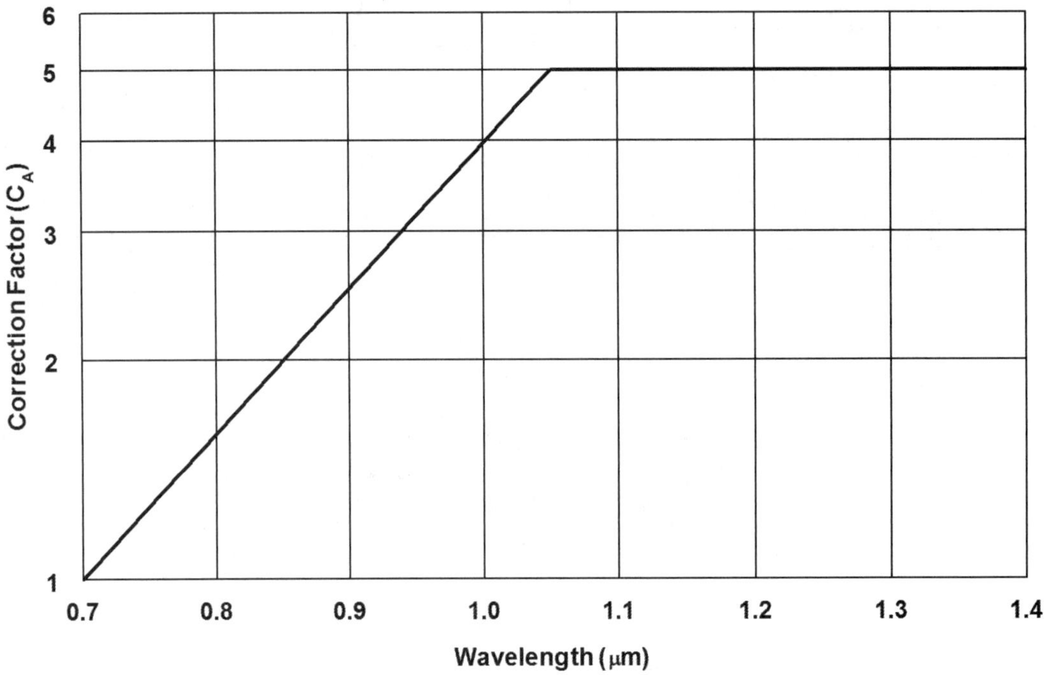

Note: $C_A = 1$ for $\lambda = 0.400$ to 0.7.00 μm
$C_A = 10^{2(\lambda-0.700)}$ for $\lambda = 0.700$ to 1.050 μm
$C_A = 5.0$ for $\lambda = 1.050$ to 1.400 μm

Figure 8a. Correction Factor C_A used to Determine the MPE for Wavelengths from 0.400 to 1.400 μm

See Table 6.

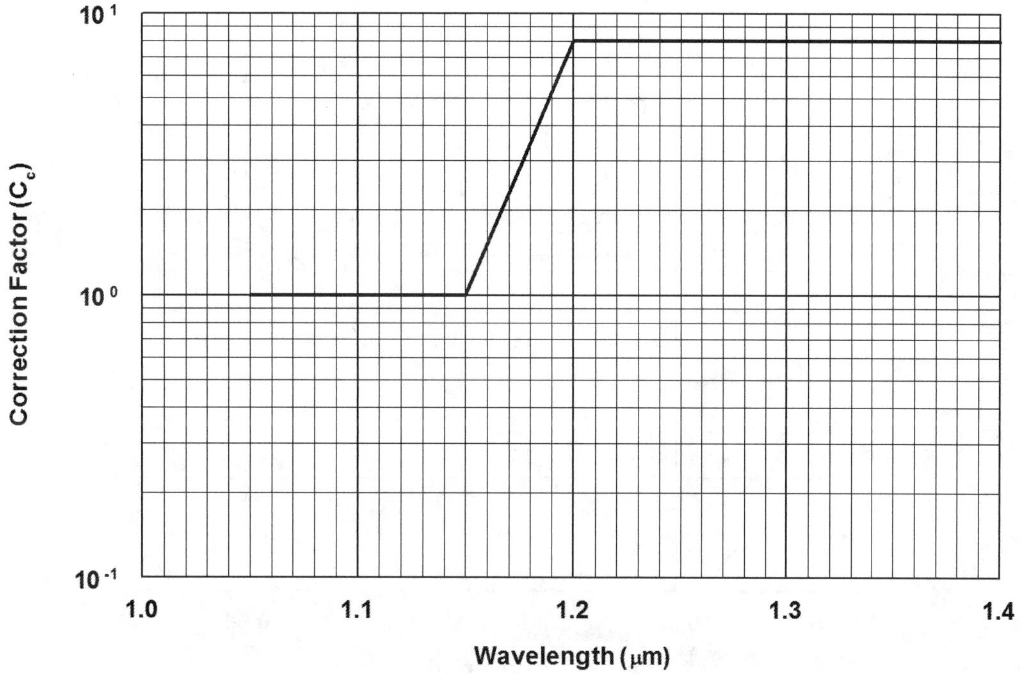

Note: $C_C = 1.0$ for $\lambda = 1.050$ to 1.150 μm
$C_C = 10^{18(\lambda-1.150)}$ for $\lambda = 1.150$ to 1.200 μm
$C_C = 8$ for $\lambda = 1.200$ to 1.400 μm

Figure 8b. Correction Factor C_C used to Determine the MPE for Wavelengths from 1.050 to 1.400 μm

See Table 6.

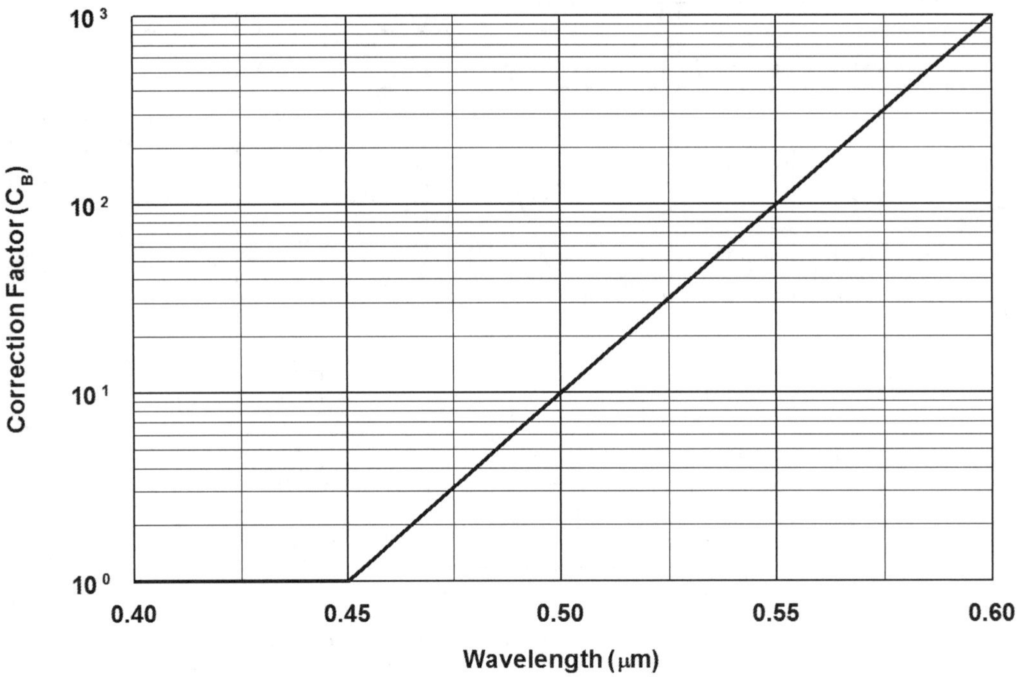

Figure 8c. Correction Factor C_B used to Determine the MPE for Wavelengths from 0.400 to 0.600 μm

See Table 6.

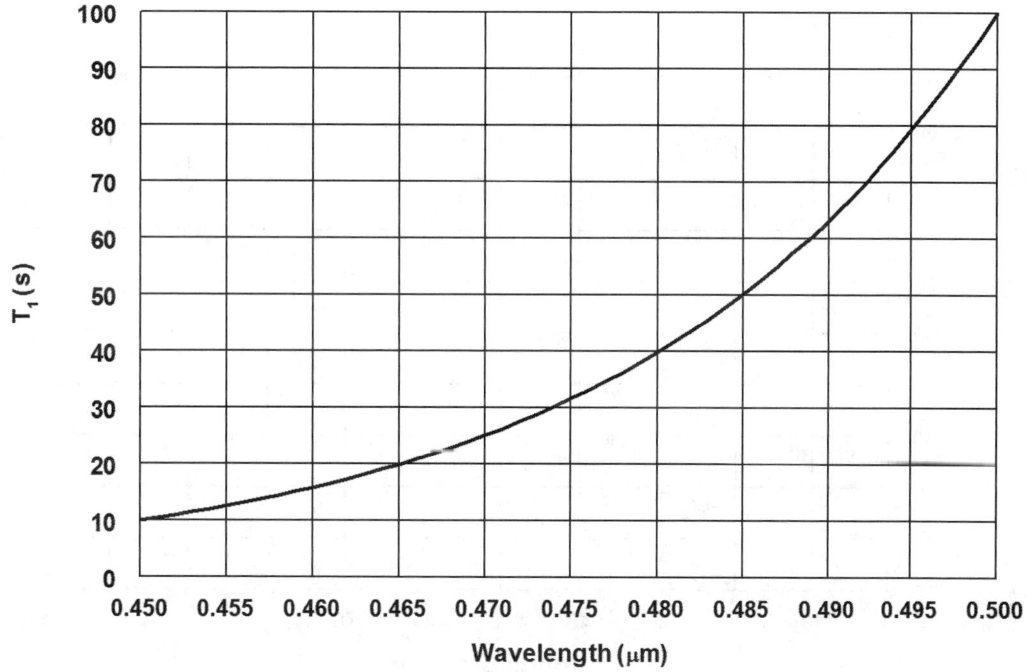

Note: $T_1 = 10 \times 10^{20(\lambda - 0.450)}$ for wavelengths from 0.450 to 0.500 μm

Figure 9a. Correction Factor T_1 Beyond which Photochemical (Rather than Thermal) Effects Determine the MPE for Point Sources for Wavelengths from 0.450 to 0.500 μm

See Tables 5a and 6.

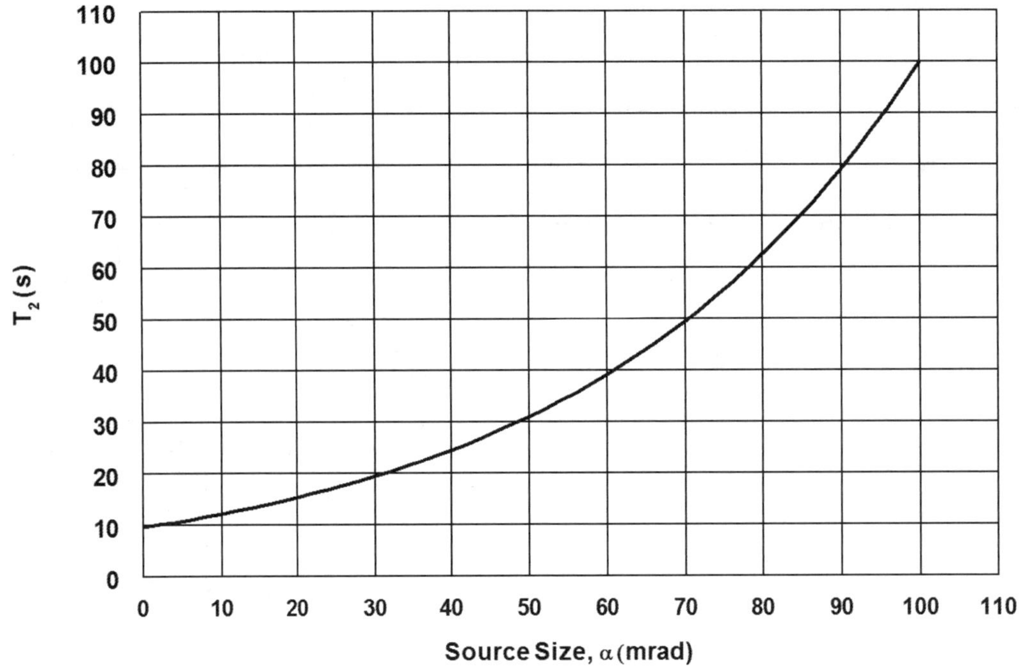

Note: $T_2 = 10 \times 10^{(\alpha-1.5)/98.5}$ for wavelengths from 0.400 to 1.400 μm (α is in milliradians)
T_2 = 10 s for point sources
T_2 = 100 s for sources equal to or exceeding 100 mrad

Figure 9b. Correction Factor T_2 used to Determine the Extended Source MPE based on Thermal Effects for Exposure Durations Greater than T_2

See Table 6.

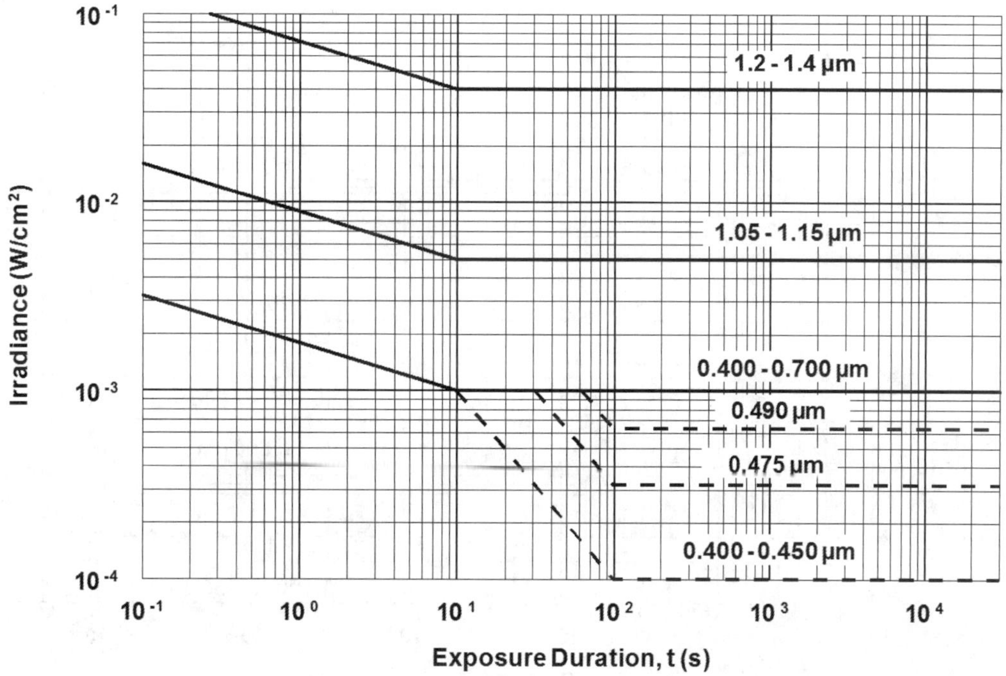

Note: Solid lines indicate the MPE based on Thermal Effects.
Dashed lines indicate the MPE based on Photochemical Effects.

Figure 10a. Ocular Point Source MPE ($\alpha \leq 1.5$ mrad) for Visible and Near Infrared Laser Radiation (Wavelengths from 0.400 to 1.400 μm)

See Table 5a.

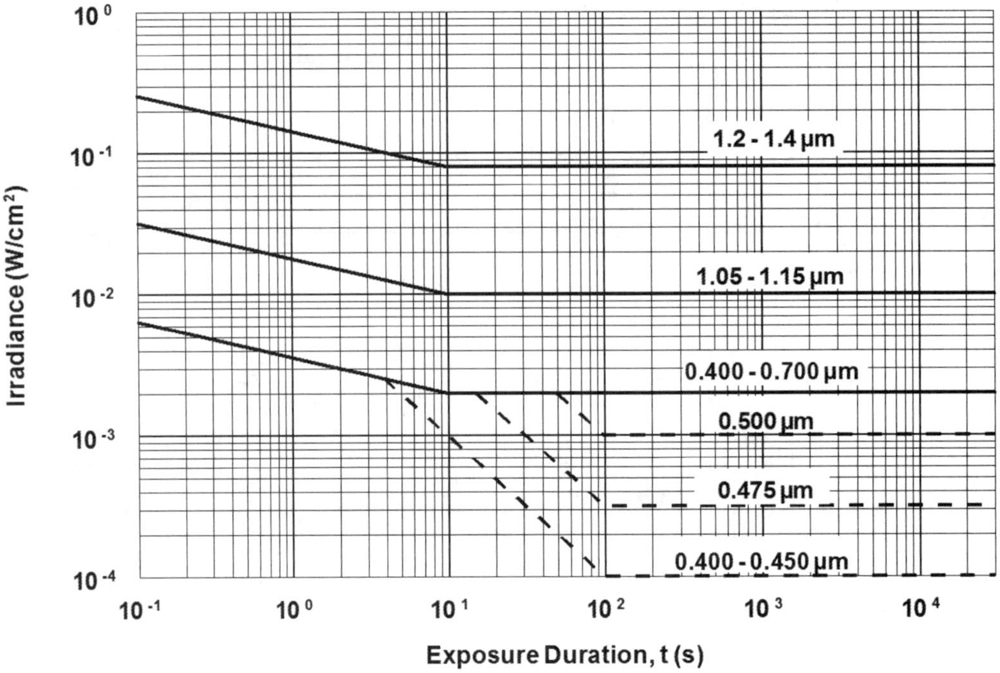

Note: Solid lines indicate the MPE based on Thermal Effects.
Dashed lines indicate the MPE based on Photochemical Effects.

Figure 10b. Ocular Extended Source MPE (α = 3.0 mrad) for Visible and Near Infrared Laser Radiation (Wavelengths from 0.400 to 1.400 μm)

See Table 5b.

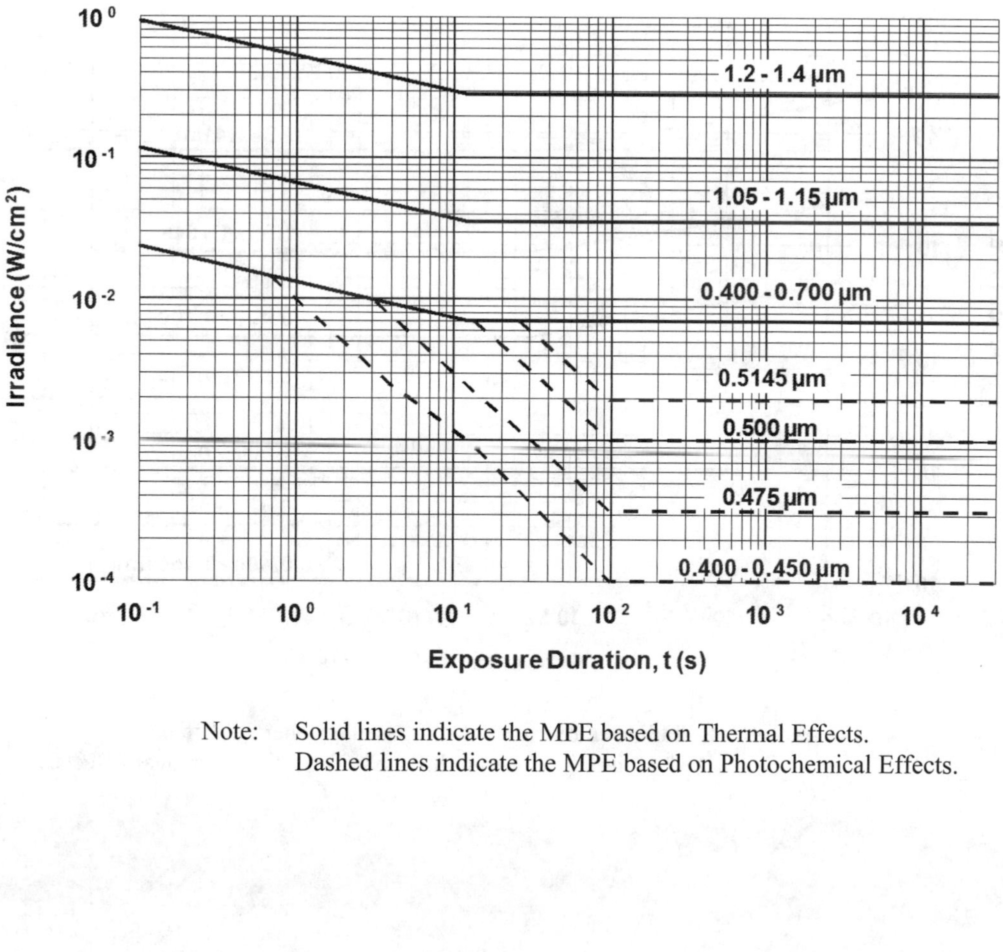

Note: Solid lines indicate the MPE based on Thermal Effects.
Dashed lines indicate the MPE based on Photochemical Effects.

Figure 10c. Ocular Extended Source MPE ($\alpha \leq 11$ mrad) for Visible and Near Infrared Laser Radiation (Wavelengths from 0.400 to 1.400 µm)

See Table 5b.

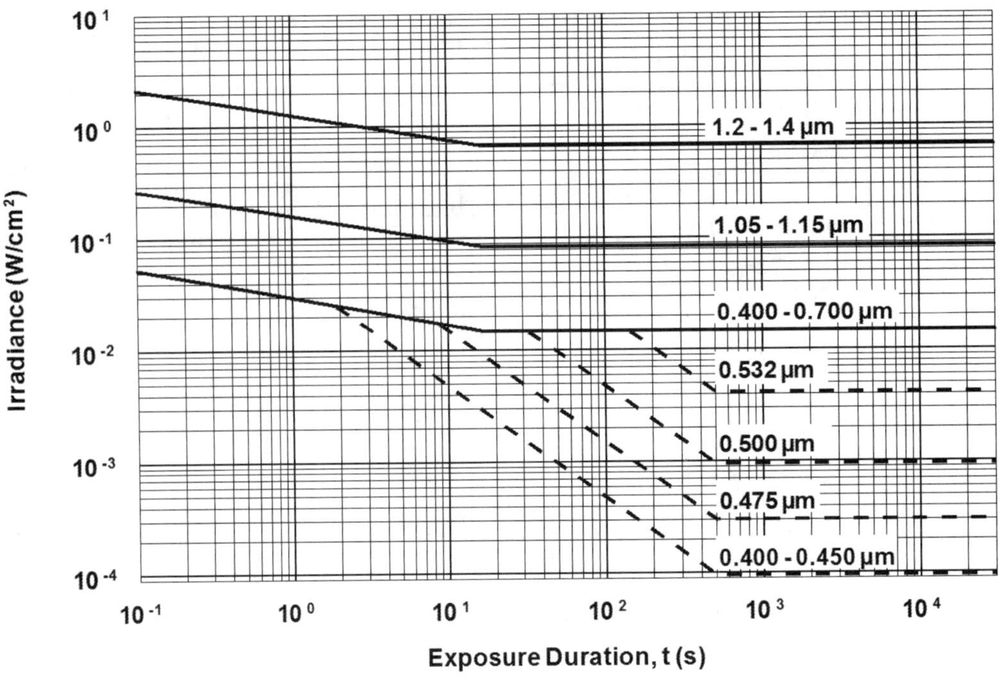

Note: Solid lines indicate the MPE based on Thermal Effects.
Dashed lines indicate the MPE based on Photochemical Effects.

Figure 10d. Ocular Extended Source MPE ($\alpha = 25$ mrad) for Visible and Near Infrared Laser Radiation (Wavelengths from 0.400 to 1.400 μm)

See Table 5b.

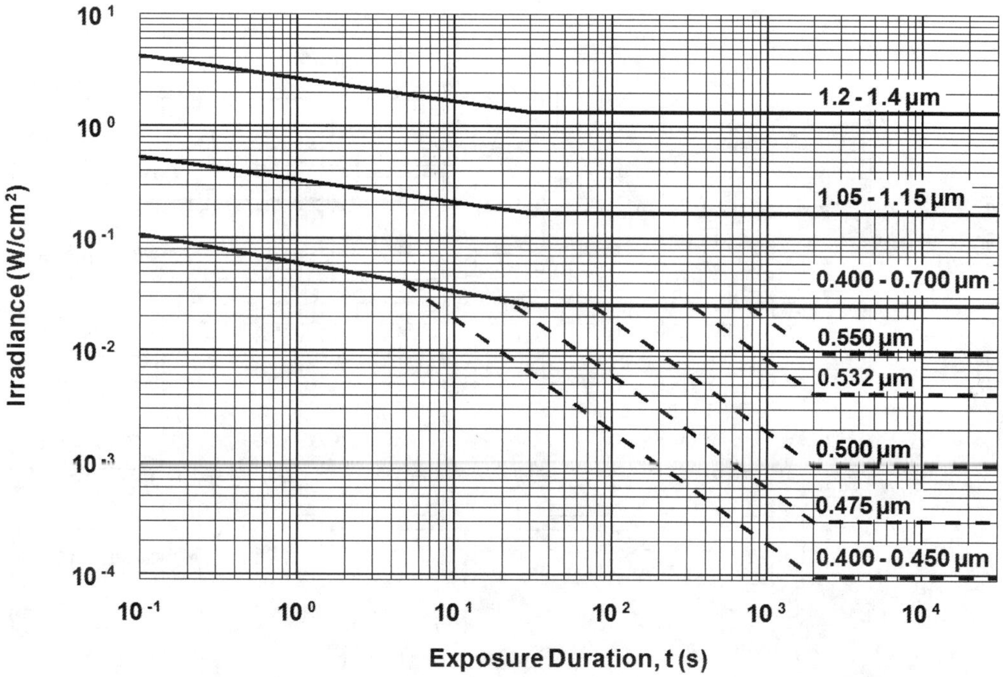

Note: Solid lines indicate the MPE based on Thermal Effects.
Dashed lines indicate the MPE based on Photochemical Effects.

Figure 10e. Ocular Extended Source MPE (α = 50 mrad) for Visible and Near Infrared Laser Radiation (Wavelengths from 0.400 to 1.400 µm)

See Table 5b.

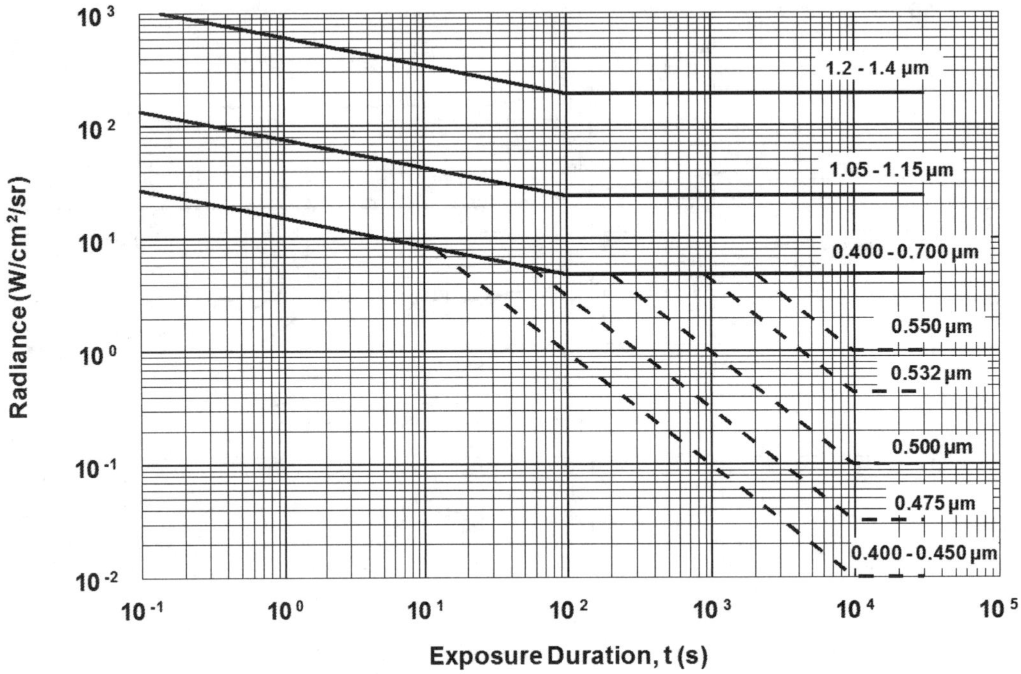

Note: Solid lines indicate the MPE based on Thermal Effects.
Dashed lines indicate the MPE based on Photochemical Effects.

Figure 11. Ocular Extended Source MPE ($\alpha \geq 110$ mrad) for Visible and Near Infrared Laser Radiation (Wavelengths from 0.400 to 1.400 µm)

See Table 5b.

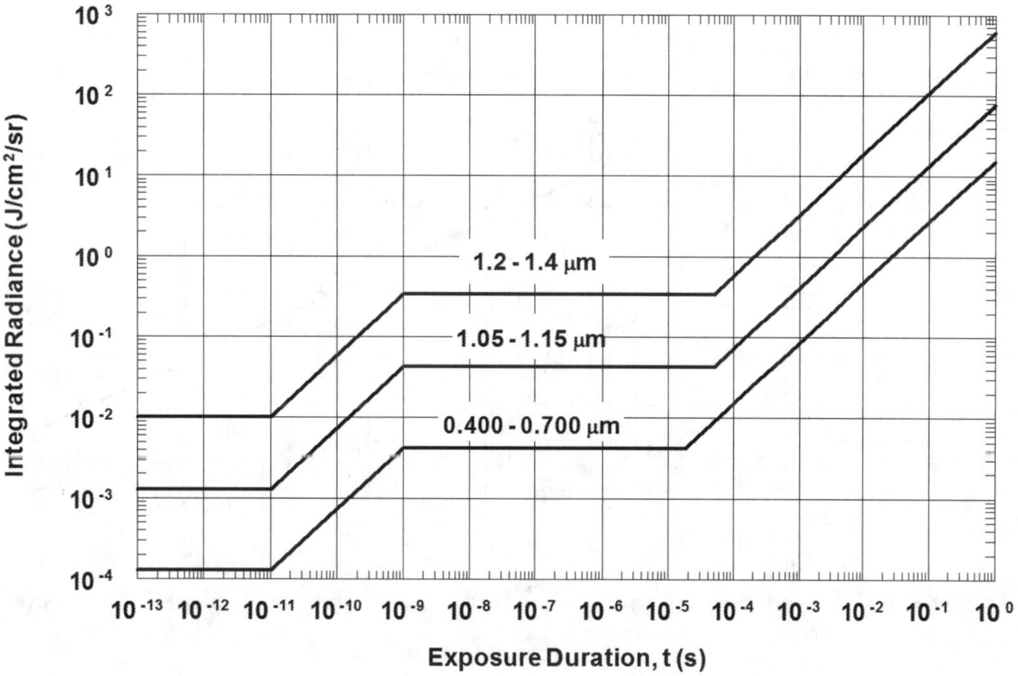

Figure 12. Ocular Extended Source Radiance MPE ($\alpha \geq 100$ mrad) for Visible and Near Infrared Laser Radiation (Wavelengths from 0.400 to 1.400 µm) for Pulsed or Continuous Exposures less than 1 s

See Table 5b.

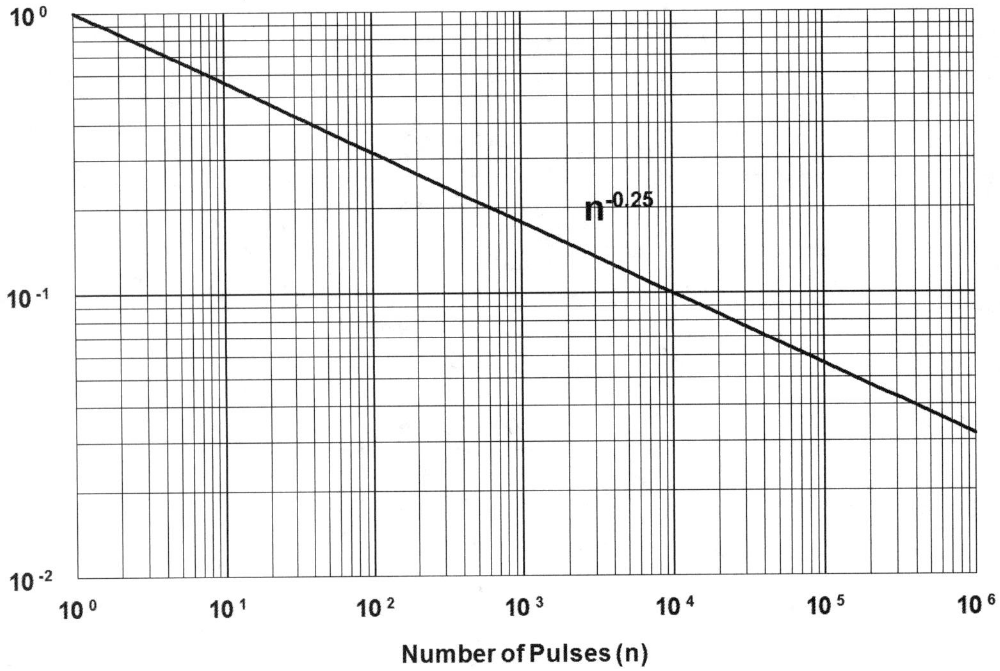

Figure 13. MPE Reduction Factor (C_P) for Repetitive-Pulse Lasers and Multiple Exposures from Scanning Lasers

Appendix A
Supplement to Section 1 – Laser Safety Programs

Note: The following material is an extension of 1.3 and, as a normative Appendix, is an integral part of the standard.

A1. Laser Safety Officer (LSO)

A1.1 General. The LSO is an individual designated by the employer with the authority and responsibility to effect the knowledgeable evaluation and control of laser hazards, and to monitor and enforce the control of such hazards. The LSO shall have authority to suspend, restrict, or terminate the operation of a laser system if he/she deems that laser hazard controls are inadequate. For the laser safety program to be effective, the LSO must have sufficient authority to accompany the responsibility. In organizations that do not permit authority to reside with non-management personnel and the LSO is a non-management position; the management shall provide protocols and reporting structure to assure adequate enforcement authority.

The LSO may be designated from among such personnel as the radiation safety officer, industrial hygienist, safety engineer, laser specialist, laser operator or user, etc. The LSO may be a part-time position when the workload for an LSO does not require a full-time effort. In some instances, the designation of an LSO may not be required. Operation and maintenance of Class 1, Class 1M, Class 2, Class 2M and Class 3R lasers and laser systems normally do not require the designation of an LSO. However, under some circumstances it may be desirable to designate an LSO, for example, if service is performed on a laser system having an embedded Class 3B, or Class 4 laser or laser system. In such instances, management may designate the service person requiring access to the embedded laser as the LSO. In any case, there shall be a designated LSO for all circumstances of operation, maintenance, and service of a Class 3B or Class 4 laser or laser system.

If necessary, a Deputy Laser Safety Officer (DLSO) shall be appointed by management or the LSO. The DLSO shall perform the functions of the LSO when the latter is not available. For institutions with multiple divisions or plant locations, a system of DLSOs may be required.

A1.2 LSO Specific Duties and Responsibilities.

(1) **Safety Program.** The LSO shall establish and maintain adequate policies and procedures for the control of laser hazards. These policies and procedures shall comply with applicable requirements, including federal, state and local regulations.

(2) **Classification.** The LSO shall classify, or verify classifications of, lasers and laser systems used under the LSO's jurisdiction. Classifications shall be consistent with classifications listed in Section 3 of this standard.

(3) **Hazard Evaluation.** The LSO shall be responsible for hazard evaluation of laser work areas. Hazard evaluation shall be conducted in accordance with Section 3 of this standard.

(4) **Control Measures.** The LSO shall be responsible for assuring that the prescribed control measures are implemented and maintained in effect. This includes avoiding unnecessary or duplicate controls, and recommending or approving substitute or alternate control measures when the primary ones are not feasible or practical.

(5) **Procedure Approvals.** The LSO shall approve Class 3B and Class 4 standard operating procedures (SOPs), and other procedures that may be part of the requirements for administrative and procedural controls.

(6) **Protective Equipment.** The LSO shall recommend or approve protective equipment, i.e., eyewear, clothing, barriers, screens, etc. as may be required to assure personnel safety. The LSO shall assure that protective equipment is audited periodically to assure proper working order.

(7) **Signs and Labels.** The LSO shall review the wording on area signs and equipment labels.

(8) **Facility and Equipment.** The LSO shall review Class 3B and Class 4 laser installations, facilities and laser equipment prior to use. This also applies to modification of existing facilities or equipment.

(9) **Training.** The LSO shall assure that adequate safety education and training are provided to laser personnel. The frequency of refresher training shall be considered on the basis of the total hazard evaluation criteria presented in Section 3.

(10) **Medical Surveillance.** The LSO shall determine the personnel categories for medical surveillance (see Section 6).

(11) **Records.** The LSO shall assure that the necessary records required by applicable government regulations are maintained. The LSO shall also submit to the appropriate medical officer the individuals' names that are obtained in accordance with A3.1(3) and A3.1(4), and shall assure that the appropriate records are maintained indicating that applicable medical examinations have been scheduled and performed. Other records documenting the maintenance of the safety program, such as training records, audits, SOP approvals, etc., shall be maintained.

(12) **Audits, Surveys and Inspections.** The LSO shall periodically audit or survey by inspection for the presence and functionality of the laser safety features and control measures required for each Class 3B and Class 4 laser or laser system in the laser facilities. The LSO shall accompany regulatory agency inspectors (such as OSHA, FDA/CDRH, state or local agencies) reviewing the laser safety program or investigating an incident and document any discrepancies or issues noted. The LSO shall assure that corrective action is taken, where required.

(13) **Accidents.** The LSO should develop a plan to respond to notifications of incidents of actual or suspected exposure to potentially harmful laser radiation. The plan should include the provision of medical assistance for the potentially exposed individual, investigation of the incident and the documentation and reporting of the investigation results.

(14) **Approval of Laser Systems Operations.** Approval of a Class 3B or Class 4 laser or laser system for operation shall be given only if the LSO is satisfied that laser hazard

control measures are adequate. These include SOPs (standard operating procedures) for maintenance and service operations within enclosed systems and operation procedures for Class 3B and 4 laser systems. The procedures should include adequate consideration of safety from non-beam hazards.

A2. Laser Safety Committee

A Laser Safety Committee may be created.

A2.1 Membership of Laser Safety Committee. The membership of the Laser Safety Committee may include members with expertise in laser technology or in the assessment of laser hazards. Management may be included in the membership. Examples of members include, but are not limited to, technical management, LSO and/or representatives of the safety/industrial hygiene organization, physician, education department member, engineer/scientist and user representative.

A2.2 Policies and Practices. The committee shall establish and maintain adequate policies and practices for the evaluation and control of laser hazards, including the recommending of appropriate laser safety training programs and materials.

A2.3 Standards. The committee shall maintain an awareness of all applicable new or revised laser safety standards.

A3. Other Personnel Responsibilities

A3.1 Laser Supervisor. The supervisor of individuals working with or having the potential for exposure to greater than Class 1 laser radiation, should have a basic overall knowledge of laser safety requirements for the lasers under the supervisor's authority.

The following responsibilities should be considered as a minimal set of responsibilities for the Laser Supervisor.

(1) The supervisor shall be responsible for the issuance of appropriate instructions and training materials on laser hazards and their control to all personnel who may work with lasers that are operated within the supervisor's jurisdiction.

(2) The supervisor shall not permit the operation of a laser unless there is adequate control of laser hazards to employees, visitors, and the general public.

(3) The supervisor shall submit the names of individuals scheduled to work with lasers to the LSO and shall submit information as requested by the LSO for medical surveillance scheduling and training completion.

(4) When the supervisor knows of, or suspects, an accident resulting from a laser operated under his or her authority, the supervisor shall immediately upon becoming aware of a suspected laser incident implement the institution's accident responsible plan and ensure it includes notification of the LSO.

(5) If necessary, the supervisor shall assist in obtaining appropriate medical attention for any employee involved in a laser accident.

(6) The supervisor shall not permit operation of a new or modified Class 3B or Class 4 laser under his or her authority without the approval of the LSO.

(7) The supervisor shall submit plans for Class 3B and Class 4 laser installations or modifications of installations to the LSO for review.

(8) For Class 3B or Class 4 lasers and laser systems, the supervisor shall be familiar with the standard operating procedures and ensure that they are provided to users of such lasers.

A3.2 Responsibility of Employees Working with Lasers. Employees working with lasers or laser systems shall have, where applicable, the following minimal responsibilities.

(1) An employee shall not energize or work with or near a laser unless authorized to do so by the supervisor for that laser.

(2) An employee shall comply with safety rules and procedures prescribed by the supervisor and the LSO. The employee shall be familiar with all applicable operating procedures.

(3) When an employee operating a laser knows or suspects that an accident has occurred involving that laser, or a laser operated by any other employee, and that such accident has caused an injury or could potentially have caused an injury, he or she shall immediately inform the supervisor. If the supervisor is not available, the employee shall notify the LSO.

A3.3 Other Personnel. Anyone involved in purchasing a laser or laser system should contact the LSO. Such personnel may also include but is not limited to purchasing, accounting, building management, etc. as may be applicable.

Appendix B
Calculations for Hazard Evaluation and Classification

B1. General

Calculations are not necessary for hazard evaluation and classification in many applications; however, in outdoor applications and other specialized uses where eye exposure is contemplated, several types of calculations permit the important quantitative study of potential hazards.

Mathematical symbols used here are defined in B2. MPE determination may require the use of formulae in B3. Hazard classification methods are discussed in B4. Formulae for computing beam irradiance and radiant exposure are contained in B5. Formulae useful in hazard evaluation and calculating nominal ocular hazard distance and nominal hazard zone are listed in B6. Methods for determining MPEs based on retinal hazards from both photochemical and thermal effects for extended visible laser sources are discussed in B7. Formulae useful in determining adequate protective eyewear or laser barriers are listed in B8. Determination of extended source sizes is discussed in B9. Applicable references are contained in B10.

Figures B1 through B9 illustrate conditions of ocular exposure to laser radiation.

B2. Symbols

The following symbols are used in the formulae of this Appendix.

a = Diameter of emergent laser beam (cm).

α = Apparent angle subtended by a source at the location of the viewer (rad).

α_{max} = Apparent angle subtended by a source above which the thermal hazard is proportional to the radiance of the source (100 mrad).

α_{min} = Apparent angle subtended by a source above which extended source MPEs apply (1.5 mrad).

b_0 = Diameter of laser beam incident on a focusing lens (cm).

b_1 = Width of rectangular beam (cm).

b = Major axis of elliptical cross-section beam (cm).

c = Minor axis of elliptical cross-section beam (cm).

c_1 = Height of rectangular beam (cm).

C_A = Wavelength correction factor ($0.700\ \mu m < \lambda < 1.050\ \mu m$).

C_B = Wavelength correction factor ($0.400\ \mu m < \lambda < 0.600\ \mu m$).

C_C = Wavelength correction factor ($1.150\ \mu m < \lambda < 1.400\ \mu m$).

C_E = Extended source correction factor (=α/α_{min} for source angles less than 100 mrad).

C_P = Repetitive-pulse correction factor[1] (= $n^{-0.25}$).

d_e = Diameter of the pupil of the eye (varies from appropriately 0.2 to 0.7 cm).

D = Barrier separation distance from the focal point of final focusing lens (cm).

D_C = Diameter of collecting aperture of optical system (cm).

D_e = Diameter of the exit pupil of an optical system (cm).

D_{exit} = Exit port diameter of a laser (cm).

D_f = Limiting aperture from Tables 8a and 8b (cm).

D_L = Diameter of laser beam at range r (cm).

D_m = Diameter of measurement aperture from Table 9 used for classification (cm).

D_0 = Diameter of objective of an optical system (cm).

D_ρ = Diameter of a reflected laser beam at the reflecting surface (cm).

D_λ = Optical density at a particular wavelength (λ).

D_s = Barrier separation distance (direct beam) (cm).

D_{SD} = Barrier diffuse reflection separation distance (cm).

D_w = Diameter of a beam waist which occurs in front of the laser exit port (cm).

e = Base of natural logarithms (2.71828).

f = Effective focal length of the eye (1.7 cm).

f_0 = Focal length of a lens (cm).

F = Pulse-repetition frequency, PRF(s^{-1}).

F_{eff} = Effective (average) PRF (s^{-1}).

γ = Limiting cone angle (field of view) for MPEs based on photochemical hazards (11 mrad for t<100 s).

G = Ratio of corneal irradiance or radiant exposure through magnifying optics to that received by the unaided eye.

G_{eff} = Ratio of ocular hazard from optically aided viewing to that for unaided viewing.

H, E = Radiant exposure (H) or irradiance (E) at range r, measured in $J \cdot cm^{-2}$ for pulsed lasers and $W \cdot cm^{-2}$ for CW lasers.

H_0, E_0 = Emergent beam radiant exposure (H_0) or irradiance (E_0) at the minimum measurement distance (10 cm) (units as for E, H).

H_{group} = Radiant exposure for the summation of all the energies in a group of pulses.

H_p = The potential eye exposure, in the appropriate units, utilized in the determination of the optical density of protective eyewear.

[1] For pulse repetition frequencies less than the critical frequency.

λ = Wavelength of source (μm).

L_e = Radiance of an extended source (W·cm^{-2}·sr^{-1}).

L_p = Integrated radiance of an extended source (J·cm^{-2}·sr^{-1}).

MPE = Maximum permissible exposure.

MPE:E = MPE expressed as irradiance. For exposure to single pulses, the MPE is for peak power, and for a group of pulses, the MPE is for the average power (W·cm^{-2}).

MPE:H = MPE expressed as radiant exposure for a single pulse or exposure (J·cm^{-2}).

MPE:H_{group} = MPE expressed as radiant exposure for the summation of all the energy in a group of pulses (J·cm^{-2}).

MPE_{large} = MPE for an extended source.

MPE:L_e = MPE expressed as radiance (W·cm^{-2}·sr^{-1}).

MPE:L_P = MPE expressed as integrated radiance (J·cm^{-2}·sr^{-1}).

MPE/Pulse = MPE expressed as radiant exposure for each pulse in a pulse train (J·cm^{-2}).

MPE_{point} = MPE for a point source.

MPE_{skin} = MPE for skin exposure.

MPE_{SP} = MPE expressed as radiant exposure (J·cm^{-2}) for exposure to a single pulse in a pulse train (without exposure to any other pulses).

n = number of pulses within total exposure duration T.

NA = Numerical aperture of optical fiber. For emission from an optical fiber, the numerical aperture is the half-angle beam divergence measured at $1/e^3$ of peak irradiance.

P = Magnifying power of an optical instrument.

ϕ = Emergent beam divergence measured at the $1/e$ peak of irradiance points (rad).

ϕ_1 = Emergent beam divergence of the major cross-sectional dimension of a rectangular or elliptical beam (rad).

ϕ_2 = Emergent beam divergence of the minor cross-sectional dimension of a rectangular or elliptical beam (rad).

Φ = Radiant power (W).

Φ_0 = Total radiant power output of a CW laser, or average radiant power of a repetitive-pulse laser (W).

Φ_d = Radiant power transmitted by an aperture (W).

Φ_{eff} = Power transmitted by the measurement aperture from Table 9 (W).

Q = Radiant energy (J).

Q_0 = Total radiant energy output of a pulsed laser (J).

Q_d = Radiant energy transmitted by an aperture (J).

Q_{eff} = Energy transmitted by the measurement aperture from Table 9 (J).

r = Distance from the viewer to the laser (cm).

r_{NHZ} = Nominal hazard zone.

r_{NOHD} = The distance along the axis of the unobstructed beam from the laser beyond which the irradiance or radiant exposure is not expected to exceed the appropriate ocular MPE (cm).

r_0 = Distance from exit port to a beam waist formed in front of the laser (cm).

r_1 = Distance from laser target to the viewer (cm).

R = Radius of curvature of a specular surface (cm).

ρ_λ = Spectral reflectance of a diffuse or specular object at wavelength λ.

S = Scan rate of a scanning laser (number of scans across eye per second).

t = Duration of single pulse or exposure (s).

τ_λ = Transmission of magnifying optics.

t_{min} = Maximum duration for which the MPE is the same as for 1 ns.

T = Total exposure duration (in seconds) of a train of pulses.

T_1 = Exposure duration depending on wavelength, beyond which the MPE for a point source is based on photochemical effects rather than thermal.

T_2 = Exposure duration beyond which the thermal MPE for an extended source is constant in terms of irradiance.

TL = Barrier threshold limit.

T_{max} = Total expected exposure duration (see Section 8.2.2).

θ_s = Maximum angular sweep of a scanning beam (rad).

θ_v = Viewing angle from the normal to a reflecting surface (see Figure B4).

ω_0 = Mode field diameter of single mode optical fiber (μm). Note that the mode field diameter is similar to the beam waist radius at $1/e^2$ peak of irradiance points (also designated ω_0) discussed in many optics text books, but is twice the value.

B3. Examples of MPE Determination

Powerful or energetic lasers can easily damage a person's vision since the cornea and lens focus the laser energy onto the retina. Direct point source exposure to a collimated visible or near infrared laser results in a small image on the retina no more than about 25 μm in diameter. The MPEs expressed as corneal exposure, are very low in order to account for this natural focusing effect of the human eye. For retinal effects, the true hazard is related to the amount of laser power or energy that enters the pupil, and is focused on the retina.

Although infrared lasers (1.400 μm to 1 mm) and ultraviolet lasers (0.180 μm to 0.400 μm) do not present a retinal hazard, these lasers can still damage the eye with sufficient power or energy. Since the cornea and lens of the eye do not focus laser energy at these wavelengths, the MPE will generally be much larger for these lasers. However, for ultraviolet exposure, photochemical effects are additive over a full day of exposure, and for some wavelengths on subsequent days, also.

The MPE may be expressed in several different ways. In Tables 5a and 5b, the MPE is provided in either $J{\cdot}cm^{-2}$ or in $W{\cdot}cm^{-2}$. Usually, the MPE provided in Tables 5a and 5b are expressed as radiant exposure ($J{\cdot}cm^{-2}$) for exposures lasting less than 10 s.

The MPEs for exposure durations exceeding 0.7 s to extended visible laser sources require concepts of radiance and integrated radiance. Techniques for determining these MPEs are provided in B7.

B3.1 Continuous-Wave Laser MPEs. For a CW laser or for an exposure lasting several milliseconds, it is natural to express the MPE as irradiance (MPE:E) in $W{\cdot}cm^{-2}$.

Example 1. **Determine the maximum irradiance permitted for a 0.25 s exposure to a visible laser (λ = 400 nm to 700 nm).**

Solution. The MPE for visible lasers from Table 5a for wavelengths between 0.4 and 0.7 μm (400 and 700 nm) for exposure durations from 18 μs to 10 s is:

$$\text{MPE:}H = 1.8\, t^{3/4}\ \text{mJ}{\cdot}\text{cm}^{-2}. \qquad \textbf{Eq B1}$$

For a 0.25 s exposure, the MPE is $1.8 \times 0.25^{0.75}\ \text{mJ}\cdot\text{cm}^{-2} = (1.8 \times 0.354)\ \text{mJ}\cdot\text{cm}^{-2} =$ 0.636 $mJ{\cdot}cm^{-2}$. For a single exposure, the irradiance may be found by dividing the radiant exposure, H, by the exposure duration, t:

$$E = \frac{H}{t}. \qquad \textbf{Eq B2}$$

For a radiant exposure (H) of 0.636 $mJ{\cdot}cm^{-2}$ for 0.25 s, the irradiance (E) is:

$$\text{MPE}: E = \frac{\text{MPE}: H}{t} = \frac{0.636\,\text{mJ}\cdot\text{cm}^{-2}}{0.25\,\text{s}}$$
$$= 2.55\ \text{mW}{\cdot}\text{cm}^{-2}.$$

Therefore the MPE may be represented either as radiant exposure when it is provided in $J{\cdot}cm^{-2}$ or as irradiance when it is provided in $W{\cdot}cm^{-2}$.

Example 2. **A helium-cadmium (HeCd) laser operating at 325 nm is used in a laboratory. Laser exposure can occur at all locations within the laboratory. A laboratory technician is required to perform tests in the laboratory which last**

10 minutes every hour. The rest of the day, the technician works elsewhere. What is the MPE for this laser for these exposure conditions?

Solution. Since the technician is only in the lab for part of the day, his total exposure time is 10 minutes (600 s) per hour multiplied by 8 hours in a day, which equals 4800 s. The MPE for 325 nm radiation is 1.0 J·cm^{-2} for exposures lasting from 10 s to 8 hours. Therefore, the MPE is 1.0 J·cm^{-2} accumulated exposure, whether the exposure is for 4800 s or 30,000 s. The MPE can also be calculated based on average power. The MPE in terms of irradiance is the MPE in terms of radiant exposure divided by the exposure duration. In this case, the MPE is:

$$\begin{aligned}\text{MPE}:E &= \frac{\text{MPE}:H}{t}.\\ &= \frac{1\,\text{J}\cdot\text{cm}^{-2}}{4800\ \text{s}} = 2.1\times10^{-4}\ \text{W}\cdot\text{cm}^{-2}\\ &= 0.21\ \text{mW}\cdot\text{cm}^{-2}.\end{aligned}$$

Example 3. **A 3 mW laser operates at a wavelength of 1.55 μm with a beam diameter of 1.1 cm. What is the MPE for a 10 s exposure?**

Solution. From Table 5a,, the MPE for a 10 s exposure at 1550 nm is 1 J·cm^{-2}. The MPE in terms of irradiance is then 1 J·cm^{-2}/10 s = 0.1 W·cm^{-2}.

B3.2 Single-Pulse Laser MPEs. MPEs for a single-pulse laser may be calculated from the information provided in Tables 5, 6 and 7 or one may extrapolate a good approximate value from Figures 4, 5, 6, 7, and 8.

Example 4. **Single-Pulse Visible Laser. Determine the MPE for a 694.3 nm, ruby laser pulse, having a pulse duration of 8 × 10^{-4} s (0.8 ms).**

Solution. The appropriate MPE is given in Table 5a, see Eq B1. Substituting the values for t in the equation yields:

$$\begin{aligned}\text{MPE}:H &= 1.8\times10^{-3}\,t^{0.75}\ \text{J}\cdot\text{cm}^{-2}\\ &= 1.8\times10^{-3}\,(8\times10^{-4})^{0.75}\\ &= 8.6\times10^{-6}\ \text{J}\cdot\text{cm}^{-2}.\end{aligned}$$

Since $E \times t = H$, the MPE may also be expressed as peak irradiance,

$$\begin{aligned}\text{MPE}:E &= \frac{\text{MPE}:H}{t} = \frac{8.6\times10^{-6}\,\text{J}\cdot\text{cm}^{-2}}{8\times10^{-4}\ \text{s}}\\ &= 1.1\times10^{-2}\ \text{W}\cdot\text{cm}^{-2}.\end{aligned}$$

Example 5. **Extremely-Short-Pulsed Laser. Find the MPE for a single 100 fs (100×10^{-15} s) pulse at 580 nm (0.58 μm).**

Solution. The MPE for a single 100 fs (100×10^{-15} s) pulse at 580 nm can be found using Table 5a.

$$\text{MPE:}H = 1.5 \times 10^{-8}\ \text{J}\cdot\text{cm}^{-2}.$$

Example 6. **Near infrared Laser. A GaAs laser operating at room temperature has a peak wavelength of 0.904 μm. What is the MPE for a single pulse of 200 ns duration?**

Solution. The MPE can be calculated from the information in Figures 4 and 8. From Figure 4, the MPE for exposure durations between 1 ns and 18 μs is 5×10^{-7} J·cm^{-2}. This MPE may be corrected for 0.9 μm by the use of C_A which is about 2.5 as read from Figure 8a. The product is 1.25×10^{-6} J·cm^{-2}.

Tables 5a and 6 can also be used to determine the MPE. From Table 5a, under "visible and near infrared," 0.700–1.05 μm, 10^{-9} to 18×10^{-6} s, the

$$\text{MPE:}H = 0.5 \times C_A \times C_E \times 10^{-6}\ \text{J}\cdot\text{cm}^{-2}. \qquad \textbf{Eq B3}$$

Since no information was provided on source size, C_E is assumed to be 1.0 (see Section B3.5). From Table 6, the value of C_A for the wavelength band of 0.7 to 1.05 μm can be calculated from the formula:

$$C_A = 10^{2(\lambda - 0.7\ \mu\text{m})} = 2.56. \qquad \textbf{Eq B4}$$

The MPE is then,

$$\begin{aligned}\text{MPE}: H &= (2.56)(5 \times 10^{-7}) \\ &= 1.28 \times 10^{-6}\ \text{J}\cdot\text{cm}^{-2}\end{aligned}$$

Example 7. **Single-Pulse Near infrared Laser. Determine the MPE for a 1.064 μm (Nd:YAG) laser having a pulse duration of 8×10^{-4} s.**

Solution. The MPE as given in Table 5a is:

$$\begin{aligned}\text{MPE:}H &= 9 \times t^{0.75} \times 10^{-3}\ \text{J}\cdot\text{cm}^{-2} \qquad \textbf{Eq B5} \\ &= 9 \times (8 \times 10^{-4})^{0.75} \times 10^{-3}\ \text{J}\cdot\text{cm}^{-2} \\ &= 4.3 \times 10^{-5}\ \text{J}\cdot\text{cm}^{-2}.\end{aligned}$$

Another way to approach this problem is to note that in Figure 8a, the MPE for this laser is five times that for a visible laser having the same exposure duration (as calculated in Example 4). Therefore, the MPE for this exposure is:

$$\begin{aligned} \mathrm{MPE}: H &= 5\times(8.6\times10^{-6}\,\mathrm{J\cdot cm^{-2}}) \\ &= 4.3\times10^{-5}\,\mathrm{J\cdot cm^{2}}. \end{aligned}$$

In terms of peak irradiance,

$$\begin{aligned} \mathrm{MPE}: E &= \frac{\mathrm{MPE}: H}{t} \\ &= \frac{4.3\times10^{-5}\ \mathrm{J\cdot cm^{-2}}}{8\times10^{-4}\ \mathrm{s}} \\ &= 5.4\times10^{-2}\ \mathrm{W\cdot cm^{-2}}. \end{aligned}$$

***Example 8.* Extremely-Short Near infrared Laser. Find the MPE for a single 20 ps (2×10^{-11} s) laser pulse at 1060 nm.**

Solution. The MPE is found using Table 5a. For exposure durations between 10 ps and 1 ns is:

$$\mathrm{MPE}{:}H \quad = 27\ C_c\, t^{\,0.75}\ \mathrm{J{\cdot}cm^{-2}}, \qquad \textbf{Eq B6}$$

where t is measured in seconds. For 1060 nm (1.06 μm), C_C is 1.0. Therefore,

$$\begin{aligned} \mathrm{MPE}{:}H \quad &= 27\ (1.0)\ (2 \times 10^{-11})^{0.75}\ \mathrm{J{\cdot}cm^{-2}} \\ &= 2.6 \times 10^{-7}\ \mathrm{J{\cdot}cm^{-2}}. \end{aligned}$$

***Example 9.* Middle Infrared Laser. What is the MPE for a single–pulse laser rangefinder operating at a wavelength of 1540 nm? The pulse width is 20 ns.**

Solution. From Table 5a, the MPE for 1540 nm (1.54 μm) is 1 $\mathrm{J{\cdot}cm^{-2}}$ for all exposure durations from 1 ns to 10 s. Therefore the MPE for this laser is 1 $\mathrm{J{\cdot}cm^{-2}}$.

B3.3 Repetitive-Pulse Laser MPE. For exposure to n pulses in a pulse train or a group of pulses, the MPE ($\mathrm{MPE}{:}H_{group}$) is expressed in radiant exposure for the sum of all the pulses. $\mathrm{MPE}{:}E_{group}$ represents the MPE expressed in average irradiance. The average irradiance is computed from the sum of the radiant exposures, for all the pulses in the group (H_{group}), divided by the length of the pulse train, T. Therefore,

$$\text{MPE}:E_{\text{group}} = \frac{\text{MPE}:H_{\text{group}}}{T}. \qquad \textbf{Eq B7}$$

The MPE for a group of pulses may be expressed in a variety of ways. Generally, several computations are necessary to determine the *MPE/Pulse* expressed in J·cm^{-2}. Usually, the first computation involves computing the MPE if a person were exposed to only one pulse, or the pulse with maximum energy, in a pulse train (MPE_{SP}). Another computation involves the MPE for the combined energy in a group of pulses or an entire pulse train (MPE:H_{group}).

To determine the applicable MPE for an exposure to a repetitive-pulse laser, the wavelength, pulse repetition frequency (F), duration of a single pulse (t), duration of any pulse groups (T), and the duration of a complete exposure must be known (T_{max}). The appropriate *MPE/pulse* is the one that indicates the greatest hazard from testing the three rules:

Rule 1. **Single-pulse limit.** The MPE is limited by the MPE_{SP} for *any* single pulse during the exposure (*assuming exposure to only one pulse*).

Rule 2. **Average-power limit.** The MPE is limited to the MPE for the duration of all pulse trains, T, divided by the number of pulses, n, during T, for all exposure durations up to T_{max}.

Rule 3. **Repetitive-pulse limit**[2]**.** The MPE is limited to MPE_{SP} multiplied by a correction factor C_P, i.e., $n^{-0.25}$, where n is the number of pulses that occur during the exposure duration T_{max}. Note that MPE_{SP} for this rule may be different than that used for Rule 1. For pulse widths less than 1 ns, MPE_{SP} must be recalculated for a width of at least 1 ns (same MPE is used for $t = t_{min}$). For this rule, all pulses that occur within a time t_{min} are considered a single pulse. If there are no spaces between pulses of a width at least as large as t_{min}, this rule need not be applied since it can be assumed that the critical frequency has been exceeded. For groups of pulses with a group width either shorter or longer than t_{min}, the time period where interpulse spacing is less than t_{min} becomes the exposure duration used to compute MPE_{SP} and all the pulses contained within that time period are counted as a single pulse.

The critical frequency is the PRF above which the MPE from Rule 2 yields the smallest MPE. For the retinal hazard region, the critical frequency[3] is generally 55 kHz for wavelengths between 0.4 to 1.05 μm and 22 kHz for wavelengths between 1.05 and 1.4 μm[4].

Example 10. **Repetitive-Pulse Visible Laser with Very High PRF. Determine the MPE for a 0.514 μm (514.5 nm) argon laser operating at a PRF of 10 MHz and a pulse width t of 10 ns (10^{-8} s). Assume an exposure duration T_{max} of 0.25 s.**

---

[2] For Rule 3, pulses that occur within t_{min} are considered a single pulse. Rule 3 does not apply for wavelengths shorter than 0.4 μm, except for the thermal limit expressed as $0.56 \times t^{0.25}$ J·cm^{-2}.

[3] When subnanosecond pulses are involved, the critical frequency could be higher. When the wavelength is outside the retinal hazard region, or the duration of the pulse train exceeds 10 s, the critical frequency is lower.

[4] For exposure durations exceeding 10 s, only those pulses contained within a time equal to T_2 are considered when computing C_P. The value of T_2 is 10 s for point sources. See Eq B88 in B7.2 for computation of T_2 for extended sources.

Solution. Since the PRF is greater than 55 kHz the average irradiance limitation from Rule 2 applies. In this case, t is actually T_{max}. From Table 5a,

$$\begin{aligned} \text{MPE:}H_{group} &= 1.8 \times t^{0.75} \times 10^{-3}\ \text{J·cm}^{-2} \qquad \textbf{Eq B8} \\ &= 1.8 \times (0.25\ \text{s})^{0.75} \times 10^{-3}\ \text{J·cm}^{-2} \\ &= 6.36 \times 10^{-4}\ \text{J·cm}^{-2}. \end{aligned}$$

This MPE is the same as for a CW laser and may be expressed in terms of average irradiance:

$$\begin{aligned} \text{MPE}: E &= \frac{\text{MPE}: H_{group}}{T} = \frac{6.36 \times 10^{-4}\ \text{J} \cdot \text{cm}^{-2}}{0.25\ \text{s}} \\ &= 2.55 \times 10^{-3}\ \text{W·cm}^{-2}. \end{aligned}$$

Example 11. **Repetitive-Pulse, Near infrared Laser with Moderate PRF. Determine the MPE for a 0.905 μm (905 nm) (GaAs) laser which has a pulse width, *t*, of 100 ns (1×10^{-7} s) and a PRF of 1 kHz.**

Solution. Since the PRF of this laser is less than the critical frequency, all three rules must be tested. Since the 905 nm wavelength will not provide a natural aversion response such as a visible wavelength laser would, assume a 10 s exposure duration (T_{max}) for this particular laser application. The total number of pulses (n) in a 10 s interval is determined from the product of the exposure duration (T) and the PRF (F), i.e.,

$$n = F \times T = 1 \times 10^{4}\ \text{pulses}. \qquad \textbf{Eq B9}$$

From Figure 13, the reduction factor $n^{-0.25}$ is found to be 0.1. From Table 6 or Figure 8a, the wavelength correction factor is 2.57 at 905 nm. The *MPE/pulse* is the most conservative (i.e., lowest value) MPE from testing the three rules. The MPE from Table 5a for a single 100 ns pulse is:

Rule 1. Single Pulse Limit:

$$\begin{aligned} MPE_{SP} &= 0.5\ C_A \times 10^{-6}\ \text{J·cm}^{-2} \\ &= 1.29 \times 10^{-6}\ \text{J·cm}^{-2}. \end{aligned}$$

Rule 2. Average Power Limit:
The MPE for a 10 s exposure is:

$$\text{MPE}: H_{group} = 1.8 \times 10^{-3} C_A t^{0.75}\ \text{J} \cdot \text{cm}^{-2}.$$

The *MPE/pulse* based on a 10 s exposure (T) is:

$$MPE/pulse = \frac{1.8\times10^{-3}\,C_A t^{0.75}\,\mathrm{J\cdot cm^{-2}}}{10^4 \text{ pulses}}$$
$$= 2.6 \times 10^{-6}\ \mathrm{J{\cdot}cm^{-2}}\,.$$

Rule 3. Repetitive Pulse Limit:
The *MPE/pulse* is the MPE_{SP} reduced by a repetitive-pulse reduction factor C_P is:

$$\begin{aligned} MPE/pulse &= n^{-0.25}\ MPE_{SP} && \textbf{Eq B10}\\ &= 10{,}000^{-0.25}\ (1.29 \times 10^{-6})\ \mathrm{J{\cdot}cm^{-2}}\\ &= 0.1 \times 1.29 \times 10^{-6}\ \mathrm{J{\cdot}cm^{-2}}\\ &= 1.3 \times 10^{-7}\ \mathrm{J{\cdot}cm^{-2}}.\end{aligned}$$

Resultant MPE (Example 11):
Rule 3 provides the *MPE/pulse* since it is the most conservative (i.e., lowest value) calculation.

Hence, the MPE expressed as a cumulative exposure for the duration of the entire pulse train is:

$$\begin{aligned} \mathrm{MPE}{:}H_{group} &= T \times F \times MPE/pulse && \textbf{Eq B11}\\ &= (10\ \mathrm{s})(10^3\ \mathrm{Hz})(1.3 \times 10^{-7}\ \mathrm{J{\cdot}cm^{-2}})\\ &= 1.3 \times 10^{-3}\ \mathrm{J{\cdot}cm^{-2}}.\end{aligned}$$

This may also be expressed in terms of average irradiance,

$$\mathrm{MPE}:E = \frac{\mathrm{MPE}:H_{group}}{T} = \frac{1.3\times10^{-3}\ \mathrm{J\cdot cm^{-2}}}{10\,\mathrm{s}}$$
$$= 1.3 \times 10^{-4}\ \mathrm{W{\cdot}cm^{-2}}.$$

Example 12. **Low-PRF, Long-Pulse, Repetitive-Pulse Visible Laser. Determine the MPE for a 0.632 μm (632.8 nm) (HeNe) laser where T_{max} = 0.25 s, pulse width, $t = 10^{-3}$ s, and F = 100 Hz.**

Solution. Since the PRF is much less than 55 kHz, the exposure duration is 0.25 s, pulses are evenly spaced, and the pulse width exceeds 1 ns, Rule 3 from paragraph 8.2.3 is the appropriate method to follow. However, all three rules will be tested.

The total number of pulses in the 0.25 s exposure is $n = F \times T$ equals 25. From Table 5a or Figure 4, the MPE for a single 1 ms pulse is:

Rule 1. Single-Pulse Limit:

$$
\begin{aligned}
MPE_{SP} &= 1.8\, t^{0.75} \times 10^{-3}\ \text{J·cm}^{-2} \\
&= 1.8 \times 5.62 \times 10^{-3} \times 10^{-3}\ \text{J·cm}^{-2} \\
&= 1.01 \times 10^{-5}\ \text{J·cm}^{-2}.
\end{aligned}
$$

This MPE in terms of average power for Rule 1 is:

$$
\begin{aligned}
\text{MPE:}E &= MPE/pulse \times F \\
&= 1.01 \times 10^{-5}\ \text{J·cm}^{-2} \times 100\ \text{Hz} = 1\ \text{mW·cm}^{-2}.
\end{aligned}
$$

Rule 2. Average-Power Limit:
The MPE found using Rule 2 is:

$$
\begin{aligned}
\text{MPE:}H_{\text{group}} &= 1.8\, t^{0.75} \times 10^{-3}\ \text{J·cm}^{-2} \\
&= 1.8\,(0.25^{0.75}) \times 10^{-3} \\
&= 6.4 \times 10^{-4}\ \text{J·cm}^{-2},
\end{aligned}
$$

for all the pulses in the train.

In terms of average irradiance, the MPE is:

$$
\begin{aligned}
\text{MPE}: E &= \frac{6.4 \times 10^{-4}\ \text{J} \cdot \text{cm}^{-2}}{0.25\ \text{s}} \\
&= 2.55 \times 10^{-3}\ \text{W} \cdot \text{cm}^{-2}
\end{aligned}
$$

Rule 3. Repetitive Pulse limit:
The *MPE/pulse* is given by the product of $n^{-0.25}$ and MPE_{SP}. From Figure 13 (or using Eq B10), the corresponding value of $n^{-0.25}$ is 0.45.

The *MPE/pulse* for a 0.25 s exposure using C_P is:

$$
\begin{aligned}
MPE/Pulse &= (n^{-0.25}) \times MPE_{SP}\ \text{J·cm}^{-2} \\
&= (0.45)\,(1.01 \times 10^{-5})\ \text{J·cm}^{-2} \\
&= 4.55 \times 10^{-6}\ \text{J·cm}^{-2}.
\end{aligned}
$$

This MPE in terms of average power for Rule 3 is:

$$
\begin{aligned}
\text{MPE:}E &= MPE/Pulse \times F\ \text{W·cm}^{-2} \\
&= (4.55 \times 10^{-6}\ \text{J·cm}^{-2}) \times (100\ \text{Hz}) \\
&= 4.55 \times 10^{-4}\ \text{W·cm}^{-2}.
\end{aligned}
$$

This MPE is then compared with the average irradiance of the laser. The effective duty factor may be used to compare the average power to the peak power. The duty factor is defined as the ratio of the pulse width t to the period ($1/F$), and can be expressed as:

$$\text{duty factor} = t \times F. \qquad \textbf{Eq B12}$$

In this example the effective duty factor is 1 ms × 100 Hz = 0.1, and, hence, the peak irradiance is 10 times the average irradiance.

Resultant MPE (Example 12):
The MPE found using Rule 3 is the correct MPE to apply, since it is the smallest.

Example 13. **A xenon chloride excimer laser operating at 308 nm is used in a medical facility. The laser emits pulses that are 20 ns in length at a PRF of 200 Hz. What is the lowest MPE for this laser, considering all three rules, for a 10 s exposure duration.**

Solution. The MPE for ultraviolet lasers is based on a dual limit of photochemical effects and thermal effects. The MPE for 308 nm is 40 mJ·cm^{-2} for exposure durations from 1 ns to 30 ks. This MPE is based on photochemical effects on the eye or skin. In addition, the MPE of 0.56 $t^{0.25}$ also cannot be exceeded. This latter MPE is based on thermal effects. In fact it is the same MPE that is used for middle and far infrared wavelengths for exposures lasting more than a few ns. The MPE can be computed by applying the three rules listed above; however, both thermal and photochemical effects must be determined for each rule.

Rule 1. Single-Pulse Limit:
For this laser, the thermal MPE limit for a single pulse is:

$$MPE_{SP} = 0.56 \times (20 \times 10^{-9})^{0.25}\ \mathrm{J{\cdot}cm^{-2}}$$
$$= 0.56 \times 1.19 \times 10^{-2}\ \mathrm{J{\cdot}cm^{-2}} = 6.66\ \mathrm{mJ{\cdot}cm^{-2}}.$$

For the photochemical limit, the MPE for a single pulse is the same as for the entire exposure (40 mJ·cm^{-2}). Therefore, the MPE for Rule 1 is based on the thermal limit.

$$MPE_{SP}\ (\text{Rule 1}) = 6.66\ \mathrm{mJ{\cdot}cm^{-2}}.$$

Rule 2. Average Power Limit:
For thermal effects, the MPE is 0.56 $t^{\,0.25}$ J·cm^{-2}, where t is now the total duration of the exposure, T_{max}, which is 10 s.

$$\text{Thermal MPE (Rule 2)} = 0.56 \times (10)^{0.25}\ \mathrm{J{\cdot}cm^{-2}} = 0.56 \times 1.78\ \mathrm{J{\cdot}cm^{-2}} = 1.0\ \mathrm{J{\cdot}cm^{-2}}.$$

In a 10 s exposure, an individual could be exposed to 200 × 10 = 2000 pulses. The thermal MPE for each pulse is then

$$1.0\ \mathrm{J{\cdot}cm^{-2}}/2000 = 0.5\ \mathrm{mJ{\cdot}cm^{-2}}.$$

The MPE based on photochemical effects for an accumulated exposure over a 10 s duration is 40 mJ·cm^{-2}. Therefore, the *MPE/pulse* based on photochemical effects is:

Photochemical *MPE/pulse* (Rule 2) = 40 mJ·cm^{-2}/2000 = 20 μJ·cm^{-2}.

Since the photochemical MPE is much less than the thermal MPE for Rule 2, the MPE for Rule 2 is:

MPE/pulse (Rule 2) = 20 μJ·cm^{-2}.

Rule 3. Repetitive-Pulse Limit:
To compute the MPE according to Rule 3, the repetitive-pulse correction factor is applied to the thermal MPE_{SP} for a single pulse, but not to the photochemical limit of 40 mJ·cm^{-2}. The thermal MPE_{SP} is 6.66 mJ·cm^{-2}. During the exposure, exposure to 2000 pulses is possible. The value of C_P is $n^{-0.25} = 0.15$.

Therefore the *MPE/pulse* for Rule 3 is:

$$MPE/pulse \text{ (Rule 3)} = 6.66 \text{ mJ·cm}^{-2} \times 0.15 = 1 \text{ mJ·cm}^{-2}.$$

Resultant MPE (Example 13):
Comparing the MPE computed according to all three rules, Rule 2 has the lowest *MPE/pulse* of 20 μJ·cm^{-2} or an average irradiance of 4 mW·cm^{-2}.

B3.4 MPEs for Repetitive-Pulse, Pulse Groups.

Example 14. **Pulse Group for Short-Pulse Laser. Find the MPE of a Q-switched ruby laser 0.6943 μm (694.3 nm) which has an output of three 200 ps pulses, each separated by 100 ns.**

Solution. This is not a repetitive-pulse laser in the usual sense (that is, one having a continuous train of pulses lasting of the order of 0.25 s or more with the pulses being reasonably equally spaced).

Rule 1. Single Pulse Limit:
From Table 5a, the MPE for a single pulse is:

$$MPE_{SP} = 2.7 \times t^{0.75} \text{ J·cm}^{-2} = 1.44 \times 10^{-7} \text{ J·cm}^{-2}.$$

Rule 2. Average Power Limit:

The duration of the pulse train is 200 ns (which is still less than t_{min} of 18 μs). The MPE:H_{group} is therefore 5×10^{-7} J·cm^{-2} for the three pulses:

$$MPE/pulse = \frac{5 \times 10^{-7}\,\text{J}\cdot\text{cm}^{-2}}{3\ \text{pulses}}$$
$$= 1.67 \times 10^{-7}\ \text{J}\cdot\text{cm}^{-2}.$$

Rule 3. Repetitive-Pulse Limit:
Since T is less than t_{min}, all the pulses are considered the same as 1 pulse, and the energies from all three pulses are summed. Therefore, C_P is 1.0. The MPE based on t_{min} is 5×10^{-7} J·cm^{-2} for the sum of the energies of all three pulses. Therefore, for this Example the *MPE/pulse* based on Rule 3 is the same as for Rule 2 (i.e., 1.67×10^{-7} J·cm^{-2}).

Resultant MPE (Example 14):
Rule 1 provides the lowest MPE. Therefore, the *MPE/pulse* for this laser is 1.44×10^{-7} J·cm^{-2}.

Example 15. **Repetitive-Pulse, Pulse Groups. Find the MPE for a mode-locked Nd:YAG, frequency-doubled laser 0.532 μm (532 nm) used in a pulse-code-modulated (PCM) communications link. The laser presents 10^4 "words" per second (that is, 10^4 pulse groups per second) and each word consists of five hundred, 2 ps pulses, spaced at coded intervals such that the average pulse separation is 100 ns. The laser is a point source when viewed from within the beam. Compute the MPE for a 0.25 s exposure.**

Solution. Since this laser involves pulses shorter than 1 ns, all three rules from paragraph 8.2.3 should be tested.

Rule 1. Single Pulse Limit:
The MPE_{SP} for a pulse less than 10 ps from Table 5a is:

$$MPE_{SP} = 1.5 \times 10^{-8}\ \text{J}\cdot\text{cm}^{-2}. \qquad \textbf{Eq B13}$$

Rule 2. Average Power Limit:
Several iterations are required for this method since the pulses are in groups.

First, consider the pulses contained within t_{min}, which is 18 μs. Since a single word of pulses (50 μs) is longer than t_{min}, the number of pulses contained within t_{min} is:

$$k = \frac{18 \times 10^{-6}\ \text{s}}{50 \times 10^{-6}\ \text{s}} \times 500\ \text{pulses} = 180\ \text{pulses}$$

For t_{min}, the MPE is the same as it is for 1 ns.

$$\text{MPE:}H_{(1\text{ ns})} = 5 \times 10^{-7}\ \text{J}\cdot\text{cm}^{-2}.$$

The MPE for each pulse is then,

$$\textit{MPE/pulse} = \frac{5\times10^{-7}\ \text{J}\cdot\text{cm}^{-2}}{180} = 2.78\times10^{-9}\ \text{J}\cdot\text{cm}^{-2}$$

Second, consider one word, a group of 500 pulses, which lasts 50 μs.

$$\text{MPE:}H_{\text{group}} = 1.8 \times 10^{-3}\ t^{\,0.75}\ \text{J}\cdot\text{cm}^{-2} = 1.07\ \mu\text{J}\cdot\text{cm}^{-2}.$$

The *MPE/pulse* is then:

$$\textit{MPE/pulse} = \frac{1.07\times10^{-6}}{500} = 2.14\times10^{-9}\ \text{J}\cdot\text{cm}^{-2}.$$

Third, consider a 0.25 s exposure. The MPE:H_{group} for 0.25 s (momentary exposure), from Table 5a is:

$$\begin{aligned}\text{MPE:}H_{\text{group}} &= 1.8\ t^{\,0.75} \times 10^{-3}\ \text{J}\cdot\text{cm}^{-2}\\ &= 6.36\times10^{-4}\ \text{J}\cdot\text{cm}^{-2}.\end{aligned}$$

This MPE is for all the pulses contained within 0.25 s. The effective PRF, F_{eff}, of the pulse train is equal to the product of the number of words per second and the number of pulses per word, or 5.0 MHz. The number of pulses contained is:

$$n = F_{\text{eff}} \times T = 1.25\times10^{6}\ \text{pulses}.$$

The *MPE/pulse* is then:

$$\begin{aligned}\textit{MPE / pulse} &= \frac{6.36\times10^{-4}\ \text{J}\cdot\text{cm}^{-2}}{1.25\times10^{6}\ \text{pulses}}\\ &= 5.1\times10^{-10}\ \text{J}\cdot\text{cm}^{-2}\end{aligned}$$

Since the latter result is less than the previous two, the *MPE/pulse* for Rule 2 is 5.1×10^{-10} J·cm^{-2}.

Rule 3. Repetitive-Pulse Limit:
Since the pulses contained within a word occur at a rate such that the separation between individual pulses is less than $t_{\min}$, a word lasting 50 μs can be considered a pulse for this rule.

The MPE for a word based on 50 μs (from Rule 2 above) is:

$$\text{MPE:}H_{\text{word}} = 1.07 \times 10^{-6}\ \text{J}\cdot\text{cm}^{-2}$$

The number of pulses (words) separated by a time at least as long as t_{min} for a 0.25 s exposure duration is:

$$n(words) = 10{,}000 \text{ words/s} \times 0.25 \text{ s}$$
$$= 2.5 \times 10^3, \text{ and therefore } C_P \text{ is then } 0.141.$$

The MPE per word is:

$$MPE/word = 1.07 \times 10^{-6} \times C_P \text{ J·cm}^{-2}$$
$$= 1.5 \times 10^{-7} \text{ J·cm}^{-2}.$$

Since there are 500 pulses in each word, the *MPE/pulse* is then:

$$MPE/pulse = \frac{MPE/word}{pulses/word}$$
$$= \frac{1.5 \times 10^{-7} \text{ J} \cdot \text{cm}^{-2}}{500 \text{ pulses}}$$
$$= 3.0 \times 10^{-10} \text{ J·cm}^{-2}.$$

Note: Another way to look at the same problem would be to consider the pulses that occur in 18 μs as a group and there would then be 3 groups/word. The value of C_P would be 0.107 and the $MPE_{(18\ \mu s)}$ is 5×10^{-7} J·cm^{-2}. For each pulse:

$$MPE/pulse = \frac{0.107 \times 5 \times 10^{-7}}{180} = 3.0 \times 10^{-10} \text{ J} \cdot \text{cm}^{-2}$$

However, the more logical method is to consider the entire pulse group as a single pulse for Rule 3 since the inter-pulse spacing is less than t_{min}.

Resultant MPE (Example 15):
Rule 3 provides the most conservative of the three rules, considering three sub-methods for Rule 2. Therefore, since the limiting aperture is constant among the three rules, the overall *MPE/pulse* for this laser is simply equal to 3×10^{-10} J·cm^{-2}.

The MPE for the entire 0.25 s train of pulses is:

$$\text{MPE}:H_{group} = 3.0 \times 10^{-10} \text{ J·cm}^{-2} \times 1.25 \times 10^6 \text{ pulses}$$
$$= 3.75 \times 10^{-4} \text{ J·cm}^{-2}.$$

This MPE can be expressed as average irradiance by dividing by the duration of the pulse train.

$$\text{MPE}: E = \frac{3.75 \times 10^{-4} \text{ J} \cdot \text{cm}^{-2}}{0.25 \text{ s}}$$
$$= 1.5 \text{ mW} \cdot \text{cm}^{-2}$$

B3.5 Determining the MPE for Extended Sources. Although most types of lasers have a point source, lasers that are formed by re-collimating diffused laser energy or from a laser diode and a collimating lens can have a source size larger than α_{min} when viewed at a close distance. For these lasers, the angular source size cannot be larger than the beam divergence. In addition, the physical source size cannot exceed the laser exit port diameter.

For determining the extended source MPE for a diffuse reflection, refer to Sections B6.6 and B7. For determining the extended source angular subtense, refer to Section B9.

***Example 16.* Find the extended source MPE for a GaAs, diode laser[5] (0.904 μm), with a pulse width of 200 ns and operating at a PRF of 2.73 kHz. The laser was made by focusing the diode into a fiber optic cable, and placing the tip of the fiber optic cable at the focal point of a short focal length lens.**

The beam is circular and has a diameter at the laser exit port of 1.5 cm. The collimating lens is 2 cm in diameter. The source size is a nearly constant 3 mrad within a distance of 667 cm, and then the exit port limits the source size to 2 cm for all viewing distances after that. Find the MPE for this laser, at a distance of 20 cm from the laser exit port.

Solution. The point source MPE for this laser is calculated from MPE_{SP} from Example 6 and Rule 3.

$$(MPE/pulse)_{point} = MPE_{SP} \times C_P \text{ J·cm}^{-2}.$$

The number of pulses that determines the value of C_P is determined from T_2, which is based on the source size. The equation for T_2 is contained in Table 6.

$$\begin{aligned} T_2 &= 10 \times 10^{(\alpha-1.5)/98.5} = 10 \times 10^{(3-1.5)/98.5} \\ &= 10.35 \text{ s.} \end{aligned}$$

The MPE_{SP} from Example 6 is 1.28×10^{-6} J·cm^{-2}. For a 10.35 s exposure duration, 28,300 pulses would be emitted. The value of C_P is then 0.077. The MPE is then:

$$\begin{aligned} MPE/pulse &= 1.28 \times 10^{-6} \text{ J·cm}^{-2} \times C_P \\ &= 1.28 \times 10^{-6} \times 0.077 \text{ J·cm}^{-2} \\ &= 9.9 \times 10^{-8} \text{ J·cm}^{-2}. \end{aligned}$$

The extended source MPE for this laser is obtained from the angular source size and the point source MPE. If this source subtends an angle greater than 1.5 mrad, the point source MPE is multiplied by C_E. For sources smaller than 100 mrad, C_E is the ratio of the angular subtense

[5] Unlike gas or solid-state lasers, some semiconductor diode lasers or laser arrays are extended sources when viewed at a close distance. The emitting stripe of the diode, or the array, may be magnified by a projection lens or a microscope.

to 1.5 mrad. Since the evaluation distance is less than 667 cm and the beam has not expanded much at this distance, the source subtends an angle of 3 mrad for this laser.

$$C_E = \frac{\alpha}{\alpha_{min}} = \frac{3 \text{ mrad}}{1.5 \text{ mrad}} = 2. \qquad \textbf{Eq B14}$$

A comparison of Table 5a and Table 5b for this wavelength and exposure duration shows that the corresponding extended source MPE is:

$$\begin{aligned}(MPE/pulse)_{extended} &= (MPE/pulse)_{point} \times C_E \\ &= 2 \times 9.9 \times 10^{-8} \text{ J·cm}^{-2} \\ &= 2.0 \times 10^{-7} \text{ J·cm}^{-2}.\end{aligned}$$

B4. Laser Classification

Laser classification is based on the potential for a laser to exceed the MPE for unaided viewing and optically aided viewing, for standard viewing conditions (when the potential use of optics exists). Example 17 through Example 24 show methods for calculating parameters necessary for classifying lasers in accordance with Section 3 of this standard. The hazard class of a laser depends on the effective output energy or effective output power of the laser and the corresponding accessible emission limit (AEL) for each class.

The effective output power or effective energy per pulse is the power or energy per pulse that is transmitted by the measurement aperture listed in Table 9. The Class 1 AEL is the product of the MPE and the area of the limiting aperture specified in Table 8b. Those lasers meeting the Class 1 AEL for power (or energy for pulsed lasers) measured through the apertures contained in Tables 8a and 8b but exceed the Class 1 AEL when the power or energy is measured through the apertures of Table 9 are Class 1M, as long as this measured power or energy does not exceed the Class 3B AEL, as discussed below.

The Class 2 AEL is based on the MPE for 0.25 s viewing of a visible laser. The Class 2 AEL is 1 mW for wavelengths between 0.4 and 0.7 μm. Those lasers meeting the Class 2 AEL for power (or energy for pulsed lasers) measured through the apertures contained in Tables 8a and 8b but exceed the Class 2 AEL when the power or energy is measured through the apertures of Table 9 are Class 2M, as long as this measured power or energy does not exceed the Class 3B AEL, as discussed below.

The Class 3 AEL is based on an acute hazard from the direct beam of the laser. The Class 3 AEL is the lesser of $0.03 \cdot C_A$ J in a single pulse, or an average power of 0.5 W during a 0.25 s exposure (125 mJ). Class 3R (formerly Class 3a) is a subset of the Class 3. The Class 3R AEL is defined as 5 times the Class 1 AEL for invisible lasers and 5 mW (5 times the Class 2 AEL) for visible lasers (λ = 0.4 to 0.7 μm). Other Class 3 lasers are classified as Class 3B.

The Class 4 AEL is based on indirect hazards of the laser such as producing a hazard from diffuse reflections, hazards to the skin, or the capacity for starting a fire, although precise values for these different effects may be difficult to determine. Class 4 lasers are those that do not meet the AELs for lesser classes.

Laser hazard classification is based on energy transmitted by the limiting aperture for either unaided viewing or optically aided viewing. This limiting aperture D_f can be 1 mm, 3.5 mm, 7 mm, or somewhere in between. When a laser beam diameter is very close to the limiting aperture or measurement aperture, the conservative approach to hazard analysis may not offer the precision desired to determine if the Class 1 AEL is exceeded near the output of the laser for classification purposes. For a Gaussian shaped beam, the fraction of the total power or energy transmitted by a measurement aperture, D_m may be determined from the following relationships:

$$\frac{\Phi_d}{\Phi_0} = 1 - e^{-\left(\frac{D_m}{D_L}\right)^2}, \qquad \textbf{Eq B15}$$

or

$$\frac{Q_d}{Q_0} = 1 - e^{-\left(\frac{D_m}{D_L}\right)^2}. \qquad \textbf{Eq B16}$$

B4.1 Classification Based on Unaided Viewing. Lasers that are used only indoors or lasers with a small beam diameter often only need to be classified for unaided viewing.

Example 17. **Classify a single-pulse (PRF < 1 Hz) Q-switched ruby laser having an output peak power specified by the manufacturer as 20 MW, a pulse duration of 25 ns, and a laser rod diameter of 5/8 inch.**

Solution. The output energy per pulse is:

$$\begin{aligned} Q &= \Phi \cdot t \qquad \textbf{Eq B17} \\ &= (2\times10^7\ \text{W})(2.5\times10^{-8}\ \text{s}) \\ &= 0.5\ \text{J}. \end{aligned}$$

where Φ represents the peak power for this laser. From Table 6, C_A is equal to 1.0 at 694.3 nm (0.69 μm). The Class 3B limit of $0.03 \cdot C_A$ J is, thus, 30 mJ. The laser is 17 times this limit, and, is therefore, Class 4 (see Section 3.3.4).

Example 18. **Classify a rhodamine 6G dye laser that has a peak output at a wavelength of 0.590 μm. The energy output is 10 mJ in a 5 mm beam for a duration of 1 μs.**

Solution. The MPE for this laser is 5×10^{-7} J·cm^{-2}, since the pulse width is less than 18 μs and the value of C_A is 1.0 at 0.590 μm (see Table 6). The Class 1 AEL is the product of the MPE and the area of the limiting aperture specified in Table 8b. At 0.590 μm, the limiting aperture diameter is 7 mm and the area of this aperture is 0.385 cm^2. The Class 1 AEL is:

$$\begin{aligned} \text{AEL} &= \text{MPE} \times \left(\frac{\pi D_f^{\,2}}{4} \right) \\ &= 5 \times 10^{-7}\,\text{J} \cdot \text{cm}^{-2} \times 0.385\ \text{cm}^2 \\ &= 1.9 \times 10^{-7}\,\text{J.} \end{aligned} \qquad \textbf{Eq B18}$$

The Class 3R AEL is 5 times the Class 1 AEL or 9.6×10^{-7} J, and the Class 3B limit is $0.03 \cdot C_A$ J = 30 mJ/pulse.

The output energy of 10 mJ is between the limits of 0.96 μJ and 30 mJ; the laser is, therefore, Class 3B.

Example 19. **Classify a tunable laser that can emit at wavelengths between 0.7 μm and 2 μm. The device has been altered to operate only at wavelengths of 0.75 μm, and 0.7 μm. The radiant energy output is 10 mJ at 0.75 μm and 1 mJ at 0.7 μm (total in 1 pulse). The beam diameter is 5 mm and the pulse duration is 1 μs. The laser is single-pulsed.**

Solution. From Figure 8a, C_A is 1.26 for 0.75 μm, and 1.0 for 0.70 μm. The MPE is:

$$MPE_{SP} = 5 \times 10^{-7}\ C_A\ \text{J·cm}^{-2}.$$

For 0.75 μm, the MPE is 6.3×10^{-7} J·cm^{-2} and for 0.7 μm, the MPE is 5.0×10^{-7} J·cm^{-2}. The laser output is well over the Class 1 or 3R AELs (see Example 18).

The Class 3B AEL ($0.03 \cdot C_A$ J/pulse) is 38 mJ for 0.75 μm, but only 30 mJ for 0.7 μm. Even if all the energy were emitted at the most hazardous wavelength, the Class 3B AEL of 30 mJ/pulse is not exceeded. Further, since the laser is single pulsed, the 11 mJ per pulse is less than the Class 3B AEL of 125 mJ total effective energy emitted within 0.25 s.

In terms of average power, the maximum average power is:

$$\Phi = \frac{Q}{t} = \frac{11\ \text{mJ}}{0.25\ \text{s}} = 44\,\text{mW},$$

which is less than the 500 mW Class 3B AEL for 0.25 s.

Example 20. **Classify a 1 W argon laser.**

Solution. The laser could fall into one of several possible classifications. The laser would be Class 1 if the entire laser beam path were enclosed, as in a sealed optical pipe. The laser is Class 4, if more than 0.5 W is emitted from the laser system as an unenclosed beam that could be collected by the measurement aperture from Table 9. The laser would be Class 3B, if after passing through beam-forming optics, the total effective optical power in the beam were greater than 5 mW but less than 0.5 W (see Section 3.3).

Example 21. **Classify a 0.6328 μm visible laser (HeNe) used as a remote control switch. The laser is electronically pulsed with 1 mW peak-power output, a pulse duration of 0.1 s (hence an energy of 1×10^{-4} J/pulse). The beam diameter is 1 cm. The recycle time of the laser is 5 s (maximum PRF = 0.2 Hz).**

Solution. Since the pulse duration of the device is 0.1 s, the exposure duration also is 0.1 s. The applicable MPE (from Table 5a or Figure 4) is 3.2×10^{-4} J·cm^{-2} or 3.2×10^{-3} W·cm^{-2} peak power. The Class 1 AEL is the product of the MPE and the area of the 7 mm limiting aperture (0.385 cm^2). Thus, the Class 1 AEL is 1.23 mW based on a single pulse.

The MPE for 5 or 10 s to a visible point source laser from Eq B1 is:

$$
\begin{aligned}
\text{MPE:}H &= 1.8 \times t^{0.75} \times 10^{-3}\ \text{J·cm}^{-2} \\
&= 6.0 \times 10^{-3}\ \text{J·cm}^{-2} \text{ for 5 s, and} \\
&= 1.0 \times 10^{-3}\ \text{J·cm}^{-2} \text{ for 10 s.}
\end{aligned}
$$

In terms of irradiance,

$$
\begin{aligned}
\text{MPE:}E &= \frac{\text{MPE}:H}{t} \\
&= 1.2\ \text{mW·cm}^{-2} \text{ for a 5 s exposure, and} \\
&= 1.0\ \text{mW·cm}^{-2} \text{ for a 10 s or longer exposure.}
\end{aligned}
$$

The Class 1 AEL based on an MPE of 1 mW·cm^{-2} is 0.385 mW.

Since the average power of 0.1 mW is less than the Class 1 AEL based on 5 or 10 s, the laser is Class 1. Exposure durations longer than 10 s would not yield a smaller Class 1 AEL for this laser.

B4.2 Classification Based on any Viewing Condition. Optically aided viewing must be considered when it is likely to occur. The transmission of ordinary viewing optics[6] is also included in the computations. Therefore, the transmission would not be expected to exceed

[6] Outside of the visible spectrum, reflection losses within the optics would reduce the transmission to 70% or less for a simple optic system, such as a pair of binoculars. For more complicated systems, less transmission would be expected. However, optics designed for human observers are antireflection coated to reduce these reflection losses.

90% throughout the visible portion of the spectrum (0.4 to 0.700 μm), and 70% in the IR (0.700 to 4.0 μm) and UV (0.302 to 0.4 μm). For other wavelengths, the transmission is assumed to be less than 2%, and therefore, would not increase the hazard over unaided viewing conditions. The larger source size and the transmission loss of the optics reduce somewhat the additional hazard associated with the use of optics.

If the laser in Example 21 were used in a locale where optically aided viewing was likely, a 50 mm measurement aperture would not increase the output energy. The internal reflection losses within the optical system would negate any increase in optical hazard. The laser is Class 1 based on any viewing condition since the peak power is 1 mW.

Extended source criteria must often be considered for optically aided viewing at close distances. In this case, a perfect 50 mm optical system is used for computations. The value of C_E is determined from the angular subtense of the magnified source.

Example 22. **A 0.905 μm, 30 W peak power, GaAs laser is used as a laser training device. The laser emits a series of coded pulses of 200 ns duration. No more than 1600 pulses occur in any 10 s interval. The intended use of the device would preclude exposure durations longer than 10 s. Optically aided viewing is possible since the device will be used outdoors. Determine the hazard class based on unaided viewing and optically aided viewing.**

The laser has a 3 cm beam diameter, which exits from a projection system that has a 4 cm lens at the exit port. The energy is emitted from a diode stack consisting of 5 diodes in an array. The divergence of the laser is 3 mrad in a somewhat square beam. The beams from each of the diodes can be separated visually with an infrared viewer, either looking at the beam striking a matte surface, or by intrabeam viewing of the actual diodes. Each diode has a divergence of 3 mrad in length, but only 0.5 mrad in width. The source size of each individual diode and also the entire diode array matches the divergence. The diode array source size is 3 mrad square.[7]

Solution. Since the PRF of the laser is much less than 55 kHz and the exposure duration is only 10 s, the *MPE/pulse* using Rule 3 of Section 8.2.3 applies. Since the peak power is 30 W and the pulse duration is 200 ns, the energy per pulse is 6.0 μJ.

The value of α_{min} is 1.5 mrad. The apparent source size is 3 mrad. Therefore, this laser may be an extended source for both unaided viewing (Condition 2) and for optically aided viewing (Condition 1). However, since the output consists of a 5-diode stack, classification, based on the worst case of either a single diode or the whole stack, determines the actual classification. A conservative solution is just to assume the laser is a point source.

Case 1 (the whole stack):
The point source MPE_{SP} is $1.28 \times 10^{-6}\ \mathrm{J \cdot cm^{-2}}$ (see Example 6). The repetitive-pulse correction factor C_P ($n^{-1/4}$) is 0.16 based on a 1600-pulse exposure. The Class 1 AEL is the

[7] For this example, the source size and beam divergence are the same, since the diode array is located at the focal point of the lens to achieve the best collimation. The source size and beam divergence are not necessarily the same value.

product of the point source MPE_{SP}, C_P, C_E, and the area of a 7 mm aperture (0.385 cm^2). The angular subtense (3 mrad) is twice α_{min}; thus, $C_E = 2.0$. Hence, the Class 1 AEL is:

$$\begin{aligned} \text{AEL} &= 1.28 \times 10^{-6}\ \text{J·cm}^{-2} \times C_P \times C_E \times 0.385\ \text{cm}^2 \\ &= 1.28 \times 10^{-6} \times 0.16 \times 2 \times 0.385 \\ &= 1.6 \times 10^{-7}\ \text{J}. \end{aligned}$$

The Class 3R AEL is 5 times the Class 1 AEL (7.9×10^{-7} J).

Unaided viewing (for Case 1).
Table 9 refers to Table 8 for the measurement aperture, D_m for unaided viewing, which is 7 mm in this case. At a 10 cm measurement distance, the energy passing through this aperture (assuming a flat-top beam profile) is:

$$\begin{aligned} Q_d &= Q_0 \times \frac{D_m^2}{D_L^2} \quad \text{for } D_m \le D_L \qquad \textbf{Eq B19} \\ &= 6\ \mu\text{J} \times \frac{(0.7\ \text{cm})^2}{(3\ \text{cm})^2} = 0.33\ \mu\text{J} \cdot \end{aligned}$$

Thus, the energy through a 7 mm aperture is less than the Class 3R AEL for unaided viewing, but exceeds the Class 1 AEL by a small amount. If the Class 1 AEL were not exceeded for unaided viewing, this laser would be Class 1M.

Optically aided viewing (for Case 1).
A 50 mm measurement aperture must be considered, simulating 7 × 50 binoculars with a 7 mm exit aperture and 70% transmission at this wavelength. All the emitted energy would be transmitted by a 50 mm aperture placed at 2 m from the laser exit port, except for transmission losses. The source will appear larger if it is not clipped by the laser exit port. The angular subtense of the laser exit port at a 2 m measurement distance is found from:

$$\begin{aligned} \alpha_{port} &= \frac{D_{exit}}{r} \qquad \textbf{Eq B20} \\ &= \frac{4\ \text{cm}}{200\ \text{cm}} = 20\ \text{mrad}, \end{aligned}$$

where D_{exit} represents the laser exit port diameter and r represents the measurement distance. Since the laser exit port subtends an angle that is much greater than the 3 mrad source size, the source is not clipped at the edges.

The optical power of the standard optical device is:

$$P = \frac{D_0}{D_e} = \frac{50\text{ mm}}{7\text{ mm}} = 7.14. \qquad \textbf{Eq B21}$$

However, the source size would be decreased slightly (2%) at a 2 m distance from the laser due to beam expansion (see Eq. B39 and Example 34). Therefore, the source would appear 7 times larger since it is not clipped by the exit port. The extended source correction factor C_E is based on the original source size multiplied by the magnifying power of the optics. C_E is then 14 instead of 2 (7 times larger). Thus,

$$\text{Class 1 AEL} = 1.6 \times 10^{-7} \times 7 = 1.12\ \mu\text{J},$$

and the Class 3R AEL is 5.6 μJ. The energy per pulse emitted from the laser is 6 μJ per pulse, but the optics would not be expected to transmit more than 70% of this energy. Thus, the laser is Class 3R based on optically aided viewing also.

Case 2 (a single diode):
For a single diode, the source size is 3 mrad by 0.5 mrad. Since the source is rectangular, each dimension must be equal to at least α_{min} before the two dimensions are averaged. Thus, the effective source size is:

$$\alpha_{eff} = \frac{\alpha_1 + \alpha_2}{2} = \frac{3\text{ mrad} + 1.5\text{ mrad}}{2} \qquad \textbf{Eq B22}$$
$$= 2.25\text{ mrad}$$

The value of C_E is then 1.5 instead of 2.0 as in Case 1. The Class 1 AEL is then 1.2×10^{-7} J and the Class 3R AEL is 6×10^{-7} J.

Since there are 5 diodes, the energy emitted by each diode is used for comparison to the Class 1 AEL for Case 2. The energy per diode passing through a 7 mm measurement aperture D_m is 1/5 that found in Case 1 (0.33 μJ/5=6.6×10^{-8} J). Thus, the energy per diode is less than the Class 1 AEL for Case 2.

The Class 1 AEL for Case 2 is slightly less than the Class 1 AEL for Case 1; however, the emitted energy per pulse for each diode is used for comparison to the AEL for Case 2, but the total emitted energy per pulse is compared with the AEL for Case 1. Thus, Case 1 indicates more of a hazard. An analysis of optically aided viewing produces a similar result.

The laser is Class 3R since the Class 3R AEL is not exceeded for the worst case, considering both Case 1 and Case 2 for the two viewing conditions: unaided and optically aided viewing.

It should be noted when evaluating hazards at various exposure distances for similar laser systems consisting of stacked arrays, the MPE that indicates the greater hazard may change with evaluation distance. For a more complicated system of a two dimensional array of sources, each possible grouping of sources must be tested in order to determine which grouping indicates the greatest hazard.

Example 23. **A 3 mW laser operates at a wavelength of 1.55 μm with a beam diameter of 1.1 cm. Determine the hazard classification, assuming that 7 × 50 binoculars are used.**

Solution. Since the laser wavelength is invisible, a 100 s exposure duration is used for classification. For exposures lasting more than 10 s, the MPE is 0.1 W·cm^{-2}. The limiting aperture for this wavelength is 3.5 mm for exposure durations greater than 10 s. The Class 1 AEL is then:

$$\text{Class 1 AEL} = \text{MPE} \times \frac{\pi D_f^{\,2}}{4} \qquad \textbf{Eq B23}$$

$$= 0.1\ \text{W} \cdot \text{cm}^{-2} \times \frac{\pi \times (0.35)^2}{4} = 9.6\ \text{mW}.$$

Since the possibility of optics exists, the measurement aperture listed in Table 9 must be used. For this wavelength, a 25 mm (2.5 cm) measurement aperture is used, which would contain the emitted power of the entire laser beam. In addition, 7 × 50 binoculars would transmit about 70% of the laser energy at this wavelength. In the case of either unaided viewing or optically aided viewing, 3 mW is less than the Class 1 AEL of 9.6 mW, and the laser is Class 1.

Example 24. **What is the hazard class of a single–pulse laser rangefinder operating at a wavelength of 1540 nm? The exit beam diameter is 2 mm and the output energy per pulse is 12 mJ. The pulse width is 20 ns.**

Solution. From Table 5a, the MPE for 1540 nm is 1 J·cm^{-2} for all exposure durations from 1 ns to 10 s. Therefore the MPE for this laser is 1 J·cm^{-2}. The Class 1 AEL is the MPE multiplied by the area of the limiting aperture. From Table 8b, the limiting aperture for this laser is 1 mm. The area of a 1 mm aperture is $\pi \times (0.1)^2/4 = 7.85 \times 10^{-3}$ cm^2. The Class 1 AEL is then 1 J·cm^{-2} × 7.85 × 10^{-3} cm^2 = 7.85 × 10^{-3} J = 7.85 mJ.

For unaided viewing (Condition 2), about ¼ of the output energy per pulse would be transmitted by the limiting aperture (from Eq B15). However, for optically aided viewing (Condition 1) all the energy would be collected by the 7 mm measurement aperture. Although 30% of the energy would not be transmitted through the optics due to reflection losses within the optics, 0.7 × 12 mJ = 8.4 mJ would exceed the Class 1 limit of 7.9 mJ, and the laser would, therefore, be Class 1M, since the Class 3B AEL for this wavelength is 125 mJ.

Example 25. **What is the hazard class of a multiple–pulse laser rangefinder operating at a wavelength of 1540 nm? The exposure duration for this device will not exceed 100 s. The exit beam diameter is 3 mm and approximately Gaussian in shape. The output energy per pulse is 10 mJ. The pulse width is 20 ns and the pulse repetition frequency is 10 Hz.**

Solution. All three rules must be tested since the device is repetitive-pulse. Since different limiting apertures are involved, the lowest MPE will not necessarily determine the hazard class. Rather the rule that indicates the greatest hazard determines the classification of the laser.

Rule 1. Single Pulse Limit:

Unaided Viewing.
From Example 24, the $MPE_{SP}{:}H$ is 1 J·cm^{-2} and the Class 1 AEL is 7.9 mJ based on a limiting aperture of 1 mm. The energy transmitted by D_f is (from Eq B15):

$$\Phi_d = \Phi_0 \left(1 - e^{-\left(\frac{D_f}{D_L}\right)^2}\right)$$

$$= \Phi_0 \times \left(1 - e^{-\left(\frac{1\ \text{mm}}{3\ \text{mm}}\right)^2}\right) = 10\ \text{mJ} \times 0.105$$

$$= 1.05\ \text{mJ}.$$

Thus, based on a single pulse exposure for unaided viewing, the laser is Class 1 since the energy transmitted by the aperture is less than the Class 1 AEL.

Optically Aided Viewing.
For optically aided viewing, the same Class 1 AEL is used but optical energy is collected through a 7 mm measurement aperture, D_m. Transmission of the optics is assumed to be 70%. From Eq B15:

$$\Phi_d = \Phi_0 \times \tau_\lambda \times \left(1 - e^{-\left(\frac{D_m}{D_L}\right)^2}\right)$$

$$= \Phi_0 \times 0.7 \times \left(1 - e^{-\left(\frac{7\ \text{mm}}{3\ \text{mm}}\right)^2}\right)$$

$$= 10\ \text{mJ} \times 0.7 \times 0.996 = 6.97\ \text{mJ}.$$

Therefore, for optically aided viewing the laser classification based on a single pulse, is also Class 1.

Rule 2. Average Power Limit:
The MPE for a 100 s exposure duration is 100 mW·cm^{-2}. For a 10 s exposure, the MPE is 1 J·cm^{-2}, the same as it is for a single pulse; however, the limiting aperture is 3.5 mm. The Class 1 AEL is the MPE multiplied by the area of a 3.5 mm aperture (9.6×10^{-2} cm^2) = 96 mJ for 10 s, or 9.6 mW. For the average power limit, the classification is the same for 10 s or for 100 s. The sum of all the pulse energies within 10 s transmitted by the measurement aperture must be summed for comparison to this MPE of 96 mJ. In 10 s, 100 pulses are emitted.

Unaided Viewing.
The measurement aperture for unaided viewing for a 10 s (or longer) exposure duration is 3.5 mm for this wavelength.

$$\Phi_d = n \times \Phi_0/\text{pulse} \times \left(1 - e^{-\left(\frac{D_m}{D_L}\right)^2}\right)$$

$$= 100 \times 10\ \text{mJ} \times \left(1 - e^{-\left(\frac{3.5\ \text{mm}}{3\ \text{mm}}\right)^2}\right)$$

$$= 1.0\ \text{J} \times 0.744 = 0.744\ \text{J} = 744\ \text{mJ}.$$

Therefore, the Class 1 AEL, based on average power of 96 mJ total energy in 10 s, is exceeded. The Class 3R AEL is 5 × 96 mJ = 480 mJ. The Class 3R AEL is also exceeded. However, a maximum of 30 mJ is emitted within 0.25 s, which is less than the 125 mJ Class 3B AEL. Therefore, the laser is Class 3B based on unaided viewing and the average power limit for a 100 s exposure duration.

Optically Aided Viewing.
The measurement aperture for optically aided viewing is 25 mm for this wavelength for a 10 s exposure duration.

$$\Phi_d = n \times \Phi_0/\text{pulse} \times \tau_\lambda \times \left(1 - e^{-\left(\frac{D_m}{D_L}\right)^2}\right)$$

$$= 100 \times 10\ \text{mJ} \times 0.7 \times \left(1 - e^{-\left(\frac{25\ \text{mm}}{3\ \text{mm}}\right)^2}\right)$$

$$= 100 \times 10\ \text{mJ} \times 0.7 = 700\ \text{mJ}.$$

Therefore, the Class 1 AEL based on average power of 96 mJ is exceeded. The Class 3R AEL is 5 × 96 mJ = 480 mJ. The Class 3R AEL is also exceeded. However, a maximum of 30 mJ is emitted within 0.25 s, which is less than the 125 mJ Class 3B AEL. Therefore, the laser is Class 3B based on both unaided viewing and optically aided viewing, and the average power limit for a 100 s exposure duration.

Rule 3. Repetitive-Pulse Limit:
The MPE for Rule 3 is based on $MPE_{SP} \times C_P$. However, all pulses contained within t_{min} are considered one pulse. The value of t_{min} for this wavelength is 10 s. Therefore for this rule, the laser is considered to only emit one pulse in 10 s. Since there are no pauses in emission lasting at least 10 s during the 100 s exposure duration, C_P need not be applied since the critical frequency has been exceeded, and the laser can be considered the same as if it were CW.

Resultant MPE (Example 25):
The laser is Class 3B based on the Class 1 AEL and MPE from Rule 2 (the average power limit) and a limiting aperture of 3.5 mm. For this example the MPE is 1 J·cm^{-2} for all 100 pulses in a 10 s exposure duration, or 10 mJ·cm^{-2}/pulse. The Class 1 AEL is 96 mJ for all 100 pulses or 0.96 mJ/pulse.

B5. Central-Beam Irradiance or Radiant Exposure

The beam irradiance or radiant exposure at the cornea is compared with the MPE (see Figure B1). Often the beam irradiance or radiant exposure is not provided in a laser's specification. Although most laser beams have a circular shape, some beams have a rectangular or elliptical shape as they leave the laser exit port. These beams then usually maintain a similar shape at a distance from the laser.

B5.1 Circular Beams. In addition to the laser beam having either a circular shape or a shape with x and y dimensions, the profile of the laser from the beam center to the edges may be different. The profile of the laser beam may be Gaussian or have a nearly top-hat profile if the laser operates multimode, uses fiber optics, or beam forming optics (see Figure B2). The Gaussian profile may also be truncated on the edges to produce a nearly top-hat appearance.

When a laser beam has a top-hat profile, the irradiance or radiant exposure are easily calculated by dividing the power or energy in the laser beam by the area of the beam. The diameter is well defined and may be determined by a variety of methods since the edges are sharp. The area is simply $\pi \times r^2$, where r is the radius of the beam. Usually the dimensions of a laser beam are provided as the full width, rather than the half-width. Therefore the area of a laser beam is $\pi \times a^2/4$, where a is the beam diameter near the laser exit port. The irradiance or radiant exposure of the laser beam is then given below:

$$E_0 = \frac{4\Phi}{\pi a^2} = \frac{1.27\Phi}{a^2} \qquad \textbf{Eq B24}$$

and

$$H_0 = 4\frac{Q}{\pi a^2} = \frac{1.27Q}{a^2} \qquad \textbf{Eq B25}$$

For safety evaluations, the center beam irradiance or radiant exposure are not used when the beam diameter is close to the limiting aperture. For visible and near infrared lasers, the limiting aperture is 7 mm, representing the pupil.

Instead of center beam values of E_0 and H_0, values of E and H averaged over the correct limiting aperture are necessary. For retinal hazards, the degree of hazard depends on the total energy reaching the retina. Rather than the actual maximum corneal irradiance, the irradiance averaged over a 7 mm pupil is more applicable to assessing retinal hazards. For wavelengths outside the retinal hazard region, a similar argument may be made for averaging the energy over a limiting aperture D_f. A reasonable approach is to calculate E and H by the following formulae:

$$E = \frac{4\Phi}{\max(D_f, a)} \qquad \textbf{Eq B26}$$

and

$$H = \frac{4Q}{\max(D_f, a)} \qquad \textbf{Eq B27}$$

where $\max(D_f, a)$ represents the maximum of the beam diameter (specified at $1/e$ of peak irradiance points) and the limiting aperture.

Example 26. **Determine whether a laser beam exceeds the MPE. A HeNe laser (632.8 nm) has a 1 mm exit beam diameter, and has a specified, maximum output power of 0.95 mW. Does this laser exceed the MPE for a 0.25 s exposure near the laser exit port?**

Solution. The MPE for a visible laser for a 0.25 s exposure is 2.55×10^{-3} W·cm^{-2} (see Example 1).

The laser beam will not increase in diameter near the laser exit port. However, for the retinal hazard region, D_f is 7 mm (0.7 cm), simulating a large pupillary diameter. The irradiance of the laser from Eq B26 is:

$$E = \frac{1.27\Phi}{[\max(a, D_f)]^2} = \frac{1.27(0.95 \times 10^{-3})}{0.7^2}$$
$$= 2.46 \text{ x } 10^{-3}\ \text{W} \cdot \text{cm}^{-2}$$

Since 2.46 mW·cm^{-2} is less than 2.55 mW·cm^{-2}, this laser does not exceed the MPE.

Example 27. **A 1 W Ar laser operating at 0.5145 μm is to be used in a communications link. Determine under what conditions the emergent beam would not be considered a skin hazard.**

Solution. The MPE for skin for exposure durations greater than 10 s is found in Table 7:

$$MPE_{\text{skin}} = 0.2 \times C_A \ \text{W·cm}^{-2}. \qquad \textbf{Eq B28}$$

The limiting aperture for the skin from Table 8a is 3.5 mm. For an Argon laser, C_A, is 1.0 and MPE_{skin} is 0.2 W·cm^{-2}. Since the total output power is greater than 0.5 W, the beam would have to be sufficiently large to reduce the irradiance below 200 mW·cm^{-2}. Thus,

$$MPE_{\text{skin}} = \text{E}_0 = \frac{4\Phi}{\pi a^2}, \qquad \textbf{Eq B29}$$

assuming that a will be larger than 3.5 mm. Therefore,

$$a = \sqrt{\frac{4\Phi}{\pi\,\text{MPE}}} \qquad \textbf{Eq B30}$$

$$= \sqrt{\frac{4(1)}{(\pi)(0.2)}} = 2.52\,\text{cm}.$$

Therefore, the beam diameter must be greater than 2.5 cm to preclude a skin hazard.

A cross-section of a Gaussian beam has an irradiance distribution similar to a normal probability curve. The beam diameter used for safety analysis is the diameter at $1/e$ of the peak irradiance, rather than the often specified beam diameter at $1/e^2$ of peak irradiance. Therefore, an aperture that is the same size as the beam diameter would collect only 63% of the laser beam power or energy when placed in the center of the beam, rather than 87.5% or 100% as would normally be thought. This difference in measured power or energy may be significant for particular laser applications.

If the laser is single mode and has a Gaussian beam profile, the central-beam irradiance, E_0, or radiant exposure, H_0, may be obtained from the beam diameter specified at the $1/e$ points and the emitted radiant power or energy from Eqs B26 and B27. For beam divergence or diameter values specified at $1/e^2$ points rather than at the $1/e$ points, the divergence or diameter specified at the $1/e^2$ points is divided by $\sqrt{2}$ to obtain the corresponding $1/e$ value.

Example 28. **Find the appropriate beam diameter to use for calculations in this standard if a laser beam diameter is specified as 3 mm as measured at $1/e^2$ of peak-irradiance points. The beam is further specified to be single-mode and Gaussian.**

Solution. Since the beam is Gaussian, the beam diameter measured at the $1/e^2$ points is greater by a factor of $\sqrt{2} = 1.41$ than the diameter measured at the $1/e$ points. Hence

$$a = \frac{0.3\ \text{cm}}{\sqrt{2}} = 0.21\ \text{cm}$$

This exercise was purely academic since the laser is in the retinal hazard region. Beam diameters less than 7 mm do not increase the retinal hazard. The value of a could, however, be used in the laser range equations (see Section B6.3).

When the laser beam diameter is nearly the same as the limiting or measurement apertures, the calculated values of H_0 or E_0, may not be relevant. The irradiance or radiant exposure must be averaged over the limiting aperture in Table 8b, before comparison to the MPE. The power or energy transmitted by various sized measurement apertures may be computed from Eqs B15 and B16. The average corneal irradiance or radiant exposure may then be determined by dividing the transmitted power or energy by the area of the limiting aperture.

Example 29. **Compare the center-beam irradiance to the beam irradiance averaged over a 0.7 cm diameter aperture for a Gaussian beam from a 5 mW laser with a 0.8 cm beam diameter.**

Solution. The center-beam irradiance is:

$$E = \frac{1.27\Phi}{a^2} = \frac{1.27\left(5 \times 10^{-3}\right)}{0.8^2}$$
$$= 9.9 \text{ x } 10^{-3}\ \text{W} \cdot \text{cm}^{-2}$$

The fraction of the laser power that would be transmitted by the aperture from Eq B15 is:

$$\frac{\Phi_d}{\Phi_0} = 1 - e^{-\left(\frac{0.7}{0.8}\right)^2} = 0.535 \cdot$$

The area of a 7 mm limiting aperture is 0.385 cm^2. The beam irradiance averaged over a 0.7 cm diameter aperture is:

$$E = \frac{5\ \text{mW} \times 0.535}{0.385\ \text{cm}^2} = 6.95\ \text{mW} \cdot \text{cm}^2$$

Although the maximum beam irradiance provides a conservative value, the latter calculation closely matches the actual exposure for a Gaussian-shaped beam.

Hazard analysis may also be accomplished through direct measurement of applicable beam parameters.

Example 30. **Find the approximate beam diameter of a Gaussian laser beam having a total output power of 5 mW and a measured power of 1 mW through a 0.7 cm diameter aperture.**

Solution. To calculate the beam diameter D_L from a measured fraction of the total power through an aperture of diameter D_f for a Gaussian beam, the following relation may be derived from Eq B15:

$$D_L = \left[\frac{-D_f^2}{\ln\left(1 - \frac{\Phi_d}{\Phi_0}\right)} \right]^{1/2} . \qquad \textbf{Eq B31}$$

Hence,

$$D_L = \left[\frac{-(0.7 \text{ cm})^2}{\ln\left(1 - \frac{1 \text{ mW}}{5 \text{ mW}}\right)} \right]^{1/2} = 1.48 \text{ cm} .$$

Example 31. **For a HeNe laser with a total output power Φ_0 of 3 mW, find the power that will pass through the limiting aperture (7 mm) if the beam diameter specified at $1/e^2$ of the peak irradiance points is 1.6 cm.**

Solution. Since the beam diameter is specified at $1/e^2$ points, the beam diameter used for laser safety calculations ($1/e$ points) is 1.6 cm/$\sqrt{2}$= 1.1 cm.

The power which passes through an aperture of diameter D_f (from Eq B15) is given by:

$$\Phi_d = \Phi_0 \left[1 - e^{-\left(\frac{D_f}{D_L}\right)^2} \right] = \qquad \textbf{Eq B32}$$

$$= 3 \text{ mW} \times \left[1 - e^{-\left(\frac{0.7 \text{ cm}}{1.1 \text{ cm}}\right)^2} \right] = 1 \text{ mW}.$$

B5.2 Axial Beam Radiant Exposure for Elliptical and Rectangular Beams. The radiant exposure for a rectangular or elliptical beam can be calculated using modifications of Eqs B26 and B27. For an elliptical beam,

$$E = \frac{1.27\Phi}{[\max(b, D_f)]\ [\max(c, D_f)]}, \qquad \textbf{Eq B33}$$

and

$$H = \frac{1.27Q}{[\max(b, D_f)]\ [\max(c, D_f)]}. \qquad \textbf{Eq B34}$$

For a rectangular beam, similar equations may be written as:

$$E = \frac{\Phi}{[\max(b_1, D_f)]\ [\max(c_1, D_f)]}, \qquad \textbf{Eq B35}$$

and

$$H = \frac{Q}{[\max(b_1, D_f)]\ [\max(c_1, D_f)]}. \qquad \textbf{Eq B36}$$

Example 32. **Find the beam irradiance at 20 cm from a GaAs laser illuminator with a rectangular beam shape and the following parameters:**

$\Phi = 2$ W, $b_1 = 2$ cm, and $c_1 = 3$ cm.

Solution. Using Eq B35,

$$E = \frac{\Phi}{[\max(b_1, D_f)]\ [\max(c_1, D_f)]} =$$

$$\frac{2\ \mathrm{W}}{(2\ \mathrm{cm}) \times (3\ \mathrm{cm})} = 0.33\ \mathrm{W \cdot cm^{-2}}$$

In addition to the basic shape of an elliptical or a rectangular beam, the profile in each dimension can resemble either a top-hat or a Gaussian profile. The beam dimensions for these beams should be measured at $1/e$ of peak irradiance points, also.

***Example 33.* Find the radiant exposure of a visible–wavelength laser emitting energy of 5 μJ/pulse with an elliptical shape, having dimensions of 1 mm × 6 cm.**

Solution. The irradiance used for safety evaluation is:

$$H = \frac{1.27Q}{[\max(b, D_f)]\ \ [\max(c, D_f)]} =$$

$$\frac{1.27 \text{ x } 5\,\mu\text{J}}{(0.7\text{ cm})\times(6\text{ cm})} = 1.5\,\mu\text{J}\cdot\text{cm}^{-2}$$

When one dimension is much smaller than the limiting aperture, an elliptical beam pattern should be assumed rather than a rectangular one, to produce a conservative estimate of irradiance or radiant exposure.

B6. Formulas and Examples Useful in Evaluation of Various Laser Applications[8]

Normally, exposure to the direct beam presents the greatest hazard from any type laser system. The direct beam of a collimated laser may extend for tens or hundreds of kilometers from the laser source when used outdoors. Generally diffuse or specular reflections present less hazard, and the hazard is somewhat localized to the laser target (see Figures B3 and B4).

B6.1 Correction for Atmospheric Attenuation. Beam irradiance E or radiant exposure H, at range r, for a non-diverging beam which is attenuated by the atmosphere[9], is given by:

$$E = E_0 e^{-\mu r}, \qquad \textbf{Eq B37}$$

and

$$H = H_0 e^{-\mu r}. \qquad \textbf{Eq B38}$$

B6.2 Beam Diameter versus Distance. The beam diameter of a Gaussian beam changes with distance according to a hyperbolic function, rather than linearly as is often thought (see Figure B2). When the beam waist occurs at or near the exit port of the laser, a good approximation for beam diameter as a function of distance is:[10]

$$D_L = \sqrt{a^2 + r^2\phi^2}. \qquad \textbf{Eq B39}$$

[8] Adapted from *Control of Hazards to Health from Laser Radiation,* US Department of the Army Technical Bulletin TB-MED-524 (1985).

[9] The attenuation coefficient μ varies from 10^{-4} cm^{-1} in thick fog to 10^{-7} cm^{-1} in air of very good visibility. The Rayleigh scatter coefficient at 0.6943 μm is 4.8×10^{-8} cm^{-1}, and 1.8×10^{-8} cm^{-1} at 0.500 μm. The effect of aerosols in even the cleanest atmospheres usually raises μ at 0.6943 μm to at least 10^{-7} cm^{-1}.

[10] These formulas are accurate only for small values of ϕ; the accuracy is better than 1% for angles less than 0.17 rad (10°) and better than 5% for angles less than 0.37 rad (21°).

The initial beam diameter is generally only necessary for computing irradiance or radiant exposure at distances close to the exit port of the laser. For distances where considerable beam expansion has occurred, the initial beam diameter may be omitted without loss of accuracy.

***Example 34.* Find the diameter of a Gaussian laser beam at 1 km where the emergent beam diameter is 10 cm and the beam divergence is 0.1 mrad.**

Solution. From Eq B39,

$$\begin{aligned} D_L &= \sqrt{a^2 + r^2\phi^2} \\ &= \sqrt{10^2 + (10^{-4})^2(10^5\ \text{cm})^2} \\ &= 14.1\ \text{cm}. \end{aligned}$$

However, in some cases, the laser beam waist is located behind the laser exit port. In these cases, the beam diameter at the laser exit port is not the waist diameter and beam expansion has already occurred. The continuing beam spread is then often more linear than hyperbolic, and the best approximation is:

$$D_L = a + r\phi. \qquad \textbf{Eq B40}$$

In other cases, the beam waist is located in front of the laser exit port (see Figure B5). The beam diameter then diminishes with distance until the location of the beam waist has been reached, and then the beam again begins to expand. The equation for this type of beam expansion for a Gaussian beam is:

$$D_L = \sqrt{D_w^2 + (r - r_0)^2\phi^2}, \qquad \textbf{Eq B41}$$

where D_w is the diameter of the beam at the waist, and r_0 is the distance from the laser exit port to the beam waist, and r is the distance from the laser to the point where the beam diameter is D_L.

For rectangular or elliptical beams, each dimension may expand independently in accordance with any of the previous methods.

B6.3 The Laser Range Equation.

B6.3.1 Circular beams. Average irradiance in the direct beam at range r (for a circular beam) is the total power in the beam at r, divided by the area of the beam at r. Likewise, the radiant exposure in a non-turbulent medium is the total energy in the beam at r divided by its total area.

When the formulae for irradiance E, and radiant exposure H,[11] are combined with the beam expansion and atmospheric attenuation equations, formulae[12] that compute the irradiance or radiant exposure at any viewer distance are formed (see Figure B6). For circular beams:[13]

$$E = \frac{\Phi e^{-\mu r}}{\pi\left[\frac{\sqrt{a^2 + r^2\phi^2}}{2}\right]^2} = \frac{1.27\Phi e^{-\mu r}}{a^2 + r^2\phi^2}, \qquad \textbf{Eq B42}$$

and

$$H = \frac{Q e^{-\mu r}}{\pi\left[\frac{\sqrt{a^2 + r^2\phi^2}}{2}\right]^2} = \frac{1.27 Q e^{-\mu r}}{a^2 + r^2\phi^2}. \qquad \textbf{Eq B43}$$

Example 35. **Find the radiant exposure for a 0.1 J, Q-switched ruby laser at 1 km (10^5 cm). The laser has a pulse length of 20 ns, and a beam divergence of 1 mrad (10^{-3} rad) and an emergent beam diameter of 0.7 cm. Assume atmospheric attenuation coefficient equal to 1×10^{-7} cm^{-1}.**

Solution. Use Eq B43 with $\mu = 10^{-7}$ cm^{-1} to provide a worst case estimate. Thus,

$$\begin{aligned} H &= \frac{1.27 Q e^{-\mu r}}{a^2 + r^2\phi^2}\ \mathrm{J\cdot cm^{-2}} \\ &= \frac{(1.27)(0.1\ \mathrm{J})e^{-(10^{-7}\ \mathrm{cm^{-1}})(10^5\ \mathrm{cm})}}{\left[(0.7\ \mathrm{cm})^2 + (10^5\ \mathrm{cm}\times 10^{-3}\ \mathrm{rad})^2\right]} \\ &= \frac{(1.27)(0.1\,\mathrm{J})(0.99)}{\left[(0.7)^2 + (100)^2\right]\mathrm{cm}^2} \\ &= 1.25\times10^{-5}\ \mathrm{J\cdot cm^{-2}}. \end{aligned}$$

A person located at or near the target would then be exposed in excess of the MPE of 5×10^{-7} J·cm^{-2}.

B6.3.2 Focused Beams. Sometimes the waist of a laser beam is located downrange from the laser exit port (see Figure B5). In this case, the location of the beam waist, r_0, and the minimum diameter of the laser beam, D_w, are of more concern than the exit beam diameter,

---

[11] The value of E is in W·cm^{-2} and the value of H is in J·cm^{-2}. All dimensions of beam diameter or distance are in cm, all angles are in radians, power is in W and energy is in J.

[12] For focused beams see B6.3.2. For rectangular or elliptical beams, see B6.3.3.

[13] The above equations assume that the smallest beam diameter (the beam waist) occurs at the exit port of the laser, and that a and ϕ are defined at the $1/e$ points of maximum irradiance.

a. When the beam is nearly collimated, only a rough approximation of the location and size of the beam waist is necessary for safety calculations. When the beam is focused, the following equations (similar to Eqs B42 and B43) may be used to determine the irradiance or radiant exposure.

$$E = \frac{1.27 \Phi e^{-\mu r}}{D_w^2 + (r - r_0)^2 \phi^2}, \qquad \textbf{Eq B44}$$

and

$$H = \frac{1.27 Q e^{-\mu r}}{D_w^2 + (r - r_0)^2 \phi^2}. \qquad \textbf{Eq B45}$$

Example 36. **Find the radiant exposure at 50 m from a low-energy Nd:YAG laser rangefinder (λ=1.064 μm) with an output radiant energy of 40 μJ, an exit beam diameter of 9 mm, a beam waist of 7 mm located 10 m in front of the laser, and a beam divergence of 0.6 mrad.**

Solution. The exit beam diameter does not appear in Eqs B44 and B45, and the atmospheric term may be neglected at short distances. The corneal radiant exposure is:

$$H = \frac{1.27 Q e^{-\mu r}}{D_w^2 + (r - r_0)^2 \phi^2}$$

$$= \frac{1.27(40 \times 10^{-6}\ \text{J})}{\left[(0.7)^2 + (5000 - 1000)^2 (0.6 \times 10^{-3})^2\right]\ \text{cm}^2}$$

$$= \frac{50.8 \times 10^{-6}\ \text{J}}{(0.49 + 5.76)\ \text{cm}^2} = 8.1 \times 10^{-6}\ \text{J} \cdot \text{cm}^{-2}.$$

Since the MPE for a single-pulse Nd:YAG laser at 1064 nm is 5×10^{-6} J·cm^{-2}, the beam radiant exposure exceeds the MPE at 50 m.

B6.3.3 Rectangular and Elliptical Beams. The radiant exposure for a rectangular or elliptical beam can be computed in a similar fashion as for a circular beam. Any of the beam expansion equations may apply to the beam expansion in each dimension.

If the beam waist is located at some distance behind the exit port of the laser, the values of b and c are not measured close to the beam waist. For this situation, the equations for the irradiance and radiant exposure for an elliptical beam are:

$$E = \frac{1.27\Phi e^{-\mu r}}{[b + r\phi_1]\ [c + r\phi_2]}, \qquad \textbf{Eq B46}$$

and

$$H = \frac{1.27 Q e^{-\mu r}}{[b + r\phi_1]\ [c + r\phi_2]}. \qquad \textbf{Eq B47}$$

For a rectangular beam, similar equations may be written as:

$$E = \frac{\Phi e^{-\mu r}}{[b_1 + r\phi_1]\ [c_1 + r\phi_2]}, \qquad \textbf{Eq B48}$$

and

$$H = \frac{Q e^{-\mu r}}{[b_1 + r\phi_1]\ [c_1 + r\phi_2]}. \qquad \textbf{Eq B49}$$

However, for many laser beams the expansion equation of the laser beam in any two orthogonal axis is different. The beam may be focused in front of the laser in one axis, while the beam is constantly expanding in the other axis.

Example 37. **Find the beam irradiance at 20 m from a GaAs laser illuminator with a rectangular beam and the following parameters: $\Phi = 2$ W; $b_1 = 2$ cm; $c_1 = 1.3$ cm; $\phi_1 = 51$ mrad; $\phi_2 = 17$ mrad.**

Solution. Using Eq B48, the initial beam dimensions or atmospheric absorption contribute little to the final irradiance. Therefore, the equation can be simplified to:

$$\begin{aligned} E &= \frac{\Phi}{[r\phi_1]\ [r\phi_2]} \\ &= \frac{2\ \text{W}}{[(2000 \times 0.051)\ \text{cm}][(2000 \times 0.017)\ \text{cm}]} \\ &= \frac{2\ \text{W}}{(102\ \text{cm})(34\ \text{cm})} = 5.77 \times 10^{-4}\ \text{W} \cdot \text{cm}^{-2}. \end{aligned}$$

Example 38. **Find the radiant exposure at 50 m from a long-range, 904 nm, infrared illuminator with a rectangular beam focused in one dimension. The laser has the following parameters: $\Phi = 30$ mW; $b_1 = 2.5$ cm; $c_1 = 0.8$ cm ; $\phi_1 = 5$ mrad; $\phi_2 = -1.7$ mrad**

(focused beam); no external waist in *b* dimension; D_w(c_l dimension) = 0.4 cm; r_0 (c_l dimension) = 4 m.

Solution. The beam expansion equations need to be modified since the beam is focused in one axis, but not the other.

$$D_{L1} = b_1 + r\phi_1$$
$$= 2.5 + (5000 \times 5 \times 10^{-3}) = 27.5 \text{ cm.}$$

$$D_{L2} = \sqrt{D_W{}^2 + (r - r_0)^2 \phi^2}$$
$$= \sqrt{(0.4)^2 + (5000 \text{ cm} - 400 \text{ cm})^2 (-1.7 \times 10^{-3})^2}$$
$$= \sqrt{0.16 + 61.2} \text{ cm} = 7.83 \text{ cm.}$$

$$E = \frac{\Phi e^{-\mu r}}{(D_{L1})(D_{L2})}$$
$$= \frac{30 \times 10^{-3} \text{ W}}{(27.5 \text{ cm})(7.83 \text{ cm})} = 0.14 \text{ mW} \cdot \text{cm}^{-2}.$$

B6.4 Nominal Ocular Hazard Distance (NOHD).

B6.4.1 Unaided Viewing. If Eqs B42 or B43 is solved for *r*, and *H* or *E* is replaced with the MPE, the corresponding value of *r* is the r_{NOHD}. Thus, if the atmospheric attenuation coefficient is neglected, a worst case estimate of the r_{NOHD} is (see Figure B6):

$$r_{\text{NOHD}} = \frac{1}{\phi}\sqrt{\frac{1.27\Phi}{\text{MPE}} - a^2} \qquad \textbf{Eq B50}$$

for CW lasers, or

$$r_{\text{NOHD}} = \frac{1}{\phi}\sqrt{\frac{1.27Q}{\text{MPE}} - a^2} \qquad \textbf{Eq B51}$$

for pulsed lasers. These equations apply mainly to large beams where the beam size is larger than the limiting or measurement aperture.

Example 39. **Find the r_{NOHD} (neglecting atmospheric effects) for the laser in Example 35.**

Solution. The MPE is 0.5 μJ·cm^{-2}.

$$
\begin{aligned}
r_{\text{NOHD}} &= \frac{1}{1\times10^{-3}}\sqrt{\frac{1.27(0.1)}{5\times10^{-7}}-(0.7)^2} \\
&= 5.04 \text{ km.}
\end{aligned}
$$

When the r_{NOHD} is very short, the beam diameter may be nearly the same size as the limiting aperture. A better equation for computing r_{NOHD} is based on the energy or power transmitted through the limiting aperture, compared with the Class 1 AEL:

From Eq B29,

$$\Phi_{\text{d}} = \Phi_0\left[1-e^{-\left(\frac{D_{\text{f}}}{D_{\text{L}}}\right)^2}\right]. \qquad \textbf{Eq B52}$$

The beam diameter, D_{L} may be written as a function of the distance from the laser according to Eqs B39, B40 or B41. When Φ_{d} is set equal to the Class 1 AEL (AEL), r becomes the distance from the laser to the point where the laser beam irradiance or radiant exposure is equal to the MPE (r_{NOHD}). For a Gaussian beam, the equation becomes:

$$\text{AEL} = \Phi_0\left[1-e^{-\left(\frac{D_{\text{f}}^2}{a^2+r_{\text{NOHD}}^2\phi^2}\right)}\right].$$

When this equation is solved for r_{NOHD}, the result is:

$$r_{\text{NOHD}} = \frac{1}{\phi}\sqrt{\frac{-D_{\text{f}}^2}{\ln\left(1-\frac{\text{AEL}}{\Phi_0}\right)}-a^2}. \qquad \textbf{Eq B53}$$

The equation for a pulsed laser may be achieved in the same manner from Eq B30, using the energy per pulse, Q_0:

$$r_{\text{NOHD}} = \frac{1}{\phi}\sqrt{\frac{-D_{\text{f}}^2}{\ln\left(1-\frac{\text{AEL}}{Q_0}\right)}-a^2}. \qquad \textbf{Eq B54}$$

***Example 40.* A low-power, visible laser has an output energy per pulse of 5 mW, an exit beam diameter of 5 mm, and a beam divergence of 1 mrad. What is the r_{NOHD} for a 0.25 s exposure?**

Solution. The MPE for a 0.25 s exposure is 2.55 mW·cm^{-2} (see Example 1). The Class 2 AEL is then about 1 mW. The limiting aperture is 7 mm for visible lasers. The r_{NOHD} from Eq B53 is therefore:

$$r_{NOHD} = \frac{1}{\phi}\sqrt{\frac{-0.49\ \text{cm}^2}{\ln\left(1-\frac{1\times10^{-3}\ \text{W}}{5\times10^{-3}\ \text{W}}\right)}-(0.5\ \text{cm})^2}$$
$$= 1.39\times10^3\ \text{cm} = 13.9\ \text{m}.$$

B6.4.2 Range Nomogram. The range nomogram[14] in Figure B8 (which includes two different attenuation coefficients) can also be used to determine r_{NOHD}.

***Example 41.* Find the r_{NOHD} for a Q-switched ruby laser with an output of 0.1 J and a beam divergence of 1 mrad.**

Solution. The MPE from Table 5a is 0.5 μJ·cm^{-2} for a single pulse from a visible Q-switched laser. A line drawn between 100 mJ and 1.0 mrad (shown as a dotted line in Figure B8) intercepts the "Integrated Radiant Intensity" scale at approximately 0.13 MJ sr^{-1}. A line from this point to 0.5 μJ·cm^{-2} on the "Radiant Exposure" scale intersects the "Range" scale at 4.9 km for a clear day, and 4 km for a hazy day.

B6.4.3 Optically Aided Viewing. When optical viewing aids are used to view the laser from within the beam (intrabeam viewing), the hazard is increased by as much as the square of the magnifying power.

Laser hazard classification is based on the characteristics of a pair of standard 7 × 50 binoculars. However, viewing with other types of magnifying optics results in various degrees of increased hazard over unaided viewing. Viewing with a Jeweler's loupe or other simple magnifying devices would usually not be more hazardous than viewing with 7 × 50 binoculars at a close distance. For evaluating the effects of binoculars or telescopes, a minimum evaluation distance of 2 m is used, since these types of magnifying devices cannot be focused at closer distances.

B6.4.3.1 Optical Gain. When a laser beam is transmitted by viewing optics, the beam diameter is reduced by the magnifying power of the optics. The gain, *G*, is the ratio of the radiant exposure or irradiance at the cornea when viewing is aided by an optical system, to that received by the unaided eye. It is defined below:

$$G = \frac{D_0^2}{D_e^2} = P^2,$$ **Eq B55**

[14] The r_{NOHD} for either pulsed or CW lasers may be calculated from the nomogram. The units for CW lasers are provided at the bottom of the scales and the units for pulsed lasers are provided at the top of the scales.

where D_0 is the entrance aperture of the optics and D_e is the exit aperture and optics transmission is 100%.

Many 7 × 50 binoculars have a power of 7.0 and an exit port diameter slightly larger than 7 mm (the limiting aperture diameter for lasers in the retinal hazard region). The gain would be 49 for these optics. For laser hazard analysis, the gain factor represents the maximum increased hazard from a laser beam due to the concentration of laser power on the cornea. However, this degree of increased hazard is usually encountered for intrabeam viewing of large-diameter, collimated laser beams. This situation would most likely occur when viewing a powerful laser beam at a long distance from the laser output port.

However, the gain factor does not account for the internal transmission losses in the optical system. All optical viewing systems transmit less than 100% of the power or energy entering the entrance aperture of the optics. For the visible portion of the spectrum (0.4 to 0.7 μm), a maximum transmission τ_λ, of 90% is assumed. For other wavelengths in the spectral region from 0.302 μm to 4.0 μm, the transmission is assumed to be about 70%, due to reflection losses within the optics (since antireflection coatings are tuned to visible wavelengths). The actual gain is then $G \times \tau_\lambda$ for large collimated beams.

Example 42. **An individual is viewing the laser source within a specularly reflected beam from a 50 mJ, visible laser rangefinder, at a distant point where the beam radiant exposure is 2×10^{-9} J·cm^{-2}. If the individual were to view the target from within the beam through a pair of 7 × 50 binoculars, (the beam diameter is larger than the objective diameter), what would be the relative hazard compared with unaided viewing?**

Solution. The magnifying power P of the binoculars is 7 and any reasonable size source would appear small at this distance, even through magnifying optics, Eq B55 provides the simplest solution when τ_λ is added:

$$G = \tau_\lambda \times P^2 = 0.9 \times 7^2 = 44.$$

Thus, the operator would be viewing an exposure 44 times greater than with the unaided eye, which is equal to a corneal radiant exposure, H, of nearly 1×10^{-7} J·cm^{-2}.

B6.4.3.2 Effective Gain. When viewing laser sources at closer distances, the hazard is usually less than that calculated from the above equation. The collecting aperture, D_C, is often the same as the measurement aperture, D_m listed in Table 9. For the retinal hazard region, this aperture diameter is 5 cm, which is much larger than most laser beams near the laser exit port.

Optical devices with a higher power than 7 usually have an exit port diameter less than 7 mm. The collecting aperture, D_C is, therefore, the minimum of the entrance diameter of the optics, D_0, and the optical power, P, multiplied by the limiting aperture diameter, D_f:

$$D_C = \min(D_0, P \times D_f). \qquad \textbf{Eq B56}$$

Therefore, for 7 × 50 binoculars with 7 power and a 7.14 cm exit aperture, the collecting aperture is 7 × 0.7 cm = 4.9 cm, since 4.9 cm is less than 5 cm.

The calculated irradiance or radiant exposure, for beam diameters less than the limiting aperture, is based on the area of the limiting aperture rather than the actual beam area. For higher-power optics, such as 10 × 50 binoculars, or for beam diameters less than D_C, the exit beam diameter from the optics will be smaller than 7 mm.

Therefore,[15]

$$G_{eff} = \tau_\lambda \times \frac{\min(D_C^2, D_L^2)}{D_f^2}. \qquad \textbf{Eq B57}$$

Example 43. **An individual is viewing a near infrared laser source from within the beam at a distance where the beam diameter is 1 m. The person has two viewing devices available: one is a 20-power optic with an 11.4 cm entrance aperture, and the other is 7 × 50 binoculars that has a 50 mm entrance aperture and an exit aperture of 7.14 mm. Determine the effective gain of each optic.**

Solution. Since the beam diameter is so large at the viewer's location, Eq B57 may be simplified:

$$G_{eff} = \tau_\lambda \times \frac{D_C^2}{D_f^2}.$$

The transmission of the optics in the near infrared is about 0.7. The measurement aperture is the product of the limiting aperture diameter and the magnifying power or the actual aperture if that is smaller. For the 1st optic, the measurement aperture is 11.4 cm since 20 × 0.7 is 14 cm. The effective gain is, therefore, $0.7 \times 11.4^2/0.49=186$.

For the 2nd optic, the collecting aperture, D_C is 4.9 cm. The effective gain is $0.7 \times 4.9^2/0.49 = 34.3$.

The effective gain is useful for calculating the hazards for lasers with wavelengths outside the retinal hazard region. Viewing optics are considered to transmit the laser wavelength, if the wavelength is between 0.302 μm and 2.8 μm. However, the hazard is to the cornea of the eye rather than to the retina. The optics will reduce the beam diameter by the magnifying power. Outside the visible portion of the spectrum, the transmission of the optics will be about 70% or less.

The limiting aperture for these wavelengths is either 1 mm or 3.5 mm. However, for a very large beam, all the energy collected by a 50 mm objective lens, D_0, would not be reduced to the size of a 1 mm aperture by a normal pair of 7 × 50 binoculars.

---

[15] The effective gain will not exceed the actual gain ($\tau_\lambda \times P^2$).

Therefore, assuming 7-power optics, the measurement aperture is about 7 times as large as the limiting aperture. For a 1 mm limiting aperture, the measurement aperture, D_m listed in Table 9 is 7 mm, and for a 3.5 mm limiting aperture, the measurement aperture is 25 mm (based on 7.14 power). For other optical systems, the collecting aperture, D_C may not match the measurement aperture.

Example 44. **An individual looks into a 1.54 μm, single-pulse, Q-switched, laser rangefinder at a distance where the beam is 1 cm in diameter. The output energy per pulse is 12 mJ and the beam profile is approximately Gaussian. Will viewing the laser through a pair of 10×50 binoculars exceed the MPE?**

Solution. From Table 5a, the MPE is 1 J·cm^{-2}, and from Tables 8a and 8b, the limiting aperture is 1 mm. The radiant exposure at the entrance of the optics is:

$$H = \frac{1.27 \times 12 \text{ mJ}}{(1 \text{ cm})^2} = 15.2 \text{ mJ} \cdot \text{cm}^{-2}$$

which is less than the MPE for unaided viewing.

From Eq B56, the collecting aperture, D_C is 10 × 1 mm = 1 cm, since D_0 is larger than 1 cm. The effective gain is:

$$\begin{aligned} G_{\text{eff}} &= \tau_\lambda \times \frac{\min(D_C^2, D_L^2)}{D_f^2} \\ &= 0.7 \times \frac{\min\left[(1.0 \text{ cm})^2, (1 \text{ cm})^2\right]}{(0.1 \text{ cm})^2} \\ &= 0.7 \times \frac{1.0}{0.01} = 70. \end{aligned}$$

The corneal radiant exposure is then 15.2 mJ·cm^{-2} × 70 = 1.06 J·cm^{-2}. Therefore, the MPE is just barely exceeded. However, this approach conservatively assumes that the radiant exposure is constant over the entire aperture diameter.

Since D_C is the same as D_L, the problem may be approached in a different way to get a more precise answer. Eq B16 may be adapted for use with actual telescopic optics:

$$\frac{Q_d}{Q_0} = \left(1 - e^{-\left(\frac{D_C}{D_L}\right)^2}\right) \times \tau_\lambda . \qquad \textbf{Eq B58}$$

Since D_C is equal to D_L in this case, 63% of the energy will be transmitted by the aperture and 30% of that will be lost due to reflection losses within the optics. Hence,

$$Q_d = Q_0\left(1-e^{-1}\right)\left(\tau_\lambda\right)$$
$$= (12\ \text{mJ})(0.63)(0.7) = 5.3\ \text{mJ}.$$

The radiant exposure averaged over the limiting aperture is then,

$$H = \frac{1.27 Q_d}{D_f^2} = \frac{1.27 \times 5.3\ \text{mJ}}{(0.1)^2}$$
$$= 0.67\ \text{J} \cdot \text{cm}^{-2}.$$

Therefore, the corneal radiant exposure averaged over the limiting aperture is not exceeded, although the maximum radiant exposure, H_0, transmitted by the optics indicates that the MPE would be exceeded.

B6.4.3.3 Viewing Extended Sources with Optics. Another effect of optical viewing devices that has not been taken into account so far is an increase in retinal image size for wavelengths in the retinal hazard region. The laser source appears larger when viewed through optical devices, and the apparent source size is increased by the optical power of the optics. For lasers with a large apparent source size already, the MPE is increased by the magnifying power of the optics. Lasers that have a small apparent point source size for unaided viewing may be extended sources when viewed through magnifying optics. For these types of laser beams, the effective gain is:

$$G_{\text{eff}} = \frac{\tau_\lambda \left[\frac{\min(D_C, D_L)}{D_f}\right]^2}{C_E(\text{aided})}, \qquad \textbf{Eq B59}$$

for $C_E < 1.0$. When the source is also extended without optics, G_{eff} is multiplied by C_E (unaided).

***Example 45.* A 1.3 μm diode laser is formed by placing the end of a fiber optic cable at the focal point of a lens, and the beam is collimated to the best achievable beam divergence without focusing, which is 2 mrad. The output of the laser is 10 mW through the lens. The beam diameter is 1.2 cm as it exits the lens.**

When viewed at a distance of 10 m, the source size is about 1 cm.[16] What is the hazard from intrabeam viewing of the laser at 10 m with a pair of 7 × 50 binoculars?

[16] The source size cannot be larger than the beam divergence. For this example, the apparent source size is close to the same size as the beam divergence (2 mrad) near the exit port, but is only 1.0 mrad at a distance of 10 m from the laser. See section B9 for additional discussion of source size.

Solution. The beam diameter at 10 m will be approximately:

$$\begin{aligned} D_{\mathrm{L}} &= \sqrt{a^2 + (r\phi)^2} \\ &= \sqrt{(1.2\ \mathrm{cm})^2 + (1000\ \mathrm{cm} \times 2 \times 10^{-3})^2} \\ &= 2.3\ \mathrm{cm}. \end{aligned}$$

The irradiance at 10 m is:

$$\begin{aligned} E &= \frac{1.27\Phi}{D_{\mathrm{L}}^2} = \frac{12.7\ \mathrm{mW}}{(2.3\ \mathrm{cm})^2} \\ &= 2.4\ \mathrm{mW} \cdot \mathrm{cm}^{-2}. \end{aligned}$$

When viewing through 7 × 50 binoculars, the corneal irradiance is increased, but the source size is also increased. For unaided viewing at this distance, the source is a point source since

$$\alpha = \frac{D_{\rho}}{r_1} \qquad \textbf{Eq B60}$$

$$= \frac{1\ \mathrm{cm}}{1000\ \mathrm{cm}} = 1\ \mathrm{mrad},$$

and $\alpha_{\min}$ is 1.5 mrad.

For optically aided viewing, the source appears 7 times larger. The extended source correction factor, C_{E}, is:

$$C_{\mathrm{E}}(\text{aided}) = \frac{7 \times (1\ \mathrm{mrad})}{1.5\ \mathrm{mrad}} = 4.7 \cdot$$

Therefore,

$$\begin{aligned} G_{\mathrm{eff}} &= \frac{\tau_{\lambda}\left[\frac{\min(5\mathrm{cm},\ 2.3\ \mathrm{cm})}{0.7\ \mathrm{cm}}\right]^2}{C_{\mathrm{E}}(\text{aided})} \\ &= 0.7 \times \left[\frac{(2.3\ \mathrm{cm})}{(0.7\ \mathrm{cm})}\right]^2 \times \frac{1}{4.7} = 1.6. \end{aligned}$$

Since the effective gain is 1.6, the corneal irradiance is 3.9 $\mathrm{mW{\cdot}cm^{-2}}$ at the exit lens of the optics. Since the point source MPE for this wavelength is about 40 $\mathrm{mW{\cdot}cm^{-2}}$, the laser does not present a hazard with viewing optics at this viewing distance.

B6.5 Scanning Lasers. The corneal radiant exposure for a single exposure from a scanning laser beam is given by Eqs B61 and B62. [Repetitive-pulse exposures depend upon distance, r (cm) scan rate, S (cm/s) and frame rate (Hz).]

$$H = \frac{1.27\Phi e^{-\mu r}}{D_L(rS\theta_s)} \text{ for } D_L > d_e, \qquad \textbf{Eq B61}$$

and

$$H = \frac{1.27\Phi e^{-\mu r}}{d_e(rS\theta_s)} \text{ for } D_L < d_e. \qquad \textbf{Eq B62}$$

The applicable MPEs depend upon the repetitive nature of the exposure duration t[17] of a single pulse, where

$$t = \frac{D_L}{rS\theta_s} \text{ for } D_L > d_e, \qquad \textbf{Eq B63}$$

and

$$t = \frac{d_e}{rS\theta_s} \text{ for } D_L < d_e. \qquad \textbf{Eq B64}$$

Example 46. **Find the exposure of a scanning HeNe system having the following parameters: a = 0.1 cm; $\phi = 5 \times 10^{-3}$ rad; Φ = 10 mW; θ_S = 0.1 rad; $S = 30\ s^{-1}$; and the intrabeam-viewing distance r is 200 cm.**

Solution. The beam diameter D_L (Eq B39) is:

$$D_L = \sqrt{a^2 + (r\phi)^2} = \sqrt{0.01 + 1} = 1.005 \text{ cm}.$$

Hence, Eq B61 applies.

[17] The maximum value of t is $1/S$ and the PRF is S if each scan passes over the eye.

The PRF at the eye is 30 pulses per second and, from Eq B63, the exposure duration for a single pulse is:

$$
\begin{aligned}
t &= \frac{D_L}{rS\theta_s} = \frac{1.005\ \text{cm}}{(200\ \text{cm})(30\ \text{s}^{-1})(0.1\ \text{rad})} \\
&= 1.68 \times 10^{-3}\ \text{s}.
\end{aligned}
$$

The radiant exposure per pulse, as found from Eq B61, is:

$$
\begin{aligned}
H &= \frac{(1.27)(10 \times 10^{-3})(1)}{(1.005)(200)(30)(0.1)}\ \text{J} \cdot \text{cm}^{-2} \\
&= 2.11 \times 10^{-5}\ \text{J} \cdot \text{cm}^{-2}.
\end{aligned}
$$

This total radiant exposure is equal to the product of the single pulse exposure and the number of pulses. The number of pulses exposure during a 0.25 s exposure is $0.25 \times 30 \approx 8$. Hence,

$$
\begin{aligned}
H_{\text{tot}} &= n(H / Pulse)\ \text{J} \cdot \text{cm}^{-2} \\
&- 8(2.11 \times 10^{-5}) \\
&= 16.9 \times 10^{-5}\ \text{J} \cdot \text{cm}^{-2}.
\end{aligned}
$$

The applicable *MPE/pulse* for a 0.25 s exposure is determined by the cumulative exposure of eight pulses (Rule 3). Thus,

$$
\begin{aligned}
MPE / Pulse &= n^{-1/4}(\text{MPE})\ \text{J} \cdot \text{cm}^{-2} \\
&= 8^{-1/4} \times 1.8 \times t^{3/4} \times 10^{-3}\ \text{J} \cdot \text{cm}^{-2} \\
&= (0.595)(1.5 \times 10^{-5})\ \text{J} \cdot \text{cm}^{-2} \\
&= 8.89 \times 10^{-6}\ \text{J} \cdot \text{cm}^{-2}.
\end{aligned}
$$

The total radiant exposure for a 0.25 s exposure duration must be compared with the MPE for a pulse train of the same duration. Thus,

$$
\begin{aligned}
MPE / Train &= n \times (MPE / Pulse)\ \text{J} \cdot \text{cm}^{-2} \\
&= 8(8.89 \times 10^{-6})\ \text{J} \cdot \text{cm}^{-2} \\
&= 7.11 \times 10^{-5}\ \text{J} \cdot \text{cm}^{-2}.
\end{aligned}
$$

Since the MPE for a 0.25 s exposure duration (7.11×10^{-5} J·cm^{-2}) is less than the radiant exposure for a train of pulses of the same duration (16.9×10^{-5} J·cm^{-2}), the exposure is not permissible for momentary (unintentional) viewing.

B6.6 Nominal Hazard Zone (NHZ). The NHZ includes all areas around a laser where the irradiance or radiant exposure would exceed the MPE. This area could include hazards from specular or diffuse reflections, the direct beam, or a modified laser beam with a lens, or a combination of these effects.

B6.6.1 Diffuse Reflection Hazards. Although the primary hazard from lasers is from the direct beam, viewing diffuse reflections from a matte surface can be hazardous from very powerful lasers (see Figure B4). However, these reflections are only hazardous when:

(1) The viewer's eye is located near the reflecting surface, and

(2) The reflecting surface is near the laser exit port.[18]

The hazard from diffuse reflections is related to the irradiance or radiant exposure at the viewer's location. The exposure at the viewer's location will be composed of both specular and diffuse components. However, from a matte surface, the reflection will be primarily diffuse. The reflected irradiance and radiant exposure for a diffuse reflection (for $r_1 > D_L$) are given by Lambert's law:

$$E = \frac{\rho_\lambda \Phi \cos\theta_v}{\pi r_1^2}, \qquad \textbf{Eq B65}$$

and

$$H = \frac{\rho_\lambda Q \cos\theta_v}{\pi r_1^2}. \qquad \textbf{Eq B66}$$

Example 47. **Find the corneal radiant exposure at 1 m from a diffuse reflection of a Q-switched ruby laser with 1 J of output energy per pulse.**

Solution. Assume that the viewing angle is at the center of the matte surface ($\cos\theta_v=1$) and the reflectance is 100%. The radiant exposure is then,

$$H = \frac{1\ \text{J}}{\pi \times (100\ \text{cm})^2} = 3.2\times10^{-5}\ \text{J}\cdot\text{cm}^{-2}.$$

Since the MPE for a single exposure to a Q-switched visible laser is 5×10^{-7} J·cm^{-2}, exposure to a diffuse reflection is probably hazardous at this distance unless the source is a very large source (see B6.6.2 for extended source MPEs).

B6.6.2 Extended source Diffuse Reflections. For very large laser beams or very close viewing distances, the hazard calculated based on a point source overstates the real hazard.

[18] Once the laser beam diameter has increased substantially, or the viewer is located beyond a few meters from the reflecting surface, the diffuse reflection hazard is greatly reduced.

Therefore, extended source MPEs should be computed. Extended source MPEs are applied only in the retinal hazard region (0.4 to 1.4 μm).

The angle, α_{min}, is used to determine when the viewing distance r_1 in a given situation may be sufficiently close to apply the extended source MPE. Figure B4 shows the relationship between r_1, D_ρ, and a. For relatively small angles (where the sine and the tangent of the angle are approximately equal to the angle expressed in radians), the angular source size is:

$$\alpha = \frac{D_\rho \cdot \cos\theta_v}{r_1} \text{ for } \theta_v \le 0.37\text{rad}, \qquad \textbf{Eq B67}$$

and therefore,

$$\alpha_{min} = \frac{D_\rho \cdot \cos\theta_v}{r_{1max}}. \qquad \textbf{Eq B68}$$

Solving Eq B68 for r_{1max}, yields:

$$r_{1max} = \frac{D_\rho \cos\theta_v}{\alpha_{min}}. \qquad \textbf{Eq B69}$$

Example 48. **Find the maximum distance r_{1max} where the extended source MPE applies for a visible laser reflection from a matte target. The illuminated spot on the target is 1 cm in diameter, and the target's reflectance is nearly 100%.**

Solution. For small viewing angles, $\cos\theta_v \approx 1$. Using Eq B69 and α_{min} (1.5 mrad):

$$r_{1max} = \frac{a}{\alpha_{min}} = \frac{(1\text{cm})}{1.5\times10^{-3}\text{ rad}} = 667 \text{ cm}$$

At distances greater than r_{1max}, there is no correction to the MPE for the source size. For sources that subtend an angle greater than α_{min}, but less than α_{max}, the extended source correction factor, C_E, is equal to α/α_{min}. Since α changes with distance, the correction factor would also decrease as a function of the viewer distance, r_1, up to the limiting distance of r_{1max}.

$$C_E = \frac{r_{1max}}{r_1} \qquad \textbf{Eq B70}$$

for $r_1 < r_{1max}$ and $\alpha < \alpha_{max}$.

Example 49. **For the laser in Example 47, the beam diameter, D_ρ, of the ruby laser beam striking the matte surface is 2 cm. Is the laser a hazard for a person standing 1 meter away?**

Solution. At a distance of 1 m, the angle subtended by the source at the viewer's eye is the diameter of the beam striking the matte target divided by the distance of the viewer from the target:

$$\alpha = \frac{D_\rho}{r_1} = \frac{2\ \text{cm}}{100\ \text{cm}} = 20\ \text{mrad}\cdot \qquad \textbf{Eq B71}$$

Therefore, for values of α less than 100 mrad (see Table 6):

$$\begin{aligned} C_E &= \frac{\alpha}{\alpha_{\min}} \\ &= \frac{20\ \text{mrad}}{1.5\ \text{mrad}} = 13.3\,. \end{aligned} \qquad \textbf{Eq B72}$$

The MPE for viewing this diffuse reflection at a distance of 1 m is $5 \times 10^{-7} \times 13.3 = 6.7 \times 10^{-6}$ J·cm^{-2}. The radiant exposure at the viewer's location is:

$$\begin{aligned} H &= \frac{\rho_\lambda Q \cos\theta_v}{\pi r_1^2} = \frac{1\ \text{J}}{\pi (100\ \text{cm})^2} \\ &= 3.18 \times 10^{-5}\ \text{J}\cdot\text{cm}^{-2}. \end{aligned}$$

The computed radiant exposure of 3.2×10^{-5} J·cm^{-2} at this distance is almost 5 times the MPE. Yes! It is still hazardous.

Example 50. **Find the minimum energy that will produce a diffuse reflection hazard from a Q-switched alexandrite laser that has a wavelength of 0.75 μm and an exit beam diameter of 1 cm. The laser is single pulsed.**

Solution. The energy that will not produce a hazardous diffuse reflection can be obtained from Table 3. For visible lasers, the value of C_A is 1.0; however, for 0.75 μm, C_A is 1.26. Therefore, the maximum energy that will not produce a hazardous diffuse reflection is 22 × 1.26 mJ = 28 mJ for a 20 cm viewing distance. For a 100 cm viewing distance, the minimum energy is 110 × 1.26 mJ = 140 mJ. For a 10 m viewing distance, incident beam energy greater than 1.6 × 1.26 = 2.0 J will produce a hazardous diffuse reflection for a 1 cm diameter spot. However, the source is small at this distance (rather than an extended source).

Example 51. **Find the minimum energy that will produce a diffuse hazard from the laser in Example 50 at a 5-m viewing distance, for a 10 s exposure, when the PRF is 10 Hz.**

Solution. For other distances, the general equation[19] from Table 3 can be used.

$$Q = \frac{\pi \mathrm{MPE}\left[r_1 + \frac{D_\mathrm{p}}{2}\right]^2}{\rho_\lambda \cos\theta} \qquad \textbf{Eq B73}$$

where D_ρ is equal to D_L at the point where the beam impacts the matte surface. Note that the MPE in the above equation must include the factors C_A, C_P, C_E, and C_C, where appropriate.

The viewing distance is 5 m (500 cm), and for a worst-case analysis, the viewing angle is assumed to be small ($\cos\theta_v \approx 1$), and the reflection coefficient (ρ_λ) is equal to 1.0. From Eq B71,

$$\begin{aligned} \alpha &= \frac{D_\mathrm{p}}{r_1} \\ &= \frac{1.0\ \mathrm{cm}}{500\ \mathrm{cm}} = 2\ \mathrm{mrad}, \end{aligned} \qquad \textbf{Eq B74}$$

which is greater than 1.5 mrad. The corresponding value of C_E is:

$$C_\mathrm{E} = \frac{\alpha}{\alpha_{\min}} = \frac{2\ \mathrm{mrad}}{1.5\ \mathrm{mrad}} = 1.33. \qquad \textbf{Eq B75}$$

The point source MPE for a visible Q-switched laser is 5×10^{-7} J·cm^{-2}. For this laser, the MPE must be multiplied by the factors of C_A, C_P, and C_E. The value of C_A is 1.26 and for a 10 s exposure, C_P is $n^{-0.25} = 0.316$. The extended source MPE is:

$$\begin{aligned} &\mathrm{MPE}: H = \mathrm{MPE}\times C_\mathrm{A}\times C_\mathrm{P}\times C_\mathrm{E} = \\ &= 5\times10^{-7}\ \mathrm{J\cdot cm^{-2}}\times1.26\times0.316\times1.33 \\ &\quad = 2.65\times10^{-7}\ \mathrm{J\cdot cm^{-2}} \end{aligned} \qquad \textbf{Eq B76}$$

The value of $D_\rho/2$ is 0.5 cm in this case. From Eq B73, the energy that will just produce a hazardous diffuse reflection is:

$$\begin{aligned} Q &= \frac{\pi\times2.65\ \mathrm{x}\ 10^{-7}\times(500+0.5\ \mathrm{cm})^2}{1.0} \\ &= 0.2\ \mathrm{J} \end{aligned}$$

[19] The $D_\rho/2$ term adds a minor correction to Lambert's law (Eqs B65 and B66) when the viewing distance is within 10 source diameters.

***Example 52.* Find the energy from the same laser (Example 51) that will produce a diffuse hazard at a 1 m viewing distance.**

Solution. The energy that will just produce a hazardous diffuse reflection at a distance of 1 m can also obtained from Eq B73. In this case,

$$\alpha = \frac{1.0 \text{ cm}}{100 \text{ cm}} = 10 \text{ mrad},$$

$$C_E = \frac{10}{1.5} = 6.7 \cdot$$

The extended source MPE is:

$$\begin{aligned} \text{MPE}: H &= \text{MPE} \times C_A \times C_P \times C_E = \\ &= 5 \times 10^{-7} \text{ J} \cdot \text{cm}^{-2} \times 1.26 \times 0.316 \times 6.7 \\ &= 1.33 \times 10^{-6} \text{ J} \cdot \text{cm}^{-2} \end{aligned}$$

and from Eq B73, Q is:[20]

$$Q = \frac{\pi\left(1.33 \text{ x } 10^{-6} \text{ J} \cdot \text{cm}^{-2}\right)\left[(100 + 0.5)\text{cm}\right]^2}{(1.0)(1.0)}$$

$$= 0.042 \text{ J}$$

B6.6.3 Optically Aided Viewing of Diffuse Reflections.

***Example 53.* The beam from a 0.1 J, visible short-pulse laser strikes a matte target with a reflectance of 0.6 (assume θ_v=1). At the location of the target, the beam diameter is 1.5 cm. What is the hazard from viewing the target at 10 m with 10 × 50 binoculars (P = 10, D_0 = 50 mm)?**

Solution. Viewing a diffuse reflection from a visible laser striking a matte target produces an angular source size of:

$$\alpha = \frac{1.5 \text{ cm}}{1000 \text{ cm}} = 1.5 \text{ mrad} \cdot$$

[20] This value could have been obtained from Table 3 by multiplying the value in the table by C_A and C_P.

Since α_{min} is also 1.5 mrad, C_E is 1.0 for unaided viewing. For the unaided eye, the radiant exposure at 10 m is:

$$H = \frac{\rho_\lambda Q \cos\theta_v}{\pi r_1^2} = \frac{(0.6)(0.1\ \text{J})(1)}{(3.14)(1000\ \text{cm})^2} = 1.9 \times 10^{-8}\ \text{J}\cdot\text{cm}^{-2}.$$

This value is less than the MPE of 5×10^{-7} J·cm^{-2} by 26 times.

For optically aided viewing, the diffusely reflected laser energy will be much larger than the viewing optics at 10 m. The reflected spot from the target will also appear 10 times larger (15 mrad); thus, increasing the MPE by C_E which is 10. The effective gain is:

$$G_{eff} = \tau_\lambda \frac{D_C^2}{D_f^2} \times \frac{1}{C_E(\text{optics})} = 0.9 \times \frac{(5\ \text{cm})^2}{(0.7\ \text{cm})^2} \times \frac{1}{10} = 4.6.$$

The hazard with optics is therefore 4.6 times greater for optically aided viewing than for unaided viewing at that distance.

B6.6.4 Medical and Industrial Applications.

Example 54. **A 50 W, CW, Nd:YAG (λ = 1.064 μm) surgical laser is used in an operating suite. It can be used either with an endoscope (where the beam is contained within the patient whenever the laser operates), or with a handpiece. The handpiece has a focal length of 10 cm, an emergent beam diameter *a* of 1 cm, and an F-number (*f/a*) of 10. Determine the NHZ, assuming a 10 s exposure duration.**

Solution. When the laser is operated with the endoscope, the NHZ is limited to the endoscope. When the handpiece is used, the beam would normally be directed downward (toward the patient and blocking the direct beam), and the diffuse reflection zone from a worst-case reflection from an anodized instrument (ρ = 0.9) could be calculated using Eq B65, by setting E equal to the MPE and r_1 equal to the r_{NHZ}. Hence,

$$\text{MPE} = \frac{\rho_\lambda \Phi \cos\theta_v}{\pi (r_{NHZ})^2}.$$

The MPE for 10 s exposure to a 1.064 μm laser is 5 mW·cm^{-2}. Assuming a worst-case viewing angle, (θ_v = 0°), the r_{NHZ} from a diffuse reflection is:

$$r_{NHZ} = \sqrt{\frac{\rho_\lambda \Phi \cos\theta_v}{\pi \, MPE}} \qquad \textbf{Eq B77}$$

$$= \sqrt{\frac{(0.9)(50\ W)(1)}{\pi(5\times10^{-3}\ W\cdot cm^{-2})}}$$

$$= \sqrt{2{,}864} = 53.5\ cm.$$

If the handpiece could be directed away from the patient, the r_{NOHD} determines the extent of the NHZ. Thus,

$$r_{NOHD} = \frac{1}{\phi}\sqrt{\frac{1.27\Phi}{MPE}}\ cm$$

$$= \left[\frac{f}{a}\right]\sqrt{\frac{1.27\Phi}{MPE}}\ cm \qquad \textbf{Eq B78}$$

$$= \frac{10\ cm}{1\ cm}\sqrt{\frac{1.27(50\ W)}{5\times10^{-3}\ W\cdot cm^{-2}}}$$

$$= 1126\ cm = 11.3\ m.$$

This above value of 11.3 m is measured from the focal point of the lens. Since the r_{NOHD} computed from Eq B78 above is measured from the focal point of the lens, 10 cm should be added to the r_{NOHD} above to account for the distance from the laser to the focal point, making the total r_{NOHD} equal to 11.4 m.

The r_{NOHD} becomes the dominant value for determining the radial extent of the NHZ if the beam can be reasonably expected to be accidentally or intentionally directed toward people. In normal surgical use, such lasers are not intentionally operated except when directed at the target tissue. Hence, the 11.3 m distance should be used to define the region wherein eye protection and other control measures (e.g., area/entryway controls) are administratively required. The r_{NHZ} during surgery is only 53 cm, and within the NHZ, stringent procedural precautions should be followed and strict enforcement of the use of eye protection is mandatory.

Example 55. **A manufacturer uses a 1000 W (1 kW) CW, CO_2 laser for a cutting process. The beam is routed through a beam conduit (pipe) to a final work station where the beam size has expanded to a diameter of 2.5 cm (1 inch). A 12.5 cm (5-inch) focal length lens is used to focus the beam. The lens determines the extent of the NHZ. Figure B9 shows the arrangement.**

Solution. First, determine the r_{NOHD} (i.e., the distance along the axis of the focal cone to that point where the beam irradiance is equal to the MPE). Although this system will operate almost continuously during a day, unintentional exposure to the direct beam could be reasonably expected to occur for up to 10 s. The 10 s MPE is 100 mW·cm^{-2}. The F-number (f/a) of the lens is:

$$f/a = (12.5)/(2.5) = 5 \qquad \textbf{Eq B79}$$

and the divergence ϕ of the unterminated beam from the focal point is:

$$\phi = \frac{1}{F-\text{number}} = \frac{1}{5} = 0.2 \text{ rad.} \qquad \textbf{Eq B80}$$

The r_{NOHD}[21] can be found from Eq B78:

$$\begin{aligned} r_{\text{NOHD}} &= \frac{1}{\phi}\sqrt{\frac{1.27\Phi}{\text{MPE}}}\ \text{cm} \\ &= \frac{1}{0.2}\sqrt{\frac{1.27(1\times 10^3\ \text{W})}{0.1\ \text{W}\cdot\text{cm}^{-2}}} \\ &= 5(113\ \text{cm}) = 565\ \text{cm} = 5.65\ \text{m.} \end{aligned}$$

This is the value used for points along the beam axis unless the beam is always terminated.

Next, determine the diffuse reflection hazard distance r_{NHZ}. The reflectance ρ_λ is probably far less than 20% and, from Eq B77 and a worst case viewing angle θ_v of 0°,

$$\begin{aligned} r_{\text{NHZ}} &= \sqrt{\frac{\Phi\rho_\lambda \cos\theta_v}{\pi\,\text{MPE}}}\ \text{cm} \qquad \textbf{Eq B81} \\ &= \sqrt{\frac{(1000\ \text{W})(0.2)(1)}{\pi(0.1\ \text{W}\cdot\text{cm}^{-2})}} \\ &= \sqrt{637\ \text{cm}^2} = 25\ \text{cm.} \end{aligned}$$

Next determine the r_{NHZ} associated with a specular reflection from the workpiece. Assume $\rho_\lambda = 0.2$ (worst case). The r_{NHZ} for a specular reflection is:

$$\begin{aligned} r_{\text{NHZ}} &= \frac{1}{\phi}\sqrt{\frac{1.27\Phi\rho_\lambda}{\text{MPE}}}\ \text{cm} \\ &= \frac{1}{0.2}\sqrt{\frac{(1.27)(1000)(0.2)}{0.1}}\ \text{cm} \\ &= 252\ \text{cm} = 2.52\ \text{m.} \end{aligned}$$

[21] The r_{NOHD} calculated in this manner is from the location where the workpiece is usually located, and not from the laser source.

The beam diameter at this distance is:

$$D_L = \phi \times r_{NHZ} = 0.2 \times 252 = 50.4 \text{ cm}.$$

The r_{NHZ} is therefore well defined near the beam path.

Finally, determine the operator exposure. After defining the NHZ one should consider long-term unavoidable exposure of the skin of the operator. Since the operator is required to manually load and unload the parts to be processed, there is a finite probability of exposure to scattered energy (from diffuse reflections) to the arms and face for periods up to 8 hours. The MPE for the skin must be reduced for large-area long-term exposures as described in Section 8.4.2. Assuming that the unprotected area A_S of both arms is approximately 400 cm^2, the corresponding MPE (see Section 8.4) is:

$$MPE_{\text{skin}} = \frac{10{,}000}{A_s} = \frac{10{,}000}{400} = 25 \text{ mW} \cdot \text{cm}^{-2}. \qquad \textbf{Eq B82}$$

This value can be used to calculate the distance along the beam axis of the focal cone to the point where the irradiance and the MPE are equal. Hence,

$$\begin{aligned} r_{\text{NHZ}} &= \frac{1}{\phi}\sqrt{\frac{1.27\Phi}{\text{MPE}}} \text{ cm} \\ &= \frac{1}{0.2}\sqrt{\frac{(1.27)(1000 \text{ W})}{0.025 \text{ W}\cdot\text{cm}^{-2}}} \\ &= 1127 \text{ cm} = 11.3 \text{ m}. \end{aligned}$$

Assume, however, that the beam is blocked by a diffusely reflecting surface located at a distance of 200 cm from the focal point. At this distance the beam diameter is $D_\rho = \phi \times r =$ 0.2(200 cm) = 40 cm. The reflection from a 100% diffusely reflecting surface can be approximated using Eq B77. Thus, the distance (r_{NHZ}) from the reflecting surface to the point at which the irradiance is equal to the *MPE* can be determined.

$$\begin{aligned} r_{\text{NHZ}} &= \sqrt{\frac{\Phi\rho_\lambda \cos\theta_v}{\pi \text{MPE}}} \text{ cm} \\ &= \sqrt{\frac{(1000 \text{ W})(1)(1)}{\pi(0.025 \text{ W}\cdot\text{cm}^{-2})}} \\ &= 113 \text{ cm} = 1.13 \text{ m}. \end{aligned}$$

Hence, the worst case ($\theta_v = 0°$) diffuse reflection hazard distance extends 113 cm from the reflecting surface.

B6.6.5 Specular Reflection Hazards. Specular reflections are more hazardous than diffuse reflections since collimation of the laser beam may be maintained and the laser power or energy can proceed in a different direction (see Figure B3). Flat glass surfaces can produce hazardous reflections directed either back at the operator or into an uncontrolled area. The percentage of the beam that is reflected depends on the angle of the beam to the reflecting surface. Flat glass will generally reflect about 4% per surface at normal incidence (reflection aimed at the laser operator). However, for near grazing angles, almost the entire laser beam can be reflected. Flat mirrors can reflect nearly 100% of the incidence beam at any angle. When beam pointing is relied upon as a safety measure, and an unexpected specular reflection occurs, the beam can be directed in an unexpected direction.

Example 56. **A ruby laser rangefinder is used in a controlled and restricted area (see Example 35). All personnel are located behind the laser during operation. A jeep located at 1000 m in front of the laser is used as a target and has a flat glass windshield. What is the radiant exposure at the operator's location from a specular reflection from the flat glass target? Assume that the atmospheric attenuation coefficient is 5×10^{-7} cm^{-1}. Would the exposure exceed the MPE?**

Solution. The jeep windshield could be considered as composed of a single piece of glass with two surfaces (front and back). Therefore a reflection would contain about 8% of the incident energy. The round-trip distance of the beam to the target and then returning from the target is 2000 m. Since the beam expands with distance, exposure to the reflected beam at the laser location would be similar to exposure to the direct beam from a laser with 8% of the energy output at 2000 m.

The calculated radiant exposure is then:

$$
\begin{aligned}
H &= \frac{1.27\rho_{\lambda} Q e^{-\mu r}}{a^2 + r^2 \phi^2} \\
&= \frac{(1.27)(0.08)(0.1\ \mathrm{J})(0.905)}{(0.7\ \mathrm{cm})^2 + \left[(2\times10^5\ \mathrm{cm})(1\times10^{-3}\ \mathrm{rad})\right]^2} \\
&= 2.3\times10^{-7}\ \mathrm{J\cdot cm^{-2}}.
\end{aligned}
$$

The computed radiant exposure is less than the MPE of 5×10^{-7} J·cm^{-2}. However, several factors in the equation are uncertain. Atmospheric scintillation may actually affect the beam radiant exposure at these distances more than absorption and scattering.

In addition, the assumption is that the glass target is perfectly flat; when in fact, the surface could be slightly curved, either convex or concave. Therefore, either an increase or decrease in the reflected radiant exposure would be possible. Since there is only about a factor of 2 between the calculated radiant exposure and the MPE, a prudent measure would be to use eye protectors designed for the ruby wavelength.

B7. The Brightness (Radiance) Units

The irradiance falling on a person's eye is reduced quickly with increased viewing distance. However, the angular source size from the viewer's perspective is also reduced, so that the radiance or luminance (brightness) remains constant with viewing distance or viewing angle. The radiometric quantities, radiance ($W \cdot cm^{-2} \cdot sr^{-1}$) and integrated radiance ($J \cdot cm^{-2} \cdot sr^{-1}$) are often useful for describing the hazards from extended sources. When the laser source exceeds an angular subtense of 0.1 rad, the MPE based on thermal effects can be written in terms of radiance or integrated radiance. The MPE for photochemical effects (Section B7.2) is expressed in terms of radiance for all source sizes.

B7.1 MPE Based on Thermal Effects.

Example 57. **Determine the MPE in terms of integrated radiance, based on thermal effects, for a laser having an angular subtense greater than 100 mrad, with a wavelength between 0.4 and 0.6 μm, and an exposure duration between 18 μs and 10 s.**

Solution. The MPE for an extended source, based on thermal effects is:

$$\text{MPE (thermal)} = MPE_{\text{point}}\,\text{(thermal)} \times C_E.$$

For a source with an angular subtense of 100 mrad (0.1 rad),

$$C_E = \frac{\alpha}{\alpha_{\min}} = \frac{100\ \text{mrad}}{1.5\ \text{mrad}} = 66.7.$$

Therefore, for a source with an angular subtense of exactly 100 mrad, the MPE is:

$$\text{MPE (thermal)} = MPE_{\text{point}}\,\text{(thermal)} \times 66.7.$$

The solid angle Ω of a laser source is approximately related to the angular subtense of a circular source by:[22]

$$\Omega = \frac{\pi\alpha^2}{4}\ \text{sr} \qquad \textbf{Eq B83}$$

The unit steradian (sr) is a measure of the solid angle, in this case, the solid angle that the source subtends. For a source with an angular subtense of 100 mrad, the solid angle is:[23]

$$\Omega = \frac{\pi\alpha^2}{4}\,\text{sr} = \frac{\pi(0.1\,\text{rad})^2}{4} = 7.85 \times 10^{-3}\ \text{sr}.$$

---

[22] The approximation yields reasonable results up to an angle α of about 0.5 radian

[23] Although the angular subtense is often expressed as mrad, it must be expressed as radians when inserted into this equation.

In terms of integrated radiance, the MPE may be expressed as:

$$\begin{aligned}\text{MPE}: L_{\text{P}} &= \frac{(MPE_{\text{small}} \times C_{\text{E}})}{\Omega \text{ sr}} \\ &= \frac{(MPE_{\text{small}} \times 66.7) \text{ J} \cdot \text{cm}^{-2}}{7.85 \times 10^{-3} \text{ sr}} \\ &= 8.5 \times 10^{3} \times MPE_{\text{small}} \text{ J} \cdot \text{cm}^{-2} \cdot \text{sr}^{-1}.\end{aligned}$$ **Eq B84**

Since the MPE for sources larger than 100 mrad is related to the integrated radiance or radiance rather than the corneal radiant exposure or irradiance, Eq B84 applies to sources larger than 100 mrad in addition to sources equal to 100 mrad.

From Eq B1, the MPE for exposure duration between 18 μs and 10 s is:

$$\text{MPE}:H \text{ (thermal)} = 1.8 \times C_{\text{E}} \times t^{0.75} \times 10^{-3} \text{ J}\cdot\text{cm}^{-2}.$$

For a 100 mrad source size, C_{E} is 66.7 and the MPE is:

$$\begin{aligned}\text{MPE}:H \text{ (thermal)} &= 1.8 \times 66.7 \times t^{0.75} \times 10^{-3} \text{ J}\cdot\text{cm}^{-2} \\ &= 0.12 \times t^{0.75} \text{ J}\cdot\text{cm}^{-2}.\end{aligned}$$

The MPE in terms of integrated radiance is then:

$$\begin{aligned}\text{MPE}: L_{\text{P}} &= \frac{H}{\Omega} = \frac{0.12 \times t^{0.75} \text{ J} \cdot \text{cm}^{-2}}{7.85 \times 10^{-3} \text{ sr}} \\ &= 15 \times t^{0.75} \text{ J} \cdot \text{cm}^{-2} \cdot \text{sr}^{-1}.\end{aligned}$$

The quantities of radiance and integrated radiance describe the source directly, and do not change with distance from the source. When viewing an extended source, the source subtends an angle greater than 0.1 rad only within a distance of 10 source diameters. Thus, for a 10 cm diameter laser beam, a diffuse reflection would exceed 0.1 rad only within 1.0 m. Within this distance, the MPE in terms of radiance or integrated radiance would be constant.

***Example 58.* Find the maximum permitted integrated radiance for a diffuse reflection (Lambertian reflector) from a matte surface illuminated by a Q-switched, visible laser with a beam diameter of 2 cm when viewed from 20 cm away.**

Solution. The maximum energy in a 2 cm diameter beam incident on a matte surface that will not exceed the MPE when viewed from a distance of 20 cm is 0.046 J (Table 3). The corresponding maximum radiant exposure at the surface is (from Eq B23):

$$\text{MPE}: H = \frac{1.27 Q_{max}}{D^2{}_L} = \frac{1.27 \times 0.046\ \text{J}}{(2\ \text{cm})^2} = 1.46 \times 10^{-2}\ \text{J} \cdot \text{cm}^{-2}$$ **Eq B85**

Since the energy reflected from a perfect Lambertian surface is radiated into π steradians, the integrated radiance L_P is found from the relation:

$$L_P = \frac{H \cdot \rho_\lambda}{\pi}\ \text{J} \cdot \text{cm}^{-2} \cdot \text{sr}^{-1}.$$ **Eq B86**

The corresponding maximum permitted integrated radiance[24] is:

$$\text{MPE}: L_p = \frac{1.46 \times 10^{-2}\ \text{J} \cdot \text{cm}^{-2} \times 100\%}{3.14\ \text{sr}}\ \text{J} \cdot \text{cm}^{-2} \cdot \text{sr}^{-1} = 4.65 \times 10^{-3}\ \text{J} \cdot \text{cm}^{-2} \cdot \text{sr}^{-1}.$$

At a distance of 20 cm, the angular subtense of the laser source (illuminated matte surface) is 2 cm/20 cm = 0.1 radian. For sources larger than 0.1 radian, the MPE is constant in terms of radiance or integrated radiance. Thus, the MPE:L_P at 10 cm is the same as the MPE:L_P at 20 cm in terms of integrated radiance since α is equal or greater than 100 mrad in both cases.

B7.2 MPE based on photochemical effects. For exposures greater than 0.7 s and for wavelengths between 0.400 μm and 0.600 μm, MPEs are based on retinal hazards consisting of both photochemical and thermal effects. Normally both effects need to be calculated to determine which effect indicates the greatest hazard, but in Table 5a, a computed time, T_1 separates the two effects for point sources ($\alpha \leq 1.5$ mrad), and determines the MPE. For extended sources ($\alpha > 1.5$ mrad), MPEs based on both effects are provided in Table 5b. The MPEs based on thermal effects are derived from the point source MPEs by the use of a correction factor, C_E. The MPE based on photochemical effects is provided as integrated radiance (100 C_B J$\cdot$cm^{-2} sr^{-1}) for exposure duration less than 10,000 s, and as radiance (0.01 C_B W$\cdot$cm^{-2} sr^{-1}) for greater exposure duration up to 30,000 s. The photochemical MPE is averaged over a cone angle γ, which is dependent on the exposure duration as defined below:

$\gamma = 11$ mrad for $t \leq 100$ s, **Eq B87**
$\gamma = 1.1 \times t^{0.5}$ mrad for $100\ \text{s} < t \leq 10{,}000$ s,
$\gamma = 110$ mrad for $10{,}000\ \text{s} < t \leq 30{,}000$ s.

[24] Assuming 100% reflectance. The MPE calculated in this manner is slightly larger than calculated from Eq B84 due to a slight correction to Lambert's law (Eqs B65 and B66) that was added to Table 3 (see Table 3).

The MPE based on photochemical effects, for sources less than 11 mrad, are provided in Table 5b as radiant exposure and irradiance, for convenience. Thus, the source size, including any hot spots (very bright areas) within the source, plays a major role in determining the hazard (see Figure B10).

Example 59. **Consider a doubled Nd:YAG laser (λ=0.532 μm) using a diffuser to create an extended source. The laser spot on the diffuser has a uniform distribution over a 5 cm spot diameter. For a 50 s exposure duration (T_{max}) at 1 m from the source, determine if the MPE based on the photochemical hazard is lower than the MPE based on the thermal hazard.**

Solution. Part 1. Thermal MPE:

When α is greater than α_{min}, the equation used to compute the thermal MPE depends on T_2, which, in turn, depends on the angular subtense, α. The value of α is (from Eq B71):

$$\alpha = \frac{D_\rho}{r_1} = \frac{5 \text{ cm}}{100 \text{ cm}} = 5 \times 10^{-2} \text{ rad} = 50 \text{ mrad}.$$

The value of T_2 is (α is expressed in milliradians):

$$T_2 = 10 \times 10^{\left(\frac{\alpha - 1.5}{98.5}\right)} = 31.1 \text{ s.} \qquad \textbf{Eq B88}$$

The extended source correction factor, C_E, is:

$$C_E = \frac{\alpha}{\alpha_{min}} = \frac{50 \text{ mrad}}{1.5 \text{ mrad}} = 33.3.$$

Since T_{max} is greater than T_2, and α is greater than α_{min}, the equation used to compute the MPE based on thermal hazards from Table 5b is:

$$\begin{aligned} \text{MPE:}E &= 1.8\, C_E\, T_2^{-0.25} \times 10^{-3} \text{ W·cm}^{-2} \qquad \textbf{Eq B89} \\ &= 1.8 \times 33.3 \times (31.1)^{-0.25} \times 10^{-3} \text{ W·cm}^{-2} \\ &= 0.0254 \text{ W·cm}^{-2} = 25.4 \text{ mW·cm}^{-2}. \end{aligned}$$

See Figure 10e for a graphical solution for the thermal MPE.

Part 2. Photochemical MPE:

Since T_{max} is less than 100 s, γ is 11 mrad. From Table 5b, the MPE for 50 s, based on photochemical hazards, for a source greater than 11 mrad is:

$$\text{MPE:}H\,(\text{photo}) = 100\; C_B\;\; \text{J}\cdot\text{cm}^{-2}\;\text{sr}^{-1}. \qquad \textbf{Eq B90}$$

Since this MPE includes a solid angle term, the solid angle subtended by the source is used to express the MPE in terms of corneal radiant exposure. For this example, the source angular subtense is 50 mrad, and the solid angle at the viewer's eye subtended by the source is (from Eq B83):

$$\begin{aligned}\Omega &= \frac{\pi\alpha^2}{4} = \frac{\pi(0.05\text{ rad})^2}{4} \\ &= 1.96\times10^{-3}\text{ sr.}\end{aligned} \qquad \textbf{Eq B91}$$

The MPE expressed as corneal radiant exposure is calculated by multiplying the MPE expressed as integrated radiance by the source solid angle:

$$\text{MPE}: H = \text{MPE}: L_e \times \Omega. \qquad \textbf{Eq B92}$$

The MPE expressed as corneal irradiance for a 50 mrad source is therefore:

$$\begin{aligned}\text{MPE}: H &= \text{MPE}: L_e \times \Omega \\ &= 100\times C_B\;\text{J cm}^{-2}\text{sr}^{-1}\times 1.96\times10^{-3}\text{ sr} \\ &= 1.96\; C_B\times10^{-1}\;\text{J cm}^{-2}\end{aligned} \qquad \textbf{Eq B93}$$

Note: If the solid angle subtended by the source had been smaller than the cone angle γ, the solid angle used in Eq B93 would have been calculated from γ rather than from the subtended angle of the source.

The value of C_B is:

$$\begin{aligned}C_B &= 10^{20(\lambda\,-\,0.45\;\mu\text{m})} \\ &= 10^{1.64} = 43.7.\end{aligned} \qquad \textbf{Eq B94}$$

Therefore, the MPE in terms of corneal radiant exposure from Eq B93 is:

$$\text{MPE:}H \;= 8.58\;\text{J}\cdot\text{cm}^{-2}$$

In terms of irradiance, the MPE for photochemical effects for this example is:

$$\begin{aligned}\text{MPE}: E(\text{photo}) &= \frac{8.58 \text{ J cm}^{-2}}{50 \text{ s}}\\ &= 0.172 \text{ W cm}^{-2} = 172 \text{ mW cm}^{-2}.\end{aligned}$$

Result (Example 59)
The MPE based on thermal effects ($25.4 \text{ mW} \cdot \text{cm}^{-2}$) is less than the MPE based on photochemical effects ($172 \text{ mW} \cdot \text{cm}^{-2}$) for this laser under these viewing conditions and exposure duration.

Example 60. **A 30 W Argon laser with a wavelength of 514.5 nm (0.5145 μm) continuously illuminates a reflective matte target. The beam is Gaussian and the beam diameter at 1/*e* of peak irradiance points striking the target is 10 cm. The target is extended enough to capture the edges of the Gaussian beam. A person is located near this target board for an entire workday, but never approaches closer than 1 m. Determine the MPE for laser exposure for 30,000 s at 1 m from the surface. Assume the reflectance is 100%.**

Solution. At 1 m, the source subtends an angle of:

$$\alpha = \frac{10 \text{ cm}}{100 \text{ cm}} = 0.1 \text{ radian}.$$

Part 1. Thermal MPE:

The thermal MPE depends on T_2, which, in turn, depends on the angular subtense, α.

The value of T_2 is from Eq B88 (α expressed in milliradians):

$$\begin{aligned}T_2 &= 10 \times 10^{\left(\frac{(100-1.5)}{98.5}\right)}\\ &= 100 \text{ s}.\end{aligned}$$

The extended source correction factor, C_E, is:

$$C_E = \frac{\alpha}{\alpha_{min}} = \frac{100 \text{ mrad}}{1.5 \text{ mrad}} = 66.7.$$

Since T_{max} is greater than T_2, and α is greater than α_{min}, the MPE based on thermal hazards from Table 5b and Eq B89 is:

$$\begin{aligned}\text{MPE:}E &= 1.8\, C_E\, T_2^{-0.25} \times 10^{-3}\ \text{W}\cdot\text{cm}^{-2}\\ &= 1.8 \times 66.7 \times (100)^{-0.25} \times 10^{-3}\ \text{W}\cdot\text{cm}^{-2}\\ &= 0.0379\ \text{W}\cdot\text{cm}^{-2} = 37.9\ \text{mW}\cdot\text{cm}^{-2}.\end{aligned}$$

From Eq B65, the corneal irradiance at 1 m from the source is [assuming 100% reflectance and a viewer located perpendicular (normal) to the matte surface]:

$$E = \frac{\Phi}{\pi r_1^2} = \frac{30\ \text{W}}{\pi (100\ \text{cm})^2} = 9.55 \times 10^{-4}\ \text{W}\cdot\text{cm}^{-2}.$$

Therefore, the corneal irradiance is about 40 times less than the thermal MPE at this distance for these exposure conditions.

Part 2. Photochemical MPE:

Since α is larger than 11 mrad, and the exposure duration is greater than 10,000 s, the MPE in terms of radiance is $C_B \times 10^{-2}$ W·cm^{-2} sr^{-1} averaged over a field of view of γ. From Eq B94, the value of C_B for 0.5145 μm is:

$$C_B = 10^{20(\lambda - 0.45\ \mu\text{m})} = 19.5$$

The MPE is then 19.5×10^{-2} W·cm^{-2} sr^{-1} averaged over a field of view of γ. Since T_{max} is larger than 10,000 s, γ is 110 mrad, which is somewhat larger than the source angle.

The radiance of the source is related to the irradiance on the target. The irradiance on the matte target from Eq B24 is:

$$E = \frac{1.27\Phi}{D_L^2} = 0.38\ \text{W}\cdot\text{cm}^{-2}.$$

The radiance is then the irradiance at the target divided by the solid angle into which the power is radiated. From a matte surface, the energy is radiated into π sr. Therefore,

$$\begin{aligned}L_e &= \frac{E}{\Omega} = \frac{0.38\ \text{W cm}^{-2}}{\pi\ \text{sr}}\\ &= 0.121\ \text{W}\cdot\text{cm}^{-2}\ \text{sr}^{-1}.\end{aligned}$$ **Eq B96**

The computed value is less than the MPE for 0.5145 μm of 0.195 W·cm^{-2} sr^{-1}. Therefore, no additional computation is necessary.

However to be precise, the radiance from Eq B96 was not averaged over a FOV of 110 mrad. Since the source is Gaussian, not all the radiated energy will originate from a cone that is less than 110 mrad although the computed angular subtense is less than 110 mrad.

Since the illuminated target is Gaussian, 63.2% of the energy would be contained within a FOV equal to α. Since γ is slightly larger than α, slightly more radiated energy will be within a cone equal to γ.

The fraction of power, Φ_d/Φ_0 contained within a FOV equal to γ is:

$$\frac{\Phi_d}{\Phi_0} = \left(1 - e^{-\left(\frac{\gamma}{\alpha}\right)^2}\right) \qquad \textbf{Eq B97}$$

$$= \left(1 - e^{-\left(\frac{110\ \text{mrad}}{100\ \text{mrad}}\right)^2}\right) = 0.7$$

The irradiance at the cornea originating from within the cone angle of 110 mrad is the computed irradiance from Part 1 (9.55×10^{-4} W$\cdot$cm^{-2}) multiplied by 0.7, which is 6.7×10^{-4} W$\cdot$cm^{-2}.

The radiance L_e is also calculated from Eq B96 by dividing the irradiance at the cornea by the solid angle subtended by the source. However since γ is larger than the source for this example, the radiance would be calculated by dividing the corneal irradiance originating within a cone angle of 110 mrad by the solid angle defined by a linear angle of 110 mrad (9.5×10^{-3} sr from Eq B91). Therefore, the radiance at a person's cornea averaged over a FOV defined by γ is:

$$L_e = \frac{6.7 \times 10^{-4}\ \text{W cm}^{-2}}{9.5 \times 10^{-3}\ \text{sr}}$$

$$= 0.07\ \text{W}\cdot\text{cm}^{-2}\cdot\text{sr}^{-1} = 70\ \text{mW}\cdot\text{cm}^{-2}\ \text{sr}^{-1}.$$

Result (Example 60)
The average radiance of 70 mW$\cdot$cm^{-2} sr^{-1} is, therefore, less than the photochemical MPE of 0.195 W$\cdot$cm^{-2} sr^{-1} by a factor of about 2.8 at this distance for these exposure conditions. From Part 1, the corneal irradiance was less than the thermal MPE by a factor of about 40. Since exposure to sources with an angular subtense greater than 110 mrad is based on integrated radiance and radiance, the exposure would not exceed the MPE at distances closer than about 90 cm since the source radiance is constant.

B8. Protective Eyewear and Barriers

B8.1 Protective Eyewear. Laser eye protection may be required when administrative or engineering controls cannot eliminate potential *accidental* hazardous exposure. Optical density D_λ is a specification that indicates the protective capability of laser eye protection. It is a value assigned at a particular wavelength and is defined as the logarithm to the base ten of the reciprocal of the transmittance. Thus,

$$D_\lambda = \log\left[\frac{1}{\tau_\lambda}\right].$$

The desired transmittance of a laser protective filter is the ratio of the MPE to the irradiance or radiant exposure at the laser exit port, at a given distance from the laser exit port or at the exit pupil of magnifying optics. The inverse of transmittance is, thus, the ratio of irradiance E or radiant exposure H to MPE (expressed in the same units as E or H). Therefore, optical density in terms of MPE is

$$D_\lambda = \log\left[\frac{E}{\text{MPE}}\right] \text{ or } \log\left[\frac{H}{\text{MPE}}\right]. \qquad \textbf{Eq B98}$$

Optical density (OD) calculations for laser eye protection are best called minimum optical density (MOD) since commercial laser eye protection rarely satisfies the calculated OD exactly. For example, the LSO may have to be satisfied with OD 4 when only OD 2 is needed because the eyewear is available only with an OD of 4. Higher OD values are permissible as long as other requirements such as visual transmission and damage thresholds are met.

There are several ways to determine the OD value. The first method or "worst-case OD" should be used when it is not known what other engineering or administrative controls may be employed and it is assumed that the entire laser output is concentrated within the limiting aperture. For visible and near-IR wavelengths this would occur if the laser beam diameter was less than 7 mm or the total beam was collected by magnifying optics.

***Example 61.* Worst-Case OD Calculation. Calculate the worst-case optical density required for a Rhodamine 6G laser that has a peak output at a wavelength of 0.590 μm. The energy output is 10 mJ in a 5 mm diameter beam and the pulse width is 1 μs.**

Solution. Worst-case optical density is calculated by averaging the radiant energy over the limiting aperture. This radiant energy is given as 10 mJ. The limiting aperture is 7 mm since the laser operates at 0.590 μm. The radiant exposure averaged over 7 mm is, therefore,

$$H = \frac{10\,\text{mJ}}{0.385\,\text{cm}^2} = 26\ \text{mJ}\cdot\text{cm}^{-2}.$$

from Table 5a, the MPE for a 1 μs, single-pulse laser operating at 0.590 μm is:

$$\text{MPE} = 0.5\ \mu\text{J}\cdot\text{cm}^{-2}.$$

The minimum worst-case optical density[25] is:

$$D_\lambda = \log\left[\frac{H}{\text{MPE}}\right] = \log\left[\frac{2.6\times10^{-2}}{5\times10^{-7}}\right] = \log\left(5.2\times10^{4}\right) = 4.72. \qquad \textbf{Eq B99}$$

Example 62. **Refer to Example 22 and determine the appropriate OD (D_λ) to protect a viewer at a distance of 10 cm from the diode array.**

Solution. For the most restrictive case, the radiant exposure was found to be 0.33 μJ and the Class 1 AEL was 0.16 μJ. An attenuation of 0.33/0.16 =2.06 ($D_\lambda = 0.3$) would be required for a protective filter, if a protective filter was deemed necessary. Alternatively, the filter could be placed in the optical train of the system to reduce the laser output to Class 1.

Example 63. **Optical Density at a Distance for Unaided Viewing. Calculate the minimum optical density required for unaided viewing at a distance of 1 km from a 0.1 J, Q-switched ruby laser with a pulse length of 20 ns, an exit beam diameter of 7 mm, and a divergence of 1 mrad (see Example 41).**

Solution. At 1 km, the beam will be about 1 m in diameter ($r \times \phi$). When the laser beam diameter is larger than the limiting aperture and optical aids are not used, the appropriate optical density is the log of the ratio of the irradiance or radiant exposure (calculated or measured at the given distance) to the corresponding MPE. The radiant exposure at 1 km is:

$$H = \frac{1.27\Phi}{D_L^2} = \frac{0.127}{(100\text{ cm})^2} = 12.7\ \mu\text{J}\cdot\text{cm}^{-2}\cdot$$

and the MPE from Table 5a is 0.5 μJ·cm^{-2}. The optical density is, thus[26],

$$D_\lambda = \log\left[\frac{H}{\text{MPE}}\right] = \log\left[\frac{1.25\times10^{-5}}{5\times10^{-7}}\right] = 1.4. \qquad \textbf{Eq B100}$$

To allow for non-uniformity in the beam caused by turbulence, etc., 1 OD unit should be added to the above. Thus, the appropriate minimum optical density for this laser at a distance of 1 km, is 2.4. (This additional safety factor is generally unnecessary for indoor laser use).

---

[25] This method should always be used for beam diameters less than the diameter of the limiting aperture.

[26] If the laser beam is smaller than the limiting aperture at the given distance, the worst-case method is used.

In general, intrabeam viewing through magnifying optics increases the potential hazard over viewing with the unaided eye. However, this is only true at wavelengths up to approximately 4.0 μm, where common glass optics cease to transmit.

Normally it is assumed that the laser beam is larger than the entrance aperture of the optics. If the beam is smaller than the entrance aperture, the worst-case technique is used and the OD must be sufficient to reduce the radiant exposure at the cornea to a level below the MPE.

Example 64. **Calculate the minimum OD for safely viewing a 50 mW HeNe laser with an initial beam diameter of 10 mm, and a divergence of 2.5 mrad. Assume 7 × 35 binoculars that transmit 85 percent at 0.633 μm are used to view the beam at a distance of 50 m.**

Solution. At 50 m, the beam diameter D_L is:

$$D_L = r \times \phi = 5000 \text{ cm} \times 2.5{\times}10^{-3} \text{ rad} = 12.5 \text{ cm}.$$ [27]

The irradiance is:

$$H = \frac{1.27 \times 50 \times 10^{-3}\ \text{W}}{(12.5\ \text{cm})^2} = 0.4\ \text{mW} \cdot \text{cm}^{-2}$$

This irradiance does not exceed the MPE for unaided viewing. For optically aided viewing, the effective gain of the optics must be considered. From Eq B57,

$$\begin{aligned} G_{\text{eff}} &= \tau_\lambda \times \frac{[\min(D_0, D_L)]^2}{D_f^2} \\ &= \frac{(0.85)(3.5\ \text{cm})^2}{(0.7)^2} = \frac{(0.85)(3.5)^2}{0.49} \\ &= 21.3. \end{aligned}$$

The corneal irradiance through the optics is then 0.4 × 21.3 mW·cm^{-2} = 8.5 mW·cm^{-2}.

The MPE from Table 5a is 2.5 mW·cm^{-2} and the minimum OD for an unintentional exposure of 0.25 s is:

$$D_\lambda = \log\left[\frac{H}{\text{MPE}}\right] = \log\left[\frac{8.5 \times 10^{-3}}{2.5 \times 10^{-3}}\right] = 0.53$$

[27] The initial beam diameter is only useful for computing beam diameter at a distance when the diameter at the distance is only slightly larger than the initial beam diameter.

B8.2 Laser Barriers. Laser barriers needed to protect personnel may need to withstand either exposure to the direct laser beam or exposure to reflections of the laser beam from a diffuse surface.

B8.2.1 Direct Intrabeam Exposure. If the irradiance at a separation distance D_s from a laser maintained at (or below) the barrier threshold limit value TL, D_s is considered the installation criteria distance for that barrier. That is, if the barrier is installed at a separation distance D_s, the irradiance on the barrier will be below the TL for the barrier. D_s may be expressed as:

$$D_s = \frac{1}{\phi}\left[\sqrt{\frac{4\Phi}{\pi \, \mathrm{TL}}} - a^2\right], \qquad \textbf{Eq B101}$$

where TL is the barrier threshold limit value in $\mathrm{W{\cdot}cm^{-2}}$.

***Example 65.* Determine the separation distance D_s for a 300 W Class 4 (open beam) industrial Nd:YAG laser materials-processing system with a beam divergence of 2.5 mrad and an exit beam diameter of 0.4 cm.**

Solution. Using Eq B101 and assuming a long term (8-hour) worst-case exposure duration and a TL of 45 $\mathrm{W{\cdot}cm^{-2}}$, D_s is:

$$D_s = \frac{1}{2.5\times10^{-3}}\left[\sqrt{\frac{4\times300}{3.14\times45}} - 0.16\right]$$
$$= 11.5 \text{ m.}$$

Thus, one would have to locate the protective barrier at a distance greater than 11.5 meters from the laser exit for the barrier to be effective. If positioned closer, the beam could penetrate the barrier and protection would no longer be afforded.

B8.2.2 Diffuse Beam Exposures. There are some instances where it is useful to calculate the distance from a point source diffuse reflector to where a specific irradiance occurs. If the MPE is replaced by TL in Eq B77, r_{NHZ} becomes the barrier diffuse reflection separation distance D_{SD}. Thus,

$$D_{\mathrm{SD}} = \sqrt{\frac{\rho\,\Phi\cos\theta}{\pi \, \mathrm{TL}}}. \qquad \textbf{Eq B102}$$

***Example 66.* Assume a 5000 W CO_2 laser is directed onto a target with a 100% reflectance at 10.6 μm. Determine D_{SD} at 45 degrees for a TL of 45 $\mathrm{W{\cdot}cm^{-2}}$.**

Solution. The value for D_{SD} obtained from Eq B102 is:

$$D_{SD} = \sqrt{\frac{1 \times 5000 \times 0.707}{3.14 \times 45}} = 0.05 \text{ m}\cdot$$

Thus, at five centimeters from the target the irradiance associated with the diffuse reflection is reduced to 45 W·cm^{-2} at 45 degrees.

B8.2.3 Laser Barriers: Lens-on-Laser Exposure. Most industrial lasers incorporate a lens as the final component in the beam path. This not only provides the increased irradiance in the focal plane of the lens to do the work intended of the laser, but it also causes the beam to spread in the space beyond the focal plane with an angle usually many times larger than the inherent laser beam divergence. Consequently, the distance D,[28] beyond which the irradiance is less than TL, is less than the intrabeam distance D_S, and is given by:

$$D = \frac{f_0}{b_0}\sqrt{\frac{4\Phi}{\pi \text{TL}}}, \qquad \textbf{Eq B103}$$

where f_0 is the lens focal length and b_0 is the beam diameter at the lens.

***Example 67.* Consider a 3000 W CO_2 laser with a 5-inch focal length lens in place. Assume the beam size at the lens is 1 inch. Determine *D*.**

Solution. Assume a long-term (8-hour) worst-case TL of 45 W·cm^{-2}, substituting into Eq B103,

$$D = \frac{5}{1}\sqrt{\frac{4 \times 3000}{3.14 \times 45}} = 0.46 \text{ m.}$$

Thus, in the direction defined by the cone of laser energy directed through the lens, the barrier could be penetrated up to a distance of 0.46 meters, beyond which point the beam has expanded sufficiently to limit E to 45 W·cm^{-2}.

B9. Determination of Extended Source Size

Although most lasers are point source emitters, some lasers have an extended source. The most common example of this type of laser is the diode laser. A diode laser is usually constructed from a laser diode and a lens, producing a beam that is fairly collimated. Depending on the size of the diode and the lens, the resulting laser may have an extended source. The MPE for these types of lasers may be increased over that used for point laser sources (see Section B3.5). Some unique situations can arise, which must be considered. For example, as the distance from the laser is increased, the hazard may increase before it decreases; the MPE for optically aided viewing may be different than that for unaided

[28] D_{lens} is measured from the focal point of the lens, not from the laser.

viewing; and the most hazardous distance from the laser may be farther than the standard measurement distances.

Example 68. **An 850 nm laser diode, 6 thousandths of an inch long (0.15 mm) and about 1 µm wide is used with a lens that is 1 cm in diameter with a 3.5 cm focal length. The diode is positioned to provide the best collimated beam. The beam diameter is about half the lens diameter. First determine the source size and then determine the MPE for this laser for a 10 s exposure near the laser exit port.**

Solution. Since this laser is well collimated, the source size near the laser exit port will be about the same dimensions as the laser divergence. Both these values will be determined from the construction characteristics of the laser. The divergence in the long dimension can be determined by,

$$\phi = \frac{D_{\text{diode}}}{f_0} \qquad \textbf{Eq B104}$$

$$\phi = \frac{D_{\text{diode}}}{f_0} = \frac{0.015\,\text{cm}}{3.5\,\text{cm}} = 4.3\,\text{mrad}$$

The divergence in the smaller dimension will be smaller than 1.5 mrad, so 1.5 mrad may be used in calculating the extended source correction factor. The arithmetic mean of the two source dimensions is then 2.9 mrad, resulting in a C_E value of 1.93. For this wavelength, C_A is 2.0. The MPE for a 10 s exposure near the exit port is then,

$$\text{MPE} = 1.8\, C_A\, C_E\, (10)^{0.75}/10\ \text{mW}\cdot\text{cm}^{-2} = 3.9\ \text{mW}\cdot\text{cm}^{-2}$$

Example 69. **The construction of the laser in Example 68 is changed so that the position of the laser diode is closer to the focusing lens, producing a beam that is 6 mrad by 6 mrad. Determine the MPE at 100 cm from the laser exit port.**

Solution. Near the exit port of the laser the source size would be about the same as for Example 68; however, at 100 cm from the laser exit port, the beam has increased in size to about 0.8 cm instead of 0.5 cm (See Eq B39 and Example 34). Therefore, the source size would be expected to be 5/8 of 4.3 mrad or 2.7 mrad. The arithmetic mean of the source is then 2.1 mrad, and the C_E value is 1.4 instead of 1.93, resulting in an MPE of 2.8 mW·cm^{-2}.

Example 70. **For the laser in Example 69 (850 nm, 5 mm beam diameter, 6 mrad beam divergence), compare the MPE for optically aided viewing at 2 m and at 10 m with 7-power telescopic optics (7 × 50 binoculars). Assume that the total output power is 1 mW and compare the corneal irradiance at both distances.**

Solution. At 2 m from the laser, the beam size is approximately 1.3 cm in diameter. Therefore, the source size is 0.5/1.3 (or 0.385) times as large. The source size is then 1.66 mrad in length and very small in width. For optically aided viewing, the source appears 7 times larger or 11.6 mrad in length. The arithmetic mean of the source is then 6.56 mrad. The C_E value is then 4.4 for optically aided viewing at 2 m. The MPE is then 8.8 $mW \cdot cm^{-2}$. Essentially all the emitted power can be collected by a 5 cm objective lens, so the corneal irradiance is,

$$E = \frac{(1 \text{ mW})(0.7)}{(0.385 \text{ cm}^2)} = 1.8 \text{ mW} \cdot \text{cm}^{-2},$$

assuming that the optics transmission is 70%.

At 10 m from the laser, the beam is 6 cm in diameter. The source size in the long dimension is 0.36 mrad for unaided viewing, but 2.5 mrad when viewing with 7-power optics. The arithmetic mean of the source is then 2.0 mrad and the C_E factor is 1.34. The MPE is then 2.7 $mW \cdot cm^{-2}$, about 5.5 times less than that at 2 m. The corneal irradiance is determined from the amount of power transmitted by the 5 cm entrance aperture of the magnifying optics (see Eq B15).

$$\Phi_d = \Phi_0 \left(1 - e^{\frac{-5^2}{6^2}} \right) = 0.5(1 \text{ mW}) = 0.5 \text{ mW}$$

$$E = \frac{(0.5 \text{ mW})(0.7)}{(0.385 \text{ cm}^2)} = 0.9 \text{ mW} \cdot \text{cm}^{-2}$$

So, for a 6 cm beam diameter, about half of the power is collected by the 5 cm lens at 10 m distance. Therefore the corneal irradiance is about half of that calculated for the 2 m distance.

Since the MPE is 5.5 times less at the 10 m distance but the corneal irradiance is only reduced by half, this laser is more hazardous when viewed with 7-power optics at 10 m from the laser than it is when viewed at 2 m. Additional computations would be necessary to determine the precise distance where the optical hazard is maximized.

B10. References

Marshall, W. J. and Conner, P. W., Field Laser Hazard Calculations, *Health Physics* 52(l), 27-37; 1987.

Marshall, W. J., Comparative Hazard Evaluation of Near infrared Diode Lasers, *Health Physics* 66(5): 532-539; 1994.

Marshall, W. J., Determining Hazard Distances from Non-Gaussian Lasers, *Appl. Opt.* 30(6), 696-698; 1991.

Marshall, W. J., Hazard Analysis on Gaussian shaped Laser Beams, *AIHA Journal* 41, 547-551; 1980.

Marshall, W. J., Laser Reflections from Relatively Flat Specular Surfaces, *Health Physics* 56(5), 753-757; 1989.

Marshall, W. J., Aldrich, R. C., and Zimmerman, S. A., Laser Hazard Evaluation Method for Middle Infrared Laser Systems, *Journal of Laser Applications*, Vol. 8, 211-216; 1996.

Marshall, W. J., Understanding Laser Hazard Evaluation, *Journal of Laser Applications*, Vol. 7, 99-105; 1995.

Marshall, W. J., Determining source size from diode laser systems, *Journal of Laser Applications*, Vol. 14, 252-259; 2002.

Sliney, D.H. and Wolbarsht, M. L., *Safety with Lasers and other Optical Sources*, New York, Plenum Press; 1980.

Thomas, R. J., Maier, D. A., Barsalou, N., McLin, L., Lambert, L. and Keppler, K., Laser Light Show Measurement Techniques, SAFE Jour 27 (2) 115-126; 1997.

Thomas R. J., Rockwell B. A., Marshall W. J., Aldrich R. C., Zimmerman S. A., Rockwell R. J. A procedure for multiple-pulse maximum permissible exposure determination under the Z136.1-2000 American National Standard for Safe Use of Lasers, *Journal of Laser Applications*, Vol. 13: 134-140; 2001.

Thomas R. J., Rockwell B. A., Marshall W. J., Aldrich R. C., Zimmerman S. A., Rockwell R. J. A procedure for laser hazard classification under the Z136.1-2000 American National Standard for Safe Use of Lasers, *Journal of Laser Applications*, Vol. 14: 57-66; 2002.

Thomas R. J., Rockwell B, A., Marshall W. J., Aldrich R. C., Gorschboth M. F., Zimmerman S. A., Rockwell R. J. A procedure for the estimation of intrabeam hazard distances and optical density requirements under the ANSI Z136.1-2000 Standard, *Journal of Laser Applications*, Vol. 16: 167-177; 2004.

U.S. Army Medical Technical Bulletin (TB MED) 524, Control of Hazards to Health from Laser Radiation, June 1985.

Van De Merwe, W. P. and Marshall, W. J., Hazardous Ranges of Laser Beams and their Reflections from Targets, *Appl. Opt.* 25(5), 605-611; 1986.

Zimmerman, S. and Aldrich, R., Comparison of Divergence Measurement Techniques for Laser Light Show Application, Proceedings of the Third International Laser Safety Conference, Laser Institute of America, 1997.

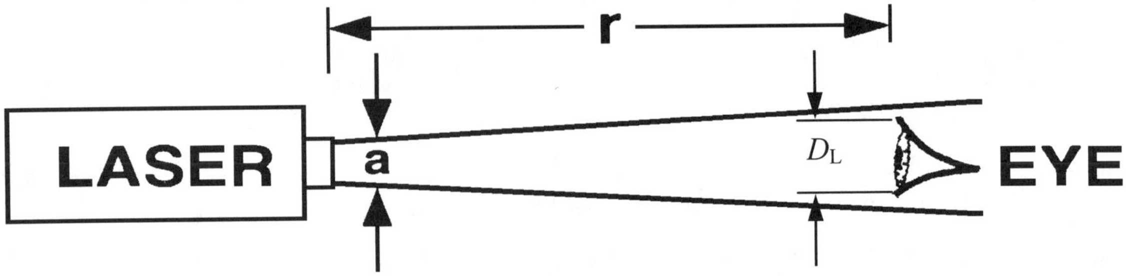

Figure B1. Intrabeam Viewing – Direct (Primary) Beam

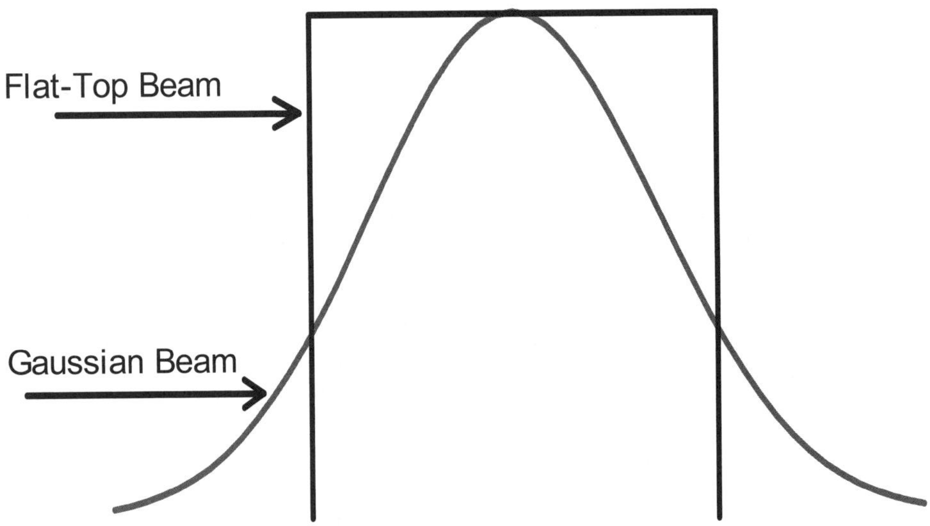

Figure B2. Flat-Top Beam Shape Compared with Gaussian Beam
Both Beams Have the Same Beam Diameter

FLAT SURFACE REFLECTION

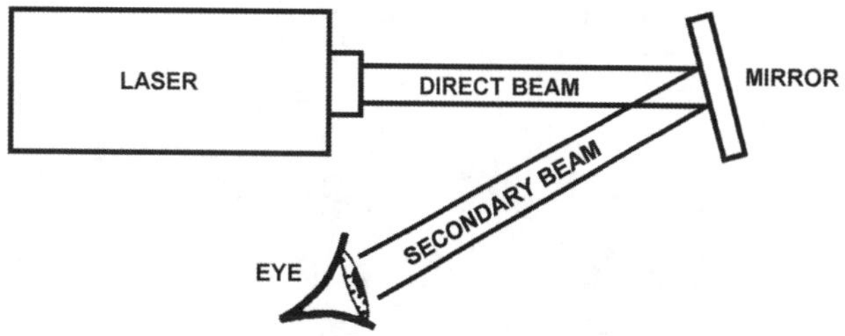

(Secondary Beam) CURVED SURFACE REFLECTION

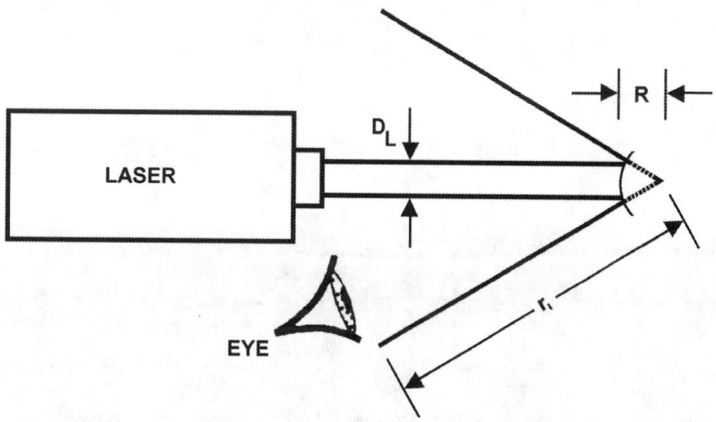

Figure B3. Intrabeam Viewing – Specularly Reflected

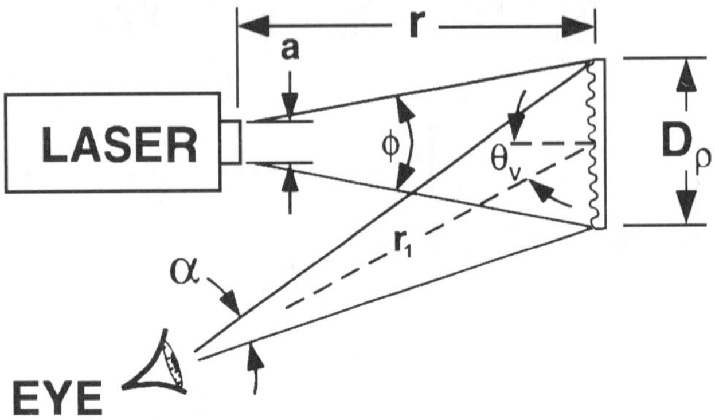

Figure B4. Viewing Diffuse Reflections

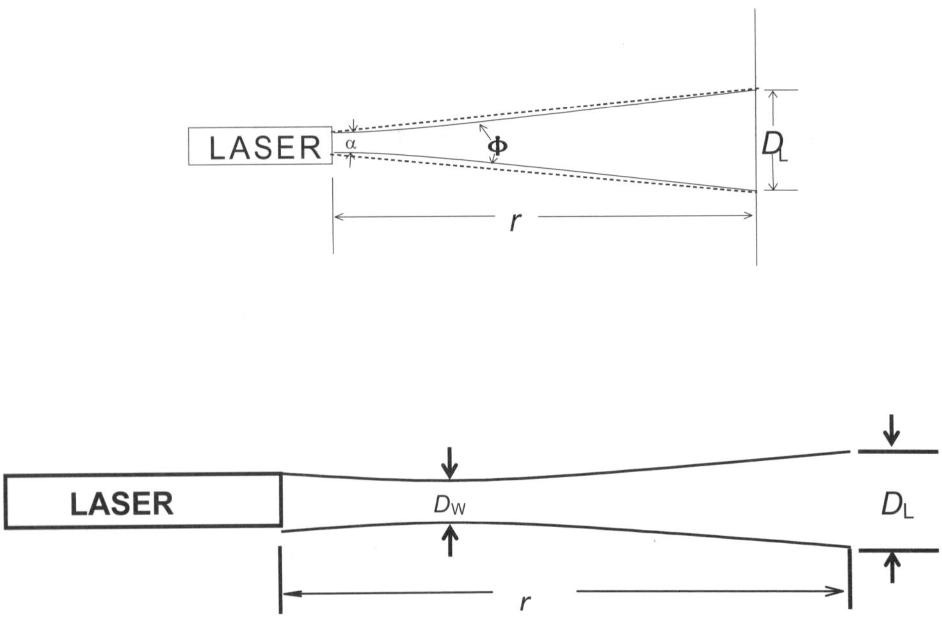

Figure B5. Beam Expansion with Distance from the Laser

Inner lines in upper diagram show beam diameter according to Eq B39 and outer dashed lines show beam diameter according to Eq B40. Lower diagram illustrates beam expansion for a focused beam (beam waist in front of laser).

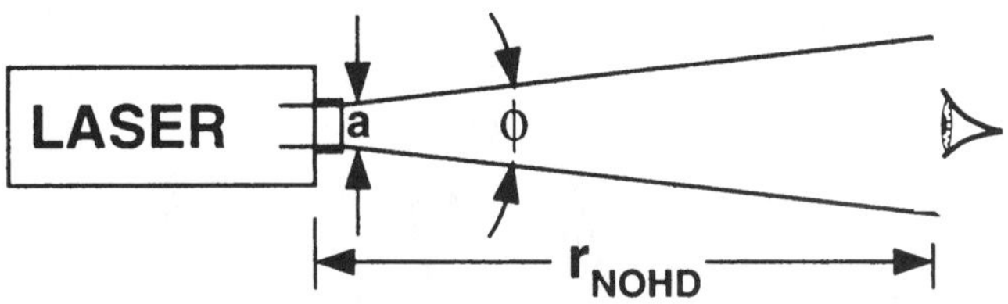

$$r_{NOHD} = \frac{1}{\phi}\left[\left(\frac{4\,\Phi}{\pi\, MPE}\right) - a^2\right]^{1/2}$$

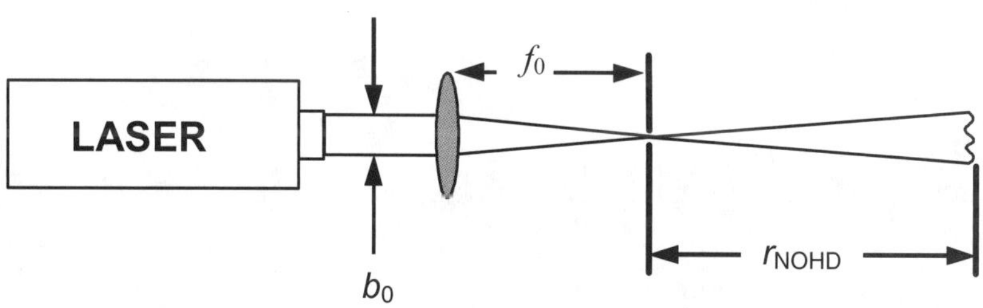

$$r_{\mathrm{NOHD}} = \left(\frac{f_0}{b_0}\right)\left(\frac{4\Phi}{\pi \mathrm{MPE}}\right)^{1/2}$$

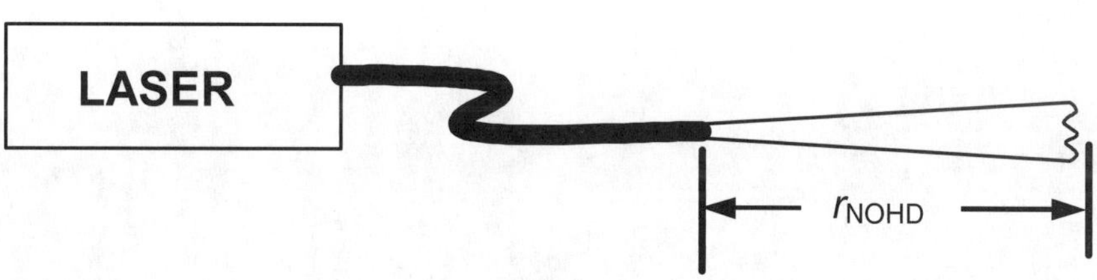

$$r_{\mathrm{NOHD}} = \frac{1.7}{NA}\left(\frac{\Phi}{\pi \mathrm{MPE}}\right)^{1/2} \quad \text{(multimode)}$$

$$r_{\mathrm{NOHD}} = \frac{\omega_o}{\lambda}\left(\frac{\pi\Phi}{2\mathrm{MPE}}\right)^{1/2} \quad \text{(single mode)}$$

Figure B6. Examples of Use of Laser Range Equations for Determining Nominal Hazard Distances

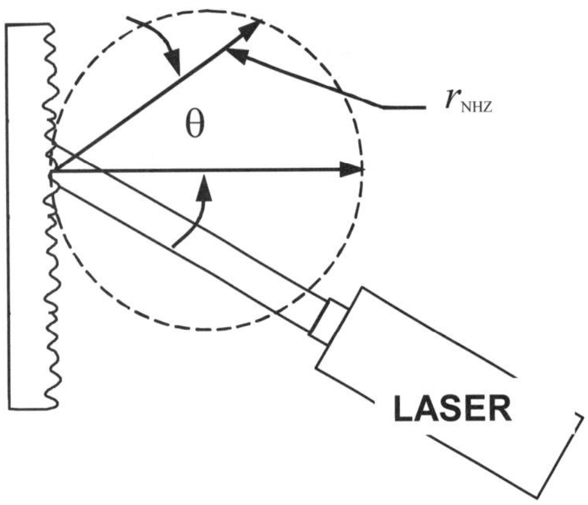

$$r_{NHZ} = \left(\frac{\rho \ \Phi \cos \theta}{\pi \ MPE} \right)^{1/2}$$

Figure B7. Nominal Hazard Zone for a Diffuse Reflection

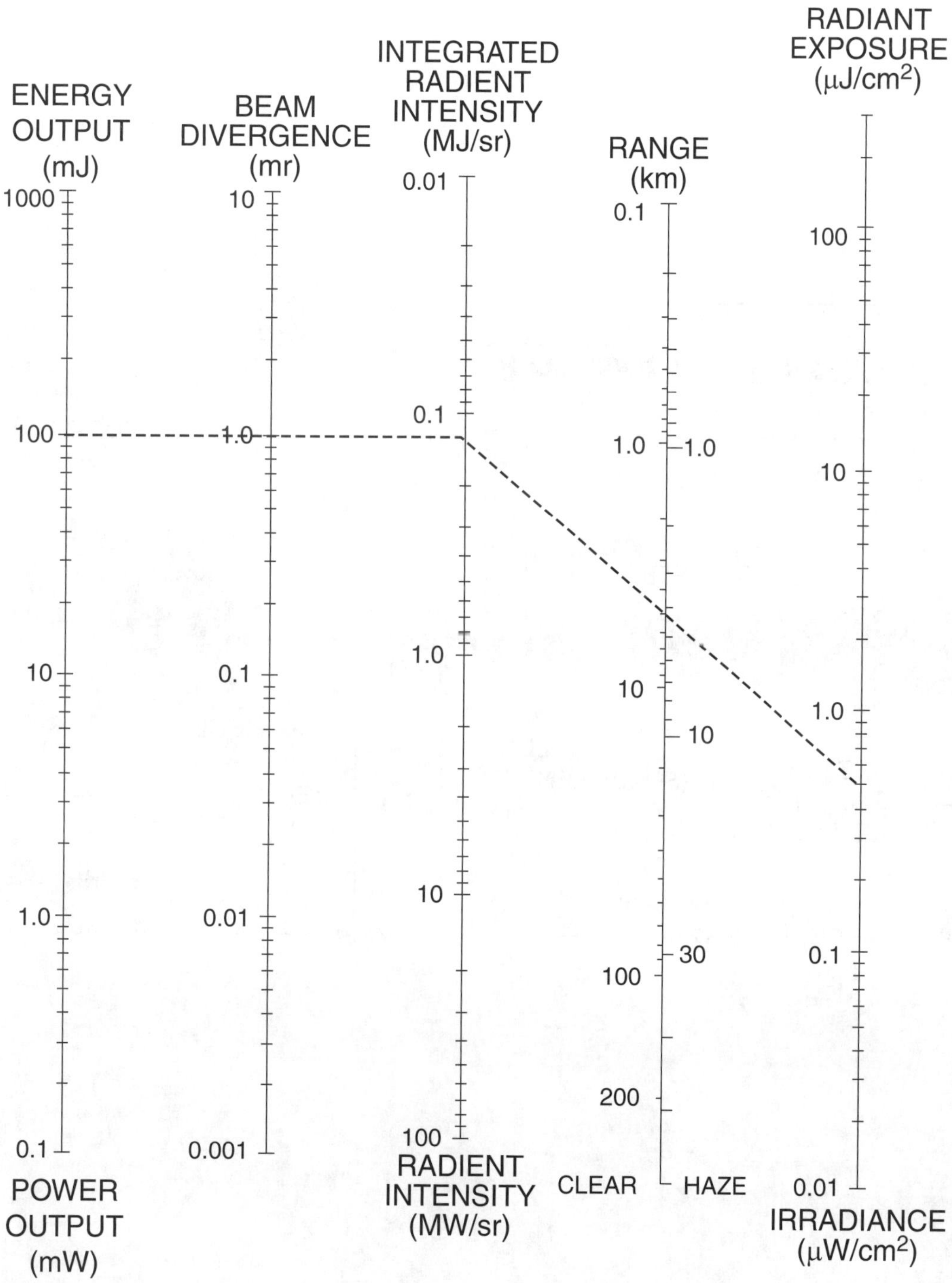

Figure B8. Laser Range Equation Nomogram

See Section B6.4.2 and Example 41.

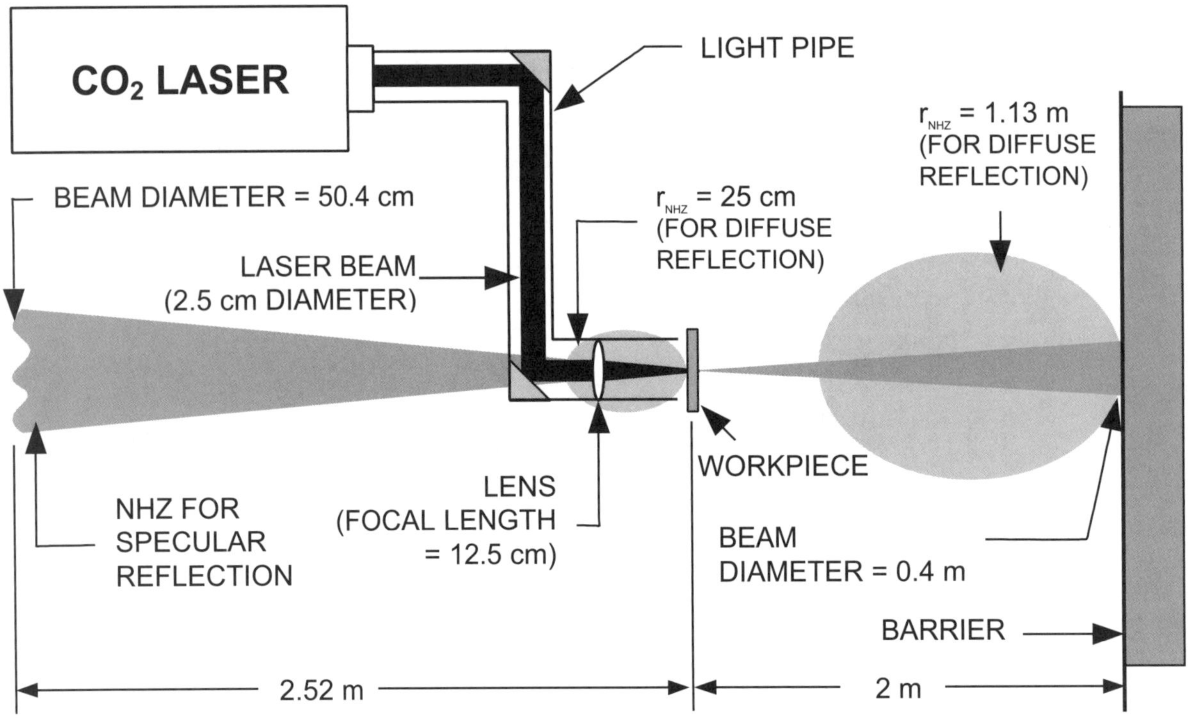

Figure B9. Diagram of the Laser Arrangement for Example 55

See Section B6.6.4.

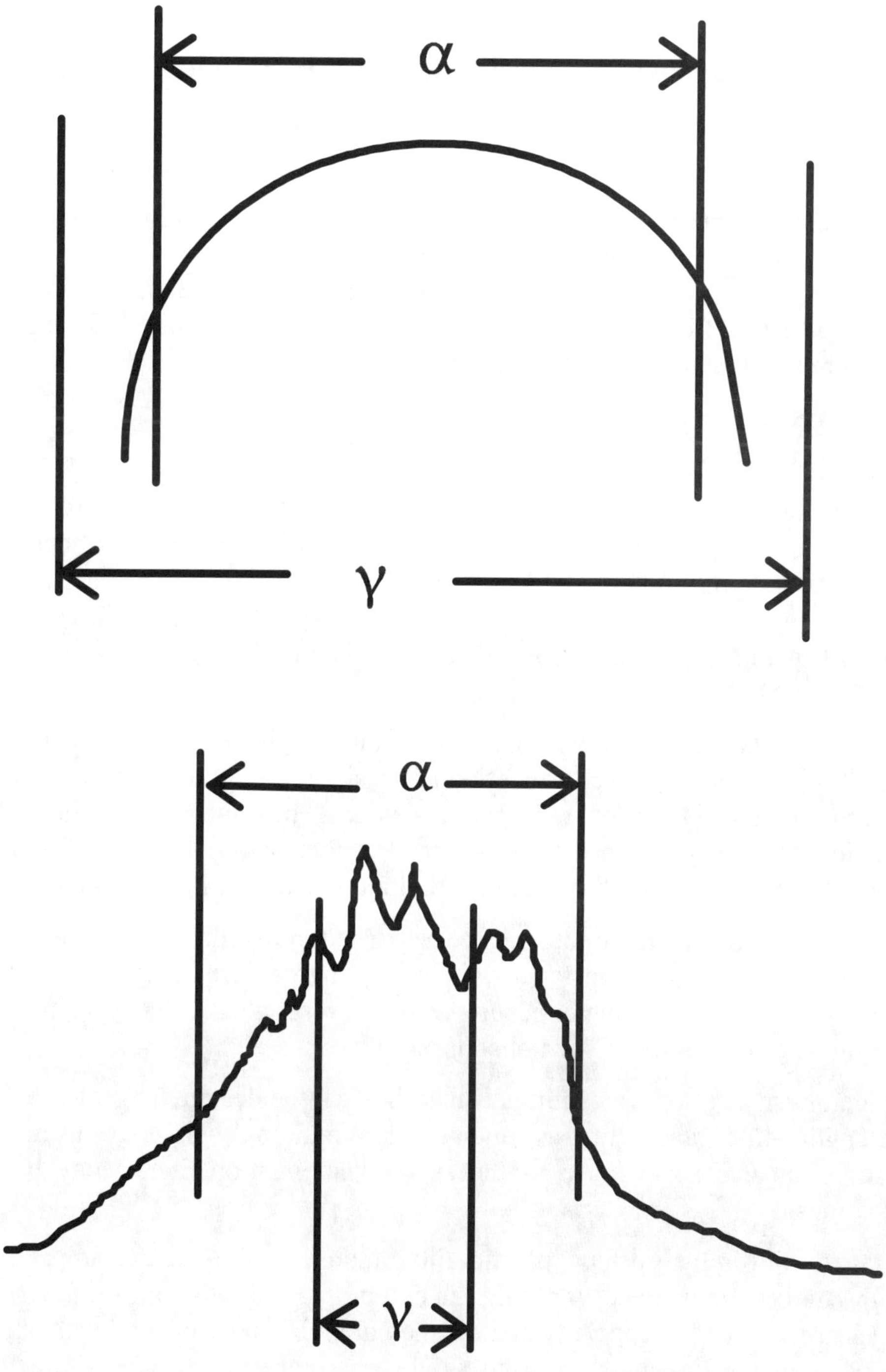

Figure B10. Determination of Limiting Cone Angle, γ

Illustration of optical sources where the source is fairly uniform and the source size, α, is less than the field or view, γ (upper). The lower figure illustrates an optical source with hot spots and the source size is larger than γ.

Appendix C
Hazard Evaluation, Classification and Control Measures

C1. Alternate Labeling

Some laser equipment manufactured outside of the USA may conform to requirements of the IEC Publication 60825, Radiation Safety of Laser Products, Equipment Classification, Requirements and User's Guide (or latest revision thereof). The IEC 60825 label style (shown in Figure 1c) is different from that required by this standard and those specified in the Federal Laser Product Performance Standard.

C2. Laser Protection Damage Threshold Evaluation

C2.1 Laser Protective Eyewear. A wide variety of commercially available optical absorbing filter materials (glass and plastics) and various coated reflecting "filters" (dielectric and holographic) are available for laser eye protection. Some are available with spectacle lenses ground to prescription specifications. Protection for multiple laser wavelengths is becoming more common as more applications involve several simultaneous wavelengths.

Each filter material has some limitations. For example, it should be noted that not all absorbing glass filters used for laser protection are easily annealed (thermally hardened) and, consequently, do not provide adequate impact resistance. In some goggles, however, impact resistant plastic filters (polycarbonate) can be used together with non-hardened glass filters in a design where the plastic is placed in front and behind of the non-hardened laser filter glass.

In some tests, glass filter plates have cracked and shattered following intense Q-switched, pulsed laser exposures. In some instances, the shattering occurred after one-quarter to one-half hour had elapsed following the exposure. Also, several glass filter types have displayed photobleaching when exposed to Q-switched laser pulses.

The advantage of using reflective coatings is that they can be designed to selectively reflect a given wavelength while transmitting as much of the remaining visible spectrum as possible. Note that some angular dependence of the spectral attenuation factor may be present in dielectric coatings.

The advantages of using absorbing plastic filter materials are greater impact resistance, lighter weight, and convenience of molding the eye protection into comfortable shapes. The disadvantages are that, unless specially coated, they are more readily scratched and the filters often age poorly as the organic dyes used as absorbers are more readily affected by heat and/or ultraviolet radiation, which eventually causes the filter to significantly darken.

It should be stressed that there are few known materials that can withstand laser exposures which exceed 10^5 W·cm^{-2} since the electric fields associated with the beam will exceed the bonding forces of matter. However, most materials will begin to degrade at levels far below these field strength levels due to thermal or shock effects.

C2.2 Laser Eyewear Filter Damage Level. At some specific beam intensity, the filter material which absorbs the laser radiation can be damaged. Plastic materials have damage thresholds much lower than glass filters and glass (by itself) is lower than glass coated with a reflective dielectric coating.

The damage threshold is especially important for those who work close to the beam interaction site where there is a much higher probability of receiving a direct exposure. Typical damage thresholds for CW lasers fall between 500 and 1000 $W{\cdot}cm^{-2}$ for dielectric coated glass, 100 to 500 $W{\cdot}cm^{-2}$ for uncoated glass and 1 to 100 $W{\cdot}cm^{-2}$ for plastics.

A 1979 FDA study, Evaluation of Commercially Available Laser Protective Eyewear [HEW Publication (FDA) 79-8086], reported limited testing of laser protective eyewear available at that time. For example, tests were reported for Q-switched ruby laser exposures (0.694 μm) on various manufacturers' protective eyewear. The plastic laser protective eyewear displayed damage thresholds (surface pitting) for Q-switched pulses ranging from 3.8 to 18 $J{\cdot}cm^{-2}$ while glass filters required a radiant exposure ranging from 93 to 1620 $J{\cdot}cm^{-2}$.

More recent analysis of polycarbonate protectors with CO_2 lasers indicated that a level of 60 $W{\cdot}cm^{-2}$ for 10 seconds was just below the penetration level. A level of 112 $W{\cdot}cm^{-2}$ for 4 s just produced penetration and 10 seconds produced significant penetration. Additional detailed damage threshold data for protective eyewear of more recent vintage is not readily available, although at least one comprehensive study is currently underway to examine these factors.

While direct intrabeam exposure of eyewear is certainly not recommended under any normal condition, it can and does occur. At least one intrabeam eye accident with thermal decomposition of plastic (non-polycarbonate) laser eyewear has been reported with a Nd:YAG laser in a research laboratory.

C2.3 Protective Viewing Windows. All viewing portals, optics, windows or display screens included as a part of the laser or laser installation shall incorporate some means to attenuate the laser radiation transmitted through the windows to levels below the appropriate MPE. This would include, for example, a viewing window into the laser facility. The filtration requirements would be based upon the level of laser radiation that would occur at the window in a typical worst-case condition in a manner identical to the eyewear evaluations discussed above.

C2.4 Laser Barriers and Protective Curtains. Area control can be effected in some cases using special barriers which have been specifically designed to withstand either direct and/or diffusely scattered beams. In this case, the barrier will exhibit a barrier threshold limit for beam penetration through the barrier during a specified exposure time (typically 60 seconds). The barrier is located at a distance from the laser source so that the threshold limit is not exceeded in the worst-case exposure scenario.

Currently available laser barriers exhibit threshold limits ranging from 10 $W{\cdot}cm^{-2}$ to 350 $W{\cdot}cm^{-2}$ for different laser wavelengths and power levels. A hazard analysis can be performed in a manner similar to the NHZ evaluations that establishes the recommended barrier type and installation separation distances between the barrier and a given laser.

Note that the factor of flammability is important in the design of a protective barrier. It is essential that the material not support combustion or be consumed by flames following the termination of the beam. Also important is the factor that decomposition products resulting from the laser interaction not be a respiratory hazard.

The purpose of a threshold limit evaluation is to define that point or distance at which the barrier must be placed so as to withstand a worst-case exposure from the laser.

C3. Examples of Typical Lasers or Laser System Classification and MPEs for Selected Lasers

Since the laser classification was designed to include all types of lasers operating at essentially any wavelength or pulse duration, the rules of classification (see Section 3.2) may appear complicated. To assist in the classification of commonly available lasers, Tables C1 and C2 have been prepared to aid the user in rapidly determining the required radiometric parameters needed to classify a laser and its applicable class once the required output parameters are known. Table C1 applies to CW lasers (potential exposure time ≥ 0.25 s), and Table C2 applies to pulsed lasers. To classify a repetitive-pulse laser, the values in Tables C1 and C2 are not generally applicable but may be used as a first step in estimating into what class the laser will fall.

In all cases the user should apply the rules given in Section 3 of the standard.

Table C1. Typical Laser Classification – Continuous Wave (CW) Point Source Lasers

Wavelength (µm)	Laser Type	Wavelength (µm)	Class 1 * (W)	Class 2 (W)	Class 3 ** (W)	Class 4 (W)
Ultraviolet						
0.180 to 0.280	Neodymium: YAG (Quadrupled)	0.266	$\le 9.6 \times 10^{-9}$ for 8 hours	None	> Class 1 but ≤ 0.5	> 0.5
	Argon	0.275				
Ultraviolet						
0.315 to 0.400	Helium-Cadmium	0.325	$\le 3.2 \times 10^{-6}$	None	> Class 1 but ≤ 0.5	> 0.5
	Argon	0.351, 0.363,				
	Krypton	0.3507, 0.3564				
Visible						
0.400 to 0.700	Helium-Cadmium	0.4416 only	$\le 4 \times 10^{-5}$	> Class 1 but $\le 1 \times 10^{-3}$	> Class 2 but ≤ 0.5	> 0.5
	Argon (Visible)	0.457	$\le 5 \times 10^{-5}$			
		0.476	$\le 1 \times 10^{-4}$			
		0.488	$\le 2 \times 10^{-4}$			
		0.514	$\le 4 \times 10^{-4}$			
	Krypton	0.530				
	Neodymium: YAG (Doubled)	0.532				
	Helium-Neon	0.543				
	Dye	0.400 - 0.500	$\le 0.4\, C_B \times 10^{-4}$			
	Helium-Selenium	0.460 - 0.500				
	Dye	0.550 - 0.700	$\le 4 \times 10^{-4}$			
	Helium-Neon	0.632				
	InGaAlP	0.670				
	Ti:Sapphire	0.350 – 0.500				
	Krypton	0.6471, 0.6764				
Near Infrared						
0.700 to 1.400	GaAlAs	0.780	$\le 5.6 \times 10^{-4}$	None	> Class 1 but ≤ 0.5	> 0.5
	GaAlAs	0.850	$\le 7.7 \times 10^{-4}$			
	GaAs	0.905	$\le 9.9 \times 10^{-4}$			
	Neodymium: YAG	1.064	$\le 1.9 \times 10^{-3}$			
	Helium-Neon	1.080	$\le 1.9 \times 10^{-3}$			
		1.152	$\le 2.1 \times 10^{-3}$			
	InGaAsP	1.310	$\le 1.5 \times 10^{-2}$			
Far Infrared						
1.400 to 10^3	InGaAsP	1.550	$\le 9.6 \times 10^{-3}$			
	Holmium	2.100				
	Erbium	2.940				
	Hydrogen Fluoride	2.600 - 3.00				
	Helium-Neon	3.390 only				
	Carbon Monoxide	5.000 - 5.500				
	Carbon Dioxide	10.6				
	Water Vapor	118	$\le 9.5 \times 10^{-2}$			
	Hydrogen Cyanide	337				

* Assumes no mechanical or electrical design incorporated into laser system to prevent exposures from lasting up to T_{max} = 8 hours (one workday); otherwise the Class 1 AEL could be larger than tabulated.

** See 3.3.3.1 for definition of Class 3R.

Table C2. Typical Laser Classification – Single-Pulse Point Source Lasers

Wavelength (μm)	Laser Type	Wavelength (μm)	Pulse Duration (s)	Class 1 (J)	Class 3B (J)	Class 4 (J)
Ultraviolet						
0.180 to 0.400	Excimer (ArF)	0.193	20×10^{-9}	$\le 2.4 \times 10^{-5}$		
	Excimer (KrF)	0.248	20×10^{-9}	$\le 2.4 \times 10^{-5}$		
	Neodymium: YAG Q-switched (Quadrupled)	0.266	20×10^{-9}	$\le 2.4 \times 10^{-5}$	> Class 1 but ≤ 0.125	> 0.125
	Excimer (XeCl)	0.308	20×10^{-9}	$\le 5.3 \times 10^{-5}$		
	Nitrogen	0.337	20×10^{-9}	$\le 5.3 \times 10^{-5}$		
	Excimer (XeF)	0.351	20×10^{-9}	$\le 5.3 \times 10^{-5}$		
Visible						
0.400 to 0.700	Rhodamine 6G (Dye Laser)	0.450-0.650	1×10^{-6}			
	Copper Vapor	0.510, 0.578	2.5×10^{-9}			
	Neodymium: YAG (Doubled) (Q-switched)	0.532	20×10^{-9}	$\le 1.9 \times 10^{-7}$	> Class 1 but ≤ 0.03	> 0.03
	Ruby (Q-switched)	0.6943	20×10^{-9}			
	Ruby (Long Pulse)	0.6943	1×10^{-3}	$\le 3.9 \times 10^{-6}$		
Near Infrared						
0.700 to 1.4	Ti: Sapphire	0.700-1.000	6×10^{-6}	$\le 1.9 \times 10^{-7}$		
	Alexandrite	0.720-0.800	1×10^{-4}	$\le 7.6 \times 10^{-7}$	> Class 1 but ≤ 0.033*	> 0.033**
	Neodymium: YAG (Q-switched)	1.064	20×10^{-9}	$\le 1.9 \times 10^{-6}$	>Class 1 but ≤ 0.125	> 0.125
Far Infrared	Erbium: Glass	1.540	10×10^{-9}	$\le 7.9 \times 10^{-3}$		
1.400 to 10^{3}	Co: Magnesium-Fluoride	1.8-2.5	80×10^{-6}	$\le 7.9 \times 10^{-4}$		
	Holmium	2.100	250×10^{-6}	$\le 7.9 \times 10^{-4}$	> Class 1 but ≤ 0.125	> 0.125
	Hydrogen Fluoride	2.600-3.000	0.4×10^{-6}	$\le 1.1 \times 10^{-4}$		
	Erbium	2.940	250×10^{-6}	$\le 5.6 \times 10^{-4}$		
	Carbon Dioxide	10.6	100×10^{-9}	$\le 7.9 \times 10^{-5}$		
	Carbon Dioxide	10.6	1×10^{-3}	$\le 7.9 \times 10^{-4}$		

* Assuming that both eye and skin may be exposed, i.e., 1.0 mm beam (area of limiting aperture = 7.9×10^{-3} cm^2).
** Class 3B AEL varies from 0.033 to 0.480 J corresponding to wavelengths that vary from 0.720 to 0.800 μm.

Table C3a. Point Source MPE for the Eye for Selected CW Lasers

Laser Type	Wavelength (μm)	Exposure Duration (s)	Maximum Permissible Exposure ($J \cdot cm^{-2}$)	($W \cdot cm^{-2}$)
Argon	0.275	10 to 3×10^4	3×10^{-3}	–
Helium-Cadmium	0.325	10 to 3×10^4	1	–
Argon	0.351	10 to 3×10^4	1	–
Helium-Cadmium	0.4416	0.25	–	2.5×10^{-3}
Argon	0.488	10 to 58	–	1×10^{-3}
	0.488	58 to 10^2	5.8×10^{-2}	
	0.488	$> 10^2$	–	5.8×10^{-4}
	0.5145	10 to 3×10^4	–	1×10^{-3}
Helium-Neon	0.632	0.25	–	2.5×10^{-3}
Helium-Neon	0.632	10 to 3×10^4	–	1×10^{-3}
Krypton	0.647	0.25	–	2.5×10^{-3}
Krypton	0.647	10 to 3×10^4	–	1×10^{-3}
InGaAlP	0.670	0.25	–	2.5×10^{-3}
GaAs	0.905	10 to 3×10^4	-	2.6×10^{-3}
Neodymium: YAG	1.064	10 to 3×10^4	-	5×10^{-3}
InGaAsP	1.310	10 to 3×10^4	-	4×10^{-2}
InGaAsP	1.550	10 to 3×10^4	-	0.1
Carbon-Dioxide	10.600	10 to 3×10^4	-	0.1

Table C3b. Point Source MPE for the Skin for Selected CW Lasers

Laser Type	Wavelength (μm)	Exposure Duration (s)	Maximum Permissible Exposure ($J \cdot cm^{-2}$)	($W \cdot cm^{-2}$)
Argon	0.275	3×10^4	3×10^{-3}	–
Helium-Cadmium	0.325	10 to 1000	1	–
	0.325	> 1000		1×10^{-3}
Argon	0.351	10 to 1000	1	–
	0.351	> 1000	–	1×10^{-3}
Helium-Cadmium	0.4416	> 10	–	0.2
Argon	0.488	>10	–	0.2
Argon	0.5145	>10	–	0.2
Helium-Neon	0.6328	>10	–	0.2
Krypton	0.647	>10	–	0.2
GaAs	0.905	>10	–	0.5
Neodymium: YAG	1.064	>10	–	1.0
Carbon-Dioxide	10.600	>10	–	0.1

Table C4. Point Source MPE for the Eye and MPE for the Skin for Selected Single-Pulse Lasers

Laser Type	Wavelength (μm)	Pulse Duration (s)	Maximum Permissible Exposure ($J \cdot cm^{-2}$) Eye	Skin
Excimer (ArF)	0.193	2×10^{-8}	3×10^{-3}	3×10^{-3}
Excimer (KrF)	0.248	2×10^{-8}	3×10^{-3}	3×10^{-3}
Excimer (XeCl)	0.308	2×10^{-8}	6.7×10^{-3}	6.7×10^{-3}
Excimer (XeF)	0.351	2×10^{-8}	6.7×10^{-3}	6.7×10^{-3}
Ruby (Normal-Pulsed)	0.6943	1×10^{-3}	1×10^{-5}	0.2
Ruby (Q-switched)	0.6943	$5 - 100 \times 10^{-9}$	5×10^{-7}	0.02
Rhodamine 6G dye laser	0.500 - 0.700	$0.5 - 18 \times 10^{-6}$	5×10^{-7}	0.03 to 0.07
Nd:YAG (Normal Pulse)	1.064	1×10^{-3}	5×10^{-5}	1.0
Nd:YAG (Q-switched)	1.064	$5 - 100 \times 10^{-9}$	5×10^{-6}	0.1
Carbon Dioxide	10.6	1×10^{-3}	0.1	0.1

C4. References

Conference of Radiation Control Program Directors: *Model State Laser Standard*, Lexington, KY.

Doyle, D. and Kokosa, J.M., Laser Processing of Kevlar. Hazardous Chemical By-products, *Proceedings of ICALEO,* Laser Institute of America, Orlando, FL, 1986.

Doyle, D. J., and Kokosa, J. M., Hazardous By-Products of Plastics Processing with Carbon Dioxide Lasers. In: *Laser Welding, Machining and Materials Processing,* C. Albright, Editor. IFS LTD., Bedford, United Kingdom, pp. 201-203; 1985.

Electronic Product Radiation and the Health Physicist, *Proceedings of the Fourth Annual Midyear Topical symposium;* 1970. Washington: U.S. Department of Health, Education, and Welfare; Bureau of Radiological Health, Division of Electronic Products; 70-26. Available from National Technical Information Service, Springfield, VA 22161.

Envall, K. R. and Murray, R., *Evaluation of Commercially Available Laser Protective Eyewear,* DHEW Publication (FDA) 79-8086, May 1979.

Goldman, L., Rockwell, R. J., Jr. *Lasers in Medicine.* 1971, chapter II; New York: Gordon and Breach Science Publishers, 1971.

Goldman, L., Rockwell, R. J., Jr., Homby, P. Laser Laboratory Design and Personnel Protection from High Energy Lasers. In: *Handbook of Laboratory Safety.* N.V. Steere, ed; 2nd ed. Cleveland: The Chemical Rubber Company: 381-389; 1971.

Guide for the Selection of Laser Eye Protection. Laser Institute of America, Orlando, FL; 1996.

International Electrotechnical Commission *Standard Radiation Safety of Laser Products, Equipment Classification, Requirements and Users Guide*, IEC Publication 825: Geneva Switzerland; 1990.

Laser Health Hazards Control. U.S. Department of the Air Force Manual AFM-161-32, 1973 (or latest revision thereof). Available from National Technical Information Service, Springfield, VA. 22161.

Laser Institute of America, *Safety Information on Electrical Hazards,* Laser News, Laser Institute of America, Vol. 6, No. 5, pp. 8-14; Sept., 1984.

Laser Product Performance Standard. Code of Federal Regulations, Title 21, Subchapter J, Part 1040, 1979.

Laser Products; Amendments to Performance Standard; Final Rule. Code of Federal Regulations, Title 21, Parts 1000 and 1040, Federal Register, Aug. 20,1985.

Marshall, W. J., Hazard analysis on Gaussian shaped laser beams. *Journal of the American Industrial Hygiene Association.* 41(8): 547-551; Aug 1980.

Rockstroh, T. J., and Mazumder, J., Spectroscopic Studies of Plasma, During CW Laser Materials Interaction. *J. Appl. Phys.,* Vol. 61, No. 3, pp. 917-923; 1987.

Rockwell, R. J., Jr. and Moss, C. E., Optical radiation hazards in laser welding processes Part 1: Neodymium - YAG Laser. *The Journal of the American Industrial Hygiene Association. 44(8);* 572-579; Aug 1983.

Rockwell, R. J., Jr., Ensuring safety in laser robotics. *Lasers and Applications. 3*(11); 65-69; Nov 1984.

Rockwell, R. J, Jr., Fundamentals of Industrial Laser Safety. In: *Industrial Laser Annual Handbook,* edited by M. Levitt and D. Belforte, Penn Well Books, Tulsa, OK., pp. 131-148; 1986.

Rockwell, R. J. Jr. and Moss, C. E., Optical Radiation Hazards of Laser Welding Processes Part H: Carbon Dioxide Laser, *The Journal of the American Industrial Hygiene Association,* Vol. 50, No. 8. pp. 419-427; August, 1989.

Rockwell, R. J. Jr., Laser Accidents: Are They All Reported and What Can Be Learned From Them?. *Journal of Laser Applications*, Laser Institute of America, Orlando, FL, pp. 53-57; 1989.

Rockwell, R. J. Jr., Analyzing Laser Hazards, *Lasers and Applications*, Vol. 5. No. 5. pp. 97-103; May, 1986.

Rockwell, R. J. Jr., Controlling Laser Hazards, *Lasers and Applications*, Vol. 5, No. 9, pp. 93-99; Sept., 1986.

Rockwell, R. J. Jr., Selecting Laser Eyewear, *Medical Laser Buyer's Guide,* Penn Well Books, Tulsa, OK., pp. 84-92; January, 1989.

Rockwell, R. J. Jr., Utilization of the Nominal Hazard Zone in Control Measure Selection, *Proceedings of the International Laser Safety Conference*, Laser Institute of America, Orlando, FL, 1991.

Sliney, D. H., Evaluating health hazards from military lasers. *Journal of the American Medical Association.* 214(6): 1047-1054; Nov., 1970.

Sliney, D. H., Laser Protective Eyewear. In: M. L. Wolbarsht, ed. *Laser Applications in Medicine and Biology.* New York. Plenum Press; v. 2, chapter 7, pp. 223-240; 1974.

Sliney, D. H., Sparks, S.D. and Wood, R.L. Jr., The Protective Characteristics of Polycarbonate Lenses Against CO_2, Laser Radiation, *Journal of Laser Applications*, Laser Institute of America, Orlando, FL, pp 49-52; Apr. 1993.

Sliney, D. H. and Wolbarsht, M. L., *Safety with Lasers and other Optical Sources.* New York.- Plenum Publishing Co; 1980.

Swope, C. H., The Eye - Protection. *Archives of Environmental Health.* 18(3): 428-433; 1969.

U.S. Department of the Army, *Control of Hazards to Health from Laser Radiation.* U.S. Department of the Army Technical Bulletin TB-MED-524; June 1985. Available from National Technical Information Service, Springfield, VA. 22161.

U.S. Army Regulation 11-9, the Army Radiation Safety Program, Headquarters, Department of the Army, Washington DC, 28 May 1999.

Appendix D
Guide for Organization and Implementation of Employee Laser Safety Training Programs

The extent to which the various parts of the following guide are applicable to a specific organization depends on the magnitude of the potential laser hazards within that organization. However, it is essential that each laser safety program include sufficient education of personnel in laser safety.

D1. Employee Training

D1.1 General. Education may be provided to users of Class 1M, Class 2, Class 2M or Class 3R lasers. Laser safety training must be provided to users of class 3B or class 4 lasers (see section 1.3.1). Training programs may be developed by the employer. Short courses and other training programs on laser safety are also commercially available.

Employers should consider awareness level training for employees operating laser systems that enclose higher power lasers. This training may be used to communicate the safety or potential hazards under conditions other than those of normal operations. An explanation of the differences of potential hazard between the classes of lasers is beneficial to the user. The employer should consider when this effort would be beneficial to the operator.

The LSO determines what, if any, training is commensurate with the laser hazards accessible at the employer's facility.

D1.2 Laser Safety Training Program Topics. Topics for a laser safety training program for Class 3B and Class 4 laser use may include, but are not necessarily limited to, the following:

(1) For user personnel routinely working with or potentially exposed to Class 3B or Class 4 laser radiation:

- (a) Fundamentals of laser operation (physical principles, construction, etc.)
- (b) Bioeffects of laser radiation on the eye and skin
- (c) Significance of specular and diffuse reflections
- (d) Non-beam hazards of lasers (see Section 7)
- (e) Laser and laser system classifications
- (f) Control measures
- (g) Overall responsibilities of management and employee
- (h) Medical surveillance practices (if applicable)
- (i) CPR for personnel servicing or working on lasers with exposed high voltages and/or the capability of producing potentially lethal electrical currents

(2) For the LSO or other individual responsible for the laser safety program, evaluation of hazards, and implementation of control measures, or any others if directed by management to obtain a thorough knowledge of laser safety:

   (a) The topics in D1.2 (1)

   (b) Laser terminology

   (c) Types of lasers, wavelengths, pulse shapes, modes, power/energy

   (d) Basic radiometric units and measurement devices

   (e) MPEs

   (f) Laser hazard evaluations and other calculations

D1.2.1 Class 2 and Class 2M Awareness Training. For optional Class 2 and Class 2M education, simple, brief programs may be developed that are designed for easy implementation by persons other than LSOs or education instructors, such as first line supervisors. Potential topics include:

(1) Simple explanation of a laser

(2) Compare difference of laser light from ordinary light

(3) Explain a Class 2 laser with the concept that it is harmless for exposure duration less than the human aversion response time of 0.25 s

(4) Explain the differences between a Class 2 and a Class 2M lasers

(5) Provide statement cautioning against intentional overcoming of the human aversion and staring into a Class 2 and Class 2M laser beam

(6) General explanation of the differences in the various laser classifications

D1.2.2 Class 1M and Class 3R Awareness Training. For optional Class 1M and Class 3R education, simple brief programs may be developed that are designed for easy implementation by persons other than LSOs or education instructors, such as first line supervisors. Potential topics include:

(1) Simple explanation of a laser

(2) Compare difference of laser light from ordinary light

(3) Describe nature of near IR beams where applicable

(4) Explanation of Class 1M and 3R lasers, and the relative potential hazard of each

(5) Explanation of the potential for collecting and focusing optics to increase the hazard

D1.2.3 Laser Pointer Awareness. If laser pointer awareness education is determined to be desirable, suggested topics can include:

(1) Simple explanation of a laser

(2) Compare difference of laser light from ordinary light

(3) Precautions for use

(4) Effects of exposures

(5) Misuse/FDA warning on misuse of pointers

(6) FDA limit of 5 mW

(7) Local ordinance limitations

D2. References

American Conference of Government Industrial Hygienists, A *Guide for Control of Laser Hazards*, ACGIH, PO Box 1937, Cincinnati, OH 45201; 1990.

Hartwig, P. A., Medical Laser Safety Programs: Management and Training. *Proceedings of the International Laser Safety Conference*, Laser Institute of America, Orlando, FL, pp. 8-31 to 8-35; 1991.

Hoffman, P., A Technical Training Approach to the Safe Operation, Maintenance and Service of Lasers in Manufacturing. *Proceedings of the International Laser Safety Conference*, Laser Institute of America, 1910.134, Respiratory Protection. Orlando, FL, pp. 7-65 to 7-74; 1991.

Johnson, J. R., Safety Audits of Industrial Laser *Facilities. Proceedings of the International Laser Safety Conference,* Laser Institute of America, Orlando, FL, pp. 5-1 to 5-4; 1991.

Kestenbaum, A. and Coyle, J., Laser System Design for Safety Manufacturing. *Proceedings of the International Laser Safety Conference*, Laser Institute of America, Orlando, FL, pp. 5-53 to 5-64; 1991.

LIA Laser Safety Guide, Laser Institute of America, Orlando, FL; 1993.

Manufacturer's accident reporting requirements are detailed in the Code of Federal Regulations, 21 CFR Subchapter J Part 1002.20.

OSHA, Guidelines for Laser Safety and Hazard Assessment, Instruction PUB 8-1.7. Chapter IX Laser Training.

Skillern, C. P., Management of a Laser Safety Program in the Research Environment. *Proceedings of the International Laser Safety Conference*, Laser Institute of America, Orlando, FL, pp. 7-1 to 7-8; 1991.

Smith, J. F., Safety Programs and Formal Training. In: Sliney and Wolbarsht. *Safety with Lasers and Other Optical Sources.* New York: Plenum Press; 1980: chapter 25.

Smith, J. F., Class 2 Laser Safety Training Programs. *Proceedings of the International Laser Safety Conference,* Laser Institute of America, Orlando, FL., pp. 7-83 to 7-86; 1991.

Smith, J. F., Murphy, J. J., Eberle, W. J., Industrial Laser Safety Program Management. Poughkeepsie, NY: IBM Corp., System Products Division.

Smith, J.F. and Jones, J.E., Laser Safety Training Operation Options for Industrial and Laboratory Environments. *Proceedings of the International Laser Safety Conference,* Laser Institute of America, Orlando, FL, 1997.

US Code of Federal Regulations: 29CFR Part 1910.132, General Requirements for Protective Equipment.

US Code of Federal Regulations: 29CFR Part 1910.133, Eye and Face Protection.

US Code of Federal Regulations: 29CFR Part 1910.134, Respiratory Protection.

US Code of Federal Regulations: 29CFR Part 1910.147, Control of Hazardous Energy (Lockout/Tagout).

US Code of Federal Regulations: 29CFR Part 1910.331, Safety Related Work Practices, Training.

US Code of Federal Regulations: 29CFR Part 1910.1200, Hazard Communication (Right to Know).

US Code of Federal Regulations: 29CFR Part 1910.1405, Occupational Exposures to Hazardous Chemicals in Laboratories.

US Code of Federal Regulations: 29CFR Part 1926.54, Nonionizing Radiation.

US Code of Federal Regulations: 29CFR Part 1926.102, Eye and Face Protection.

Appendix E
Medical Examinations

E1. Medical Referral Following Suspected or Known Laser Injury

Any employee with an actual or suspected laser-induced injury should be evaluated by a medical professional as soon as possible after the exposure. Referral for medical examinations shall be consistent with the medical symptoms and the anticipated biological effect (see Appendix G)based upon the laser system in use at the time of the incident. For laser-induced injury to the retina, the medical evaluation shall be performed by an ophthalmologist. Employees with skin injuries should be seen by a physician.

E1.1 Medical Examinations for Exposure Incidents. Recommended medical examinations for actual or suspected exposure include but are not limited to those specified in Section E3.

E2. Medical Surveillance Examinations

E2.1 Rational for Surveillance Examinations. The basic reasons for performing medical surveillance of personnel working in a laser environment are the same as for other potential health hazards. Medical surveillance examinations may include assessment of physical fitness to safely perform assigned duties, biological monitoring of exposure to a specific agent, and early detection of biological damage or effect.

Physical fitness assessments are used to determine whether an employee would be at increased or unusual risk in a particular environment. For workers using laser devices, the need for this type of assessment is most likely to be determined by factors other than laser radiation per se. Specific information on medical surveillance requirements that might exist because of other potential exposures, such as toxic gases, noise, ionizing radiation, etc., are outside the scope of this appendix.

Direct biological monitoring of laser radiation is impossible, and practical indirect monitoring through the use of personal dosimeters is not available.

Early detection of biological change or damage presupposes that chronic or subacute effects may result from exposure to a particular agent at levels below that required to produce acute injury. Active intervention must then be possible to arrest further biological damage or to allow recovery from biological effects. Although chronic injury from laser radiation in the ultraviolet, near ultraviolet, blue portion of the visible, and near infrared regions appears to be theoretically possible, risks to workers using laser devices are primarily from accidental acute injuries. Based on risks involved with current uses of laser devices, medical surveillance requirements that should be incorporated into a formal standard appear to be minimal.

Other arguments in favor of performing extensive medical surveillance have been based on the fear that repeated accidents might occur and the workers would not report minimal acute injuries. The limited number of laser injuries that have been reported in the past 30 years and the excellent safety records with laser devices do not provide support to this argument.

E3. Medical Examinations

E3.1 Rationale for Examinations. Past experience has shown that pre-incident examinations would normally not be as extensive as a post incident examination. Therefore, the medical-legal value of pre-examination has been shown to be of limited value with litigation tending to be driven by biophysical measurements of the accident site and the exposure geometry. Individual institutions may provide pre-exposure screening and even continuing surveillance; however, that surveillance was not deemed to be a requirement for safe laser usage.

E3.1.1 Preassignment Medical Examinations. Except for examination following suspected injury, these are the only examinations required by this standard. One purpose is to establish a baseline against which damage (primarily ocular) can be measured in the event of an accidental injury. A second purpose is to identify certain workers who might be at special risk from chronic exposure to selected continuous wave lasers. For incidental workers (e.g., custodial, military personnel on maneuvers, clerical and supervisory personnel not working directly with lasers) only visual acuity measurement is required. For laser workers' medical histories, visual acuity measurement, and selected examination protocols are required. The wavelength of laser radiation is the determinant of which specific protocols are required (see Section E3.2). Examinations should be performed by, or under the supervision of, an ophthalmologist or optometrist or other qualified physician. Certain examination protocols may be performed by other qualified practitioners or technicians under the supervision of a physician. Although skin damage from chronic exposure to laser radiation has not been reported, and indeed seems unlikely, this area has not been adequately studied. Limited skin examinations are suggested to serve as a baseline until future epidemiologic studies indicate whether they are needed or not.

E3.1.2 Periodic Medical Examinations. Periodic examinations are not required by this standard. At present, no chronic health problems have been linked to working with lasers. Also, most uses of lasers do not result in chronic exposure of employees even to low levels of radiation. A large number of these examinations have been performed in the past, and no indication of any detectable biological change was noted. Employers may wish to offer their employees periodic eye examinations or other medical examinations as a health benefit. However, there does not appear to be any valid reason to require such examinations as part of a medical surveillance program.

E3.1.3 Termination Medical Examinations. The primary purpose of termination examinations is for the legal protection of the employer against unwarranted claims for damage that might occur after an employee leaves a particular job. The decision on whether to offer or require such examinations is left to individual employers.

E3.2 Examination Protocols.

E3.2.1 Ocular History. The past eye history and family history are reviewed. Any current complaints concerned with the eyes are noted. Inquiry should be made into the general health status with a special emphasis upon systemic diseases which might produce ocular problems in regard to the performance cited in Section 6.1. The current refraction prescription and the date of the most recent examination should be recorded.

Certain medical conditions may cause the laser worker to be at an increased risk for chronic exposure. Use of photosensitizing medications, such as phenothiazines and psoralens, lower the threshold for biological effects in the skin, cornea, lens and retina of experimental animals exposed to ultraviolet and near ultraviolet radiation. Aphakic individuals would be subject to additional retinal exposure from blue light and near ultraviolet and ultraviolet radiation. Unless chronic viewing of these wavelengths is required, there should be no reason to deny employment to these individuals.

E3.2.2 Visual Acuity. Visual acuity for far and near vision should be measured with some standardized and reproducible method. Refraction corrections should be made if required for both distant and near test targets. If refractive corrections are not sufficient to change acuity to 20/20 (6/6) for distance and near vision, a more extensive examination is indicated as defined in Section 6.3.

E3.2.3 Macular Function. An Amsler grid or similar pattern is used to test macular function for distortions and scotomas. The test should be administered in a fashion to minimize malingering and false negatives. If any distortions or missing portions of the grid pattern are present, the test is not normal.

E3.2.4 Color Vision. Color vision discrimination can be documented by Ishihara or similar color vision tests.

E3.2.5 Examination of the Ocular Fundus with an Ophthalmoscope or Appropriate Fundus Lens at a Slit Lamp. This portion of the examination is to be administered to individuals whose ocular function in any of Section E.3.2.1 through E.3.2.4 is not normal. The points to be covered are: the presence or absence of opacities in the media; the sharpness of outline of the optic disc; the color of the optic disc; the depth of the physiological cup, if present; the ratio of the size of the retinal veins to that of the retinal arteries, the presence or absence of a well defined macula and the presence or absence of a foveal reflex; and any retinal pathology that can be seen with an ophthalmoscope (hyper-pigmentation, depigmentation, retinal degeneration, exudate, as well as any induced pathology associated with changes in macular function). Even small deviations from normal should be described and carefully localized. Dilation of the pupil is required.

E3.2.6 Skin Examination. Not required for preplacement examinations of laser workers; however, it is suggested for employees with history of photosensitivity or working with ultraviolet lasers. Any previous dermatological abnormalities and family history are reviewed. Any current complaints concerned with the skin are noted as well as the history of medication usage, particularly concentrating on those drugs which are potentially photosensitizing.

Further examination should be based on the type of laser radiation, above the appropriate MPEs, present in the individual's work environment.

E3.2.7 Other Examinations. Further examinations should be done as deemed necessary by the examiner.

E4. Records and Record Retention

Complete and accurate records of all medical examinations (including specific test results) should be maintained for all personnel included in the medical surveillance program. Records should be retained for at least 30 years.

E5. Access to Records

The results of medical surveillance examinations should be discussed with the employee.

All non-personally identifiable records of the medical surveillance examinations acquired in Section E.4 of these guidelines should be made available on written request to authorized physicians and medical consultants for epidemiological purposes. The record of individuals will, as is usual, be furnished upon request to their private physician.

E6. Epidemiologic Studies

Past use of lasers has generally been stringently controlled. Actual exposure of laser workers has been minimal or even nonexistent. It is not surprising that acute accidental injury has been rare and that the few reports of repeated eye examinations have not noted any chronic eye changes. For these reasons, the examination requirements of this standard are minimal. However, animal experiments with both laser and narrow-band radiation indicate the potential for chronic damage from both subacute and chronic exposure to radiation at certain wavelengths. Lens opacities have been produced by radiation in the 0.295 to 0.45 μm range and are also theoretically possible from 0.75 to 1.4 μm.

Photochemical retinitis appears to be inducible by exposure to 0.35 to 0.5 μm radiation. If laser systems are developed that require chronic exposure of laser workers to even low levels of radiation at these wavelengths, it is recommended that such workers be included in the long-term epidemiologic studies and have periodic examinations of the appropriate eye structures.

Epidemiologic studies of workers with chronic skin exposure to laser radiation (particularly ultraviolet) are suggested.

E7. References

Friedman, A. L. The ophthalmic screening of laser workers. *Ann Occup Hyg.* 21: 277-279; 1978.

Hathaway, J. A., Stern, N., Soles, E. M., Leighton, E. Ocular medical surveillance on microwave and laser workers. *J. Occup Med.* 19: 683-688; 1977.

Hathaway, J. A. The Need for Medical Surveillance of Laser and Microwave Workers. Current Concepts in Ergophthalmology. *Societas Ergophthalmologica Internationalis.* Sweden: 139-160; 1978.

Wolbarsht, M. L., and Landers, M. B., Testing visual capabilities for medical surveillance or to ensure job fitness. *J. Occup Med.* 27: 897-901; 1985.

Mainster, M.A., Sliney, D.H., Marshall, J., Warren, K.A., Timberlake, G.T., Trokel, S.L . But Is It Really Light Damage? *Ophthalmol.* 104(2): 179-180; 1997.

Mainster, M.A., Timberlake, G.T., Sliney, D.H., Pointers on Laser Pointers. Ophthalmol. 104(8): 1213-1214;1997.

Mainster, M.A., Stuck, B.E., Brown J., Assessment of Alleged Retinal laser Injuries, Arch. of Ophthalmol. 122: 1210-1217; Aug 2004.

Green, R.P., Cartledge, R.M., Cheney, F.E., Menendez, A.R. Medical Management of Combat Laser Eye Injuries. USAFSAM-TR-88-21, Brooks Air Force Base, TX. October 1988

Department of the Army Field Manual 8-50. Prevention and Medical Management of Laser Injuries, Headquarters, Department of the Army, Washington, D.C. August 1990.

http://www.adtdl.army.mil/cgibin/atdl.dll/fm/8-50/toc.htm

Appendix F
Non-Beam Hazards

Non-beam hazards may be categorized into physical, chemical, or biological agents. Physical agents include, but are not limited to electrical hazards, collateral and plasma radiation, noise, and mechanical hazards. Chemical agents may be subdivided into laser generated airborne contaminants (LGAC), compressed gases, dyes, and solvents. Biological agents include blood borne materials such as blood components and microorganisms.

F1. Physical Agents

F1.1 Electrical Hazards.

F1.1.1 Grounding. The frames, enclosures and other accessible non-current-carrying metallic parts of laser equipment should be grounded. Grounding should be accomplished by providing a reliable, continuous metallic connection between the part or parts to be grounded and the grounding conductor of the power wiring system.

F1.1.2 Electrical Fire Hazards. Components in electrical circuits should be evaluated with respect to potential fire hazards. Enclosures, barriers or baffles of nonmetallic material should comply with Underwriters Laboratory Standard, UL 746C, Polymeric Materials - Use in Electrical Equipment Evaluations.

F1.1.3 Electrical Hazards from Explosion. Gas laser tubes and flash lamps should be supported to ensure that their terminals cannot make any contact which will result in a shock or fire hazard in the event of a tube or lamp failure. Components such as electrolytic capacitors may explode if subjected to voltages higher than their ratings, with the result that ejected metallic material may bridge live electrical parts. Such capacitors should be rated to withstand the highest probable voltage should other circuit components fail, unless the capacitors are adequately contained so as not to create a hazard.

F1.1.4 Marking. The user should ensure that each laser or laser system is permanently marked with its primary electrical rating in volts, frequency, and power or current. The user should also determine if the system has electrical components that operate at other frequencies, such as radio frequencies. This is important because the threshold for current-induced biological effects will vary with frequency. If the laser is intended for use by the public or by personnel untrained in laser safety, and is provided with electrical safety interlocks, warning notices instructing the user not to defeat the interlock should be applied to the device.

F1.1.5 Other. Where applicable, the user should comply with provisions of OSHA Standards for Electrical Safety-Related Work Practices (29 CFR 1910 Subpart S) and the Control of Hazardous Energy (lockout/tagout; 29 CFR 1910.147).

F1.2 Plasma and Collateral Radiation. Plasma radiation is produced when the output from an energetic laser beam interacts with target materials. This has been demonstrated most often for pulsed emissions from carbon dioxide lasers when welding, drilling or otherwise treating metallic materials. Such plasma radiation is rich in actinic UV (UV-C and UV-B) and contains UV-A and visible wavelengths. Of greatest concern for visible wavelengths is the blue-light component and the total luminance (photometric brightness) of the plasma. Some studies have demonstrated potential overexposures to actinic radiation and blue light at distances around 1 meter from the beam-material interaction site. Luminance may exceed exposure criteria at this distance, too. The acceptable exposure duration for actinic radiation during some evaluations has been shown to be less than a minute, but this depends on a number of factors including beam power, shield gas, and base material. Other lasers used in material processing may also produce plasma radiation and should be evaluated to determine exposure. Hence, when specifying control measures for material processing lasers, plasma radiation must be a consideration.

Collateral radiation includes those wavelengths emitted by the laser or laser system other than laser radiation. An example of this is x-radiation emitted by a high-energy switch, such as a thyratron, in a pulsed laser. Collateral x-radiation is produced by the process known as bremsstrahlung, or braking radiation. This occurs when electrons, under a high difference in electric potential, are sharply accelerated resulting in the emission of x-rays. Broadband optical radiation may be produced by lamps used to energize (optically-pumped) solid-state lasers. Radio-frequency radiation may be generated from energy-pumping components in some gas lasers, such as sealed plasma-tube CO_2 lasers, or from pulse-forming components in pulsed lasers. Power-frequency electric and magnetic fields (50 or 60 Hz and harmonics) are produced by electrical power supplies, wiring, and circuit components, for all alternating current lasers. As with plasma radiation, collateral radiation should be evaluated to determine the potential for overexposure, and appropriate control measures utilized as necessary.

F1.2.1 Control Measures. These include distance, shielding, and personal protective equipment. The intensity of the electromagnetic energy decreases with distance, usually decreasing with the second or third power of distance, which can effectively decrease exposure. Shielding is effective for optical, microwave, RF radiation and power-frequency electric fields. Much of the optical radiation band may be shielded with plastics such as polycarbonate and poly(methyl methacrylate)-type plastics, although additives (dyes) may be necessary for visible and some IR wavelengths. Microwaves and electric fields may be shielded with conductive materials (e.g., metals such as aluminum or copper). Shielding is more difficult for low-frequency RF and power-frequency magnetic fields, which may require the use of special shielding materials, such as ferrous alloys containing nickel or cobalt. Personal protective equipment, for the eyes and skin, is useful for optical radiation. In general, personal protective equipment is not useful for RF and power-frequency fields.

F1.3 Noise. Some pulsed lasers may present a potential noise hazard. This has occurred with certain excimer lasers and transversely-excited atmospheric (TEA) carbon dioxide lasers. The LSO should request information on potential noise exposure or equipment sound levels from the laser product manufacturer. In many cases, sound levels will not result in overexposure to noise, but may be a nuisance that must be addressed.

F2. Chemical Agents

F2.1 Laser Generated Airborne Contaminants (LGAC). LGAC may be aerosols, gases or vapors. Factors important in the generation of LGAC include the base material, shield gas, and beam irradiance. In general, if the beam irradiance exceeds 10^7 W/cm^2, the intensity is sufficiently high to produce LGAC from most target materials, as shown in Table F1(a), although beam irradiance values as low as hundreds of W/cm^2 have been reported to produce LGAC (see Table F1(b)).

Aerosols, generated by absorption of laser radiation, will vary in their size distribution, composition, morphology and toxicity. For the most part, the size distribution is usually weighted towards aerosols that are small in size, and are, therefore, respirable. An important type of LGAC aerosol, metallic oxide fumes, comes from laser processing of metals. If the metal is mild steel, the major aerosol will be iron oxides. If the metal is certain stainless steels, the aerosol will include oxides of iron, nickel, and chromium.

Gases and vapors that form during laser beam interaction may be representative of the base material, such as the monomer from which a polymer is synthesized. In other cases, the base material may dissociate and reactions may produce new compounds. Some of the compounds from various materials include: polycyclic aromatic hydrocarbons (PAH) from mode burns on poly (methyl methacrylate)-type polymers; hydrogen cyanide and benzene from cutting of aromatic polyamide fibers; fused silica from cutting quartz; and hydrogen chloride and benzene from cutting polyvinyl chloride. A more complete list is included in Table F1(b). Possible biological effects and control measures are in Table F1(c).

F2.1.1 Control Measures. Engineering control measures should be given priority for LGAC control measures. Foremost among these are isolation, the use of local exhaust ventilation, and the substitution of substances that produce less toxic by-products (see Section 7.3.1).

F2.2 Compressed Gases. Common laser gases may be inert (helium-neon, argon), flammable (hydrogen), toxic (chlorine, fluorine), corrosive (hydrogen chloride), or oxidizing (oxygen). The potential hazard(s) associated with a specific gas or gas mixture must be addressed, and some potential hazards may not be obvious. For example, toxic gases may be diluted (typically less than a few percent) in biologically inert gases. However, if released to the atmosphere, the dilute concentration may result in airborne concentrations that are immediately dangerous to life and health (IDLH). Consider that a gas mixture for some carbon dioxide lasers includes 2% carbon monoxide, which equals 20,000 parts per million (ppm). If released to the atmosphere, this would be well above the IDLH level for CO, which is 1200 ppm. Also, in sufficient quantity, the inert gases may produce an adverse biologic effect, simple asphyxiation by displacement of the available oxygen.

F.2.2.1 Control Measures. Prior to installation of a gas system, the LSO should consider elements of design and control. This includes, but is not limited to, cylinder location, cylinder security, regulator selection, purge system, ventilation requirements, remote operation including emergency shutoff, personal protective equipment, labeling, and employee training.

F2.3 Laser Dyes and Solvents. In general, there is potential exposure to dyes during weighing and mixing, and during decontamination of the system. There is potential exposure to solvents during transfer processes. The potential for exposure to both dyes and solvents exists during mixing, spill clean up, and disposal.

Laser dyes include xanthenes, polymethines, coumarins, and stilbenes. Acute toxicity studies have demonstrated that a number of these dyes are poisons, where the dose lethal to 50% of the test animals (LD_{50}) was less than 50 mg/kg. Additionally, bioassays have shown that some dyes are mutagenic. The solvents used with dyes are organic compounds that are relatively common in industry and research. These solvents may pose a wide variety of possible health hazards, including those of both a chemical (e.g., toxicity) and physical (e.g., fire) nature.

F.2.3.1 Control Measures. If more than one solvent can be used for a given application, the solvents should be compared with ensure that the safest is selected. The information necessary to aid in this determination is often contained in the material safety data sheet (MSDS). For example, the user should compare acute toxicity data (often in the form of the LD_{50}), exposure limits (e.g., threshold limit values = ACGIH TLVs; or permissible exposure limits = OSHA PELs), volatility (vapor pressure), and flammability (flash point).

The LSO must address control measures appropriate for mixing and use of dyes and solvents, too. This includes, but is not limited to, methods of solvent transfer, adequate ventilation, personal protective equipment, process isolation, provision of secondary containment, path and construction of tubing or piping, labeling and employee training. Some useful information on control measures for dye/solvent systems has been developed by Lawrence Livermore National Laboratory and is included in the reference section, below.

F3. Biological Agents

Lasers may be used in surgery in the medical, dental and veterinary environments. This creates the potential for the generation of LGAC and airborne infectious materials, when the laser beam interacts with tissues.

F3.1 LGAC. As discussed above, LGAC in the laser plume may be aerosols, gases or vapors. Gaseous materials generated by laser-tissue interaction may be numerous, but of special interest are benzene, formaldehyde, and hydrogen cyanide. The condensable phase may include PAHs such as benzo(a)pyrene. Additionally, LGAC may be generated if the laser beam contacts articles in the health care environment, such as tubing or swabs.

F3.2 Infectious Materials. The laser plume may contain aerosolized blood (plasma and blood cells or fragments of cells) and blood borne pathogens. Blood borne pathogens may include bacteria and viruses. Viral organisms that have been found include a bacteriophage and human papillomavirus. In vitro studies of bacterial targets demonstrated viable *Escherichia coli* and *Staphylococcus aureus* in the laser plume.

F3.3 Control Measures. The primary control measure is exhaust ventilation; specifically smoke evacuation. Most smoke evacuation units are movable units that include a small, high-velocity nozzle (hood) that can be located very near the laser-tissue interaction site. The collected effluent is conveyed to the filtration system which includes an activated carbon bed for organic LGACs and a HEPA (high efficiency particulate air-) or ULPA (ultra-low particulate air-) filter for aerosols. In some cases, the source of exhaust ventilation may be a house vacuum system. Regardless of the type of system, the LSO should ensure that the filtration system is on a preventative maintenance schedule so that filter penetration does not occur.

F4. References

F4.1 Electrical Hazards.

Dalziel, C.F.: Effects of electric shock on man. IRE Trans. Med. Elec. PGME-5: 44-62; 1956.

Dalziel, C.F.: Electric shock hazard. IEEE Spectrum 9(2): 41-50; 1972.

Larkin, W.D., J.P. Reilly, and L.B. Kittler: Individual differences in sensitivity to transient electrocutaneous stimulation. IEEE Trans. Biomed. Eng. BME-33: 495-504; 1986.

Lee, R.H.: Electrical safety in industrial plants. IEEE Spectrum 8(6): 51-55; 1971.

Thomas, D.K.: Often overlooked electrical hazards common in many lasers. In Proceedings of the 1992 International Laser Safety Conference. Orlando, FL: Laser Institute of America, 4I-41 - 4I-44; 1993.

Sliney, D.H. and M.L. Wolbarsht: Safety with Lasers and Other Optical Sources. New York: Plenum Publishing, (chapter 28); 1985.

Varanelli, A.G.: Electrical hazards associated with lasers. Journal of Laser Applications 7: 62-64; 1995.

F4.2 Plasma and Collateral Radiation.

F4.2.1 X-radiation.

Carroll, F.E.: Generation of "soft x-rays" by using the free electron laser as a proposed means of diagnosing and treating breast cancer. Lasers Surg. Med. 11: 72-78; 1991.

Chen, H. et al.: Study of x-ray emission from picosecond laser-plasma interaction. SPIE 1413: 112-119; 1991.

Kuhnle, G. et al.: X-ray production by irradiation of solid targets with sub-picosecond excimer laser pulses. Appl. Phys. B 47: 361-366; 1988.

Shmaenok, L.A., et al.: Soft x-rays emitted by a laser plasma created by two consecutive laser pulses. Tech. Phys. Lett. 21: 920-922; 1995.

F4.2.2 Optical Radiation.

Abbott, D.H. and C.E. Albright: CO2 shielding gas effects in laser welding mild steel. Journal of Laser Applications 6(2): 69-80 (1994).

Bos, A.J.J. and M.P. de Haas: On the safe use of a high power ultraviolet laser. In Human Exposure to Ultraviolet Radiation: Risks and Regulations, edited by W.F. Passchier and B.F.M. Bosnjakovic. New York: Elsevier Science Publishers, pp. 377-382; 1987.

Hietanen, M. and P. Von Nandelstadh: Scattered and plasma-related optical radiations associated with industrial laser processes. In Proceedings of the International Laser Safety Conference. Orlando, FL: Laser Institute of America, pp. 3-105 - 3-108; 1991.

Hietanen, M., et al.: Evaluation of hazards in CO2 laser welding and related processes. Ann. Occup. Hyg. 36:183-188; 1992.

Hitchcock, R.T.: Ultraviolet Radiation (Nonionizing Radiation Guide Series). Akron, OH: American Industrial Hygiene Association, 49 pp; 2001.

Rockwell, R.J., Jr. and C.E. Moss: Optical radiation assessment of laser welding. In Proceedings of the Medicine and Biology Symposium. Laser Institute of America: ICALEO (vol 32), pp. 100-108; 1982.

Rockwell, R.J., Jr.. and C.E. Moss: Optical radiation hazards of laser welding processes part 1: neodymium-YAG laser. Am. Ind. Hyg. Assoc. J. 44: 572-579; 1983.

Rockwell, R.J., Jr. and C.E. Moss: Optical radiation hazards of laser welding processes part 2: CO2 laser. Am. Ind. Hyg. Assoc. J. 50: 419-427; 1989.

Schulmeister, K., et al.: Hazardous ultraviolet and blue-light emissions of CO2 laser beam welding. In Proceedings of the International Laser Safety Conference. Orlando, FL: Laser Institute of America, pp. 229-232; 1997.

F4.2.3 Radio-frequency Radiation.

Bioelectromagnetics, Supplement 6, Wiley-Liss, 2003

Hitchcock, R.T.: Radio-Frequency and Microwave Radiation (Nonionizing Radiation Guide Series). Fairfax, VA: American Industrial Hygiene Association, 33 pp; 2004.

Seitz, T.A. and C.E. Moss: RF-excited carbon dioxide lasers: concerns of RF occupational exposures. In Proceedings of the International Laser Safety Conference. Orlando, FL: Laser Institute of America, pp. 3-35 - 3-40; 1991.

F4.2.4 Power-frequency (Extremely low frequency, ELF) Fields.

Bowman, J.D. et al.: Exposures to extremely low frequency (ELF) electromagnetic fields in occupations with elevated leukemia rates. Appl. Ind. Hyg. 3: 189-194; 1988.

Hitchcock, R.T., S. McMahan, and G.C. Miller: Extremely Low Frequency (ELF) Electric and Magnetic Fields (Nonionizing Radiation Guide Series). Fairfax, VA: American Industrial Hygiene Association, 59 pp; 1995.

Reilly J. P. Applied Bioelectricity: From Electrical Stimulation To Electropathology, Springer, NY, 1998.

F4.3 Fires and Explosions.

Bos, A.J.J. and M.P. de Haas: On the safe use of a high power ultraviolet laser. In Human Exposure to Ultraviolet Radiation: Risks and Regulations, edited by W.F. Passchier and B.F.M. Bosnjakovic. New York: Elsevier Science Publishers, pp. 377-382; 1987.

Caldwell, C.: Laser fire protection. In Proceedings of the 1992 International Laser Safety Conference. Orlando, FL: Laser Institute of America, 4I-1 - 4I-8; 1993.

Cozine, K. et al.: Laser-induced endotracheal tube fire. Anesthesiology 55: 583-585; 1981.

Domin, M.A.: Ignition potential of surgical appliances and materials. In Proceedings of the 1992 International Laser Safety Conference. Orlando, FL: Laser Institute of America, 4M-5 - 4M-12; 1993.

Dubaniewicz, T.H., et al.: Laser ignition of flammable gas. In Proceedings of the International Laser Safety Conference ILSC 1999. Orlando, FL: Laser Institute of America, pp. 309-318; 2003.

Engel, D.: Laser generated metal dust explosive potential. In Proceedings of the 1992 International Laser Safety Conference. Orlando, FL: Laser Institute of America, 4I-21 - 4I-24; 1993.

Fried, M.P. et al.: Laser resistant stainless steel endotracheal tube: experimental and clinical evaluation. Lasers Surg. Med. 11: 301-306; 1991.

Hirshman, C.A. and D. Leon: Ignition of an endotracheal tube during laser microsurgery. Anesthesiology 53: 177; 1980.

Hughes, R.: Fire in the hole: an endotracheal tube fire. In ILSC 2003 Conference Proceedings & Program. Orlando, FL: Laser Institute of America, pp. 307-314; 2003.

Kashiwagi, T.: Ignition of a liquid fuel under high intensity radiation. Combustion Sci. Technol. 21: 131-139; 1980.

Lavid, M., S.K. Gulati, and W.R. Lempert: Laser ignition of ball power (nitrocellulose base). Proc. SPIE 2122: 129-143; 1994.

Lavid, M. and J.G. Stevens: Photochemical ignition of premixed hydrogen/oxidizer mixtures with excimer lasers. Combust. Flame 60: 195-202; 1985.

Pashayan, A.G. and J.S. Gravenstein: Airway fires during surgery with the carbon dioxide laser. Anesthesiology 71L: 478; 1989.

Sosis, M.: Polyvinylchloride endotracheal tubes are hazardous for CO2 laser surgery (letter); Pashayan, A.G. et al. (reply). Anesthesiology 69: 801-802; 1988.

Sosis, M.B. and F.X. Dillon: Comparison of CO2 laser ignition of the Xomed plastic and rubber tracheal tubes. In Proceedings of the 1992 International Laser Safety Conference. Orlando, FL: Laser Institute of America, 4M-13 - 4M-16; 1993.

F4.4 Chemical Agents.

F4.4.1 LGAC.

Busch, H. et al.: Aerosol formation during laser cutting of fibre reinforced plastics. J. Aerosol Sci. 20: 1473-1476 (1989).

Dahmen, M., et al.: Degradation of optical components in laser machines for manufacturing. In Proceedings of SPIE 2428: 248-254; 1995.

Doyle, D.J.: Spectroscopic evaluation of toxic by-products produced during industrial laser processing. In Proceedings of the International Laser Safety Conference. Orlando, FL: Laser institute of America, pp. 3-109 - 3-114; 1991.

Doyle, D.J. and J.M. Kokosa: Chemical by-products of laser cutting of Kevlar. Polymer Preprints 27: 206-207; 1986.

Fleeger, A. and C.E. Moss: Airborne emissions produced by the interaction of a carbon dioxide laser with glass, metals, and plastics. In Proceedings of the International Laser Safety Conference. Orlando, FL: Laser Institute of America, pp. 3-23 - 3-33; 1991.

Haferkamp. H., et al.: Hazardous emissions: characterization of CO2 laser material processing. Journal of Laser Applications 7: 83-88; 1988.

Haferkamp, H., et al.: Air contaminants generated during laser processing of organic materials and protective measures. In Proceedings of the International Laser Safety Conference. Orlando, FL: Laser Institute of America, pp. 209-218; 1997.

Hietanen, M., et al.: Evaluation of hazards in CO2 laser welding and related processes. Ann. Occup. Hyg. 36:183-188; 1992.

Kiefer, M. and C.E. Moss: Laser generated air contaminants released during laser cutting of fabrics and polymers. Journal of Laser Applications 9: 7-13; 1997.

Klein, R.M., et al.: Workplace exposure during laser-machining. In Proceedings of the International Laser Safety Conference. Orlando, FL: Laser Institute of America, pp. 252-261; 1997.

Kokosa, J.M.: Hazardous chemicals produced by laser materials processing. Journal of Laser Applications 6(4): 195-201; 1994.

Kokosa, J.M. and D.J. Doyle: Condensed phase pyrolysates produced by CO2 laser processing of polymers I: polycyclic aromatic hydrocarbons obtained from polyvinyl chloride. Polymer Preprints 26: 255-256; 1985.

Kwan, J.K.: Toxicological characterization of chemicals produced from laser irradiation of graphite composite materials. In Proceedings of the International Laser Safety Conference. Orlando, FL: Laser Institute of America, pp. 3-69 - 3-96; 1991.

Moss, C.E. and T. Seitz: Hazard evaluation and technical assistance report No. HETA-90-102-L2075, Ebtec East, Agawam, Massachusetts. Springfield, VA: National Technical Information Service, 1990.

Pena, A.C., J.G. Soler, and G.R. Caicedo : The characterization of aerosols generated during the cutting of metallic materials with lasers. Environ. Technol. 19:83-90; 1998.

Powell, J., A. Ivarson, and C. Magnusson: Laser cutting of steels: a physical and chemical analysis of the particles ejected during cutting. Journal of Laser Applications 5(1): 25-31; 1993.

Rockwell, R.J., Jr., et al.: Occupational hazards of laser material processing (Final Report Prepared for NIOSH). Springfield, VA: National Technical Information Service (Order No. PB89-186-530); 1976.

Schroder, K. et al.: UV-radiation induced ozone and nitrogen oxide emission during CO2 laser welding. In Proceedings of the 3rd EUREKA Industrial Laser Safety Forum, pp. 317-322; 1995.

Steiner, H., D. Windelberg, and B. Georgi: Aerosol generation during cutting of various materials with plasma, laser and consumable electrode. J. Aerosol Sci. 19: 1381-1384; 1988.

Tarroni, G., et al.: Characterization of aerosols produced in cutting steel components and concrete structures by means of a laser beam. J. Aerosol Sci. 17: 587-591; 1986.

Thomas, D.W. and M. Scott: Assessment of material particle sizes generated during excimer laser processing. In Proceedings of the 3rd EUREKA Industrial Laser Safety Forum, pp. 173-181; 1995.

Tonshoff, H.K., R. Egger, and F. Klocke: Environmental and safety aspects of electrophysical and electrochemical processes. CIRP Annals - Manufacturing Techno. 45(2): 553-568; 1996.

Troutman, K.R. and R.A. Froehlich: Case studies of laser generated air pollution. In Proceedings of the 1992 International Laser Safety Conference. Orlando, FL: Laser Institute of America, 4I-25 - 4I-32; 1993.

F4.4.2 Compressed Gases.

Benoit, H., J. Clark, and W.J. Keon: Installation of a commercial excimer laser in the operating room. Journal of Laser Applications 1(3): 45-50; 1989.

Bos, A.J.J. and M.P. de Haas: On the safe use of a high power ultraviolet laser. In Human Exposure to Ultraviolet Radiation: Risks and Regulations, edited by W.F. Passchier and B.F.M. Bosnjakovic. New York: Elsevier Science Publishers, pp. 377-382; 1987.

Dietz, A. and E. Bradford: Safe handling of excimer gases. In The Photonics Design and Applications Handbook (Book 3). Pittsfield, MA: Laurin Publishing Co., pp. H-240 - H-243; 1991.

Lorenz, A.K.: Gas handling safety for laser makers and users. Lasers and Applications 6(3): 69-73; 1987.

Sliney, D.H. and T.N. Clapham: Safety of medical exicmer lasers with an emphasis on compressed gases. Journal of Laser Applications 3(3): 59-62; 1991.

F4.4.3 Dyes and Solvents.

Austin, L. and U. Brackman: Dye lasers and laser dyes. In The Photonics Design and Applications Handbook (Book 3). Pittsfield, MA: Laurin Publishing Co., pp. H-204 - H-207; 1991.

Chiarella, W.: Cleaning and handling of optical components. In The Photonics Design and Applications Handbook (Book 3). Pittsfield, MA: Laurin Publishing Co., pp. H-317 - H-320; 1991.

Kues, H.A. and G.A. Lutty: Dyes can be deadly. Laser Focus 11(4): 69-60; 1975.

Lawrence Livermore National Lab: Laser Dyes. Section 14.11, LLNL Environment, Safety and Health Manual http://www.llnl.gov/es_and_h/hsm/doc_14.11/doc14-11.html

Miller, G.: Industrial hygiene concerns of laser dyes. In Proceedings of the International Laser Safety Conference. Orlando, FL: Laser institute of America, pp. 3-97 - 3-103; 1991.

Miyazoe, Y. and M. Maeda: Stimulated emission from 19 polymethine dyes--laser action over the continuous range of 710-1060 mμ. Appl. Phys. Letters 12: 206-208; 1968.

Mosovsky, J.A.: Laser dye toxicity, hazards, and recommended controls (Report No. UCRL-89148). Livermore, CA: Lawrence Livermore National Laboratory; 1983.

Wuebbles, B.J.Y. and J.S. Felton: Evaluation of laser dye mutagenicity using the Ames/Salmonella microsome test. Environ. Mut. 7: 511-522; 1985.

F4.5 Biological.

F4.5.1 LGAC.

Albrecht, H. and W. Waesche: Evaluation of potential health hazards caused by laser and RF surgery. Proc. SPIE 2624:200-204; 1996.

Felten, R.P.: Summary of laser plume effects and safety session. Journal of Laser Applications 1(2): 4-5; 1989.

Freitag, L., et al.: Laser smoke effect on the bronchial system. Lasers Surg. Med. 7: 283-288; 1987.

Kokosa, J.M. and M.D. Benedetto: Probing plume protection problems in the health care environment. Journal of Laser Applications 4(3): 39- 43; 1992.

Kokosa, J.M. and J. Eugene: Chemical composition of laser-tissue interaction smoke plume. Journal of Laser Applications 1(3): 59-63; 1989.

Moss, C.E., et al.: NIOSH Health Hazard Evaluation Report HETA 88-101-2008, University of Utah Health Sciences Center, Salt Lake City, Utah. Springfield, VA: National Technical Information Service (PB91-107789); 1990.

Occupational Safety and Health Administration (OSHA): Laser/Electrosurgery Plume web page: http://www.osha.gov/SLTC/laserelectrosurgeryplume/index.html

Wasche, W. and H. Albrecht: Investigation of the distribution of aerosols and VOC in plume produced during laser treatment under OR conditions. Proc. SPIE 2624: 270-275; 1996.

Weber, L. and T. Meier: Concepts of risk assessment of complex chemical mixtures in laser pyrolysis fumes. Proc. SPIE 2624: 259-269; 1996.

Weigmann, H.-J., et al.: Permanent gases and highly volatile organic compounds in laser plume. Proc. SPIE 2923: 164-167; 1996.

Ziegler, B.L., et al.: Generation of infectious retrovirus aerosol through medical laser irradiation. Lasers Surg. Med. 22: 37-41; 1998.

F4.5.2 Infectious Agents.

Abramson, A.L., T.P. DiLorenzo, and B.M. Steinberg: Is Papillomavirus detectable in the plume of laser-treated laryngeal Papilloma? Arch. Otolaryngol. Head Neck Surg. 116: 604-607; 1990.

Baggish, M.S., et al.: Presence of human immunodeficiency virus DNA in laser smoke. Lasers Surg. Med. 11: 197-203; 1991.

Bellina, J.H., R.L. Stjernholm, and J.E. Kurpel: Analysis of plume emissions after Papovavirus irradiation with the carbon dioxide laser. J. Reprod. Med. 27: 268-270; 1982.

Benedetto, M.D. and J.M. Kokosa: Laser plume hazards in the healthcare environment. Proc. SPIE 1892: 188-194; 1993.

Byrne, P.O. et al.: Carbon dioxide laser irradiation of bacterial targets in vitro. J. Hosp. Infect. 9: 265-273; 1987.

Capizzi, P.J., R.P. Clay, and M.J. Battey: Microbiologic activity in laser resurfacing plume and debris. Lasers Surg. Med. 23: 172-174; 1998.

Ediger, M.N. and L.S. Matchette: In vitro production of viable bacteriophage in a laser plume. Lasers Surg. Med. 9: 296-299; 1989.

Felten, R.P.: Summary of laser plume effects and safety session. Journal of Laser Applications 1(2): 4-5; 1989.

Ferenczy, A., C. Bergeron, and R.M. Richart: Human Papillomavirus DNA in CO2 laser generated plume of smoke and its consequences to the surgeon. Obstet. Gynecol. 75: 114-118; 1990.

Furzikov, N.P., et al.: Relative efficiency and products of atherosclerotic plaque destruction by pulsed laser radiation. Lasers Life Sci. 1(4): 265-274; 1987.

Lobraico, R.V., M.J. Schifano, and K.R. Brader: A retrospective study on the hazards of the carbon dioxide laser plume. Journal of Laser Applications 1(1): 6-8; 1988.

Matchette, L.S., et al.: In vitro production of viable bacteriophage in carbon dioxide and argon laser plumes. Lasers Surg. Med. 11: 380-384; 1991.

Matchette, L.S., T.J. Vegella, and R.W. Faaland: Viable bacteriophage in CO2 laser plume: aerodynamic size distribution. Lasers Surg. Med. 13: 18-22; 1993.

Nezhat, C., et al.: Smoke from laser surgery: is there a health hazard? Lasers Surg. Med. 7: 376-382; 1987.

Sawchuk, W.S. and R.P. Felten: Infectious potential of aerosolized particles. Arch. Dermatol. 125: 1689-1692; 1989.

Sawchuk, W.S. et al.: Infectious Papillomavirus in the vapor of warts treated with carbon dioxide laser or electrocoagulation: detection and protection. J. Am. Acad. Dermatol. 21: 41-49; 1989.

Treffler, B., et al.: Investigations of pulsed laser tissue ablation by short-time exposure video recording and image processing. Proc. SPIE 2624:226-233; 1996.

Walker, N.P.J., J. Matthews, and S.W.B. Newsom: Possible hazards from irradiation with the carbon dioxide laser. Lasers Surg. Med. 6: 84-86; 1986.

Weber, L.: Spreading of infectious materials from the laser interaction zone: viruses and bacteria. Proc. SPIE 2923: 178-181; 1996.

Ziegler, B.K., et al.: Generation of infectious retrovirus aerosol through medical irradiation. Lasers Surg. Med. 22: 37-41; 1998.

F4.6 Control Measures.

American Conference of Governmental Industrial Hygienists: Industrial Ventilation--A Manual of Recommended Practice. Cincinnati, OH: ACGIH (or latest revision thereof).

Baggish, M.S., P. Baltoyannis, and E. Sze: Protection of the rat lung from the harmful effects of laser smoke. Lasers Surg. Med. 8: 248-253; 1988.

Ball, R.D., B. Kulik, and S.L. Tan: The assessment and control of hazardous by-products from materials processing with CO2 lasers. In Industrial Laser Handbook. Pennwell Publishing Co., pp. 154-164; 1989.

Benoit, H., J. Clark, and W.J. Keon: Installation of a commercial excimer laser in the operating room. Journal of Laser Applications 1(3): 45-50; 1989.

Caldwell, C.: Laser fire protection. In Proceedings of the 1992 International Laser Safety Conference. Orlando, FL: Laser Institute of America, 4I-1 - 4I-9; 1993.

Council on Scientific Affairs, American Medical Association: Lasers in medicine and surgery. J. Am. Med. Assoc. 256: 900-907; 1986.

ECRI: Laser smoke evacuators. Health Devices 1: 1990.

Fleeger, A. and C.E. Moss: NIOSH Health Hazard Evaluation Report HETA 89-331-2078, Photon Dynamics Ltd., Inc., Longwood, Florida. Springfield, VA: National Technical Information Service (PB91-188946); 1990.

Fried, M.P. et al.: Laser resistant stainless steel endotracheal tube: experimental and clinical evaluation. Lasers Surg. Med. 11: 301-306; 1991.

Garner, R.K.: Research, development and future of filtration methods. In Proceedings of the 1992 International Laser Safety Conference. Orlando, FL: Laser Institute of America, 4M 21 - 4M-24; 1993.

Haferkamp, H., et al.: Air contaminants generated during laser processing of organic materials and protective measures. In Proceedings of the International Laser Safety Conference. Orlando, FL: Laser Institute of America, pp. 209-218; 1997.

Hitchcock, R.T. (ed.): LIA Guide to Non-beam Hazards Associated with Laser Use. Orlando, FL: Laser Institute of America; 1999.

Hitchcock, R.T. and R..M. Patterson: Radio-Frequency and ELF Electromagnetic Energies - A Handbook for Health Professionals. New York: Van Nostrand Reinhold; 1995.

Itoh, K.: Environmental protection in laser processing in Japan. In ICALEO '92 Laser Materials Processing. Orlando, FL: Laser Institute of America, pp. 348-353; 1992.

Kestenbaum, A., R.J. Coyle, and P.P. Solan: Safe laser system design for production. Journal of Laser Applications 7: 31-37; 1995.

Kokosa, J.M. and M.D. Benedetto: Probing plume protection problems in the health care environment. Journal of Laser Applications 4(3): 39-43; 1992.

Kumar, A. and E. Frost: Prevention of fire hazard during laser microsurgery. Anesthesiology 54: 350; 1981.

Lawrence Livermore National Lab: Laser Dyes. Section 14.11, LLNL Environment, Safety and Health Manual http://www.llnl.gov/es_and_h/hsm/doc_14.11/doc14-11.html

Liu, B.Y.H., K.L. Rubow, and D.Y.H. Pui: Performance of HEPA and ULPA filters. Paper presented at the 31st Annual Technical Meeting of the Institute of Environmental Sciences, Las Vegas, NV; April 29-May 2, 1985.

Lobraico, R.V.: Laser safety in health care facilities. Journal of Laser Applications 4(1): 37-41; 1992.

Lorenz, A.K.: Gas handling safety for laser makers and users. Lasers and Applications 6(3): 69-73; 1987.

Miller, R.L.: Characteristics of blood-containing aerosols generated by common powered dental instruments. Am. Ind. Hyg. Assoc. J. 56:670-676; 1995.

Milstein, H.G.: A simple solution to decreasing the hazards of carbon dioxide laser plume in the operating room (letter); Groot, D. (reply). J. Am. Acad. Dermatol. 20: 708; 1989.

Moss, C.E.: Control measures necessary for limiting occupational exposures in laser surgical procedures. In Proceedings of the International Laser Safety Conference. Orlando, FL: Laser institute of America, pp. 3-1 - 3-21; 1991.

Moss, C.E., et al.: NIOSH Health Hazard Evaluation Report HETA 88-101-2008, University of Utah Health Sciences Center, Salt Lake City, Utah. Springfield, VA: National Technical Information Service (PB91-107789); 1990.

Moss, C.E. and T. Seitz: Hazard Evaluation and Technical Assistance Report No. HETA-90-102-L2075, Ebtec East, Agawam, Massachusetts. Springfield, VA: National Technical Information Service (PB91-146233); 1990.

National Fire Protection Association: Standard for Laser Fire Protection (NFPA 115). Qunicy, MA: NFPA; 2003.

National Institute of Occupational Safety and Health (NIOSH): Control of smoke from laser/electric surgical procedures, (http://www.cdc.gov/niosh/hc11.html).

Ott, D.E.: Proposal for a standard for laser plume filter technology. Journal of Laser Applications 6(2): 108-110; 1994.

Pashayan, A.G., et al.: The helium protocol for laryngotracheal operations with CO2 laser: a retrospective review of 523 cases. Anesthesiology 68: 801-804; 1988.

Sawchuk, W.S. et al.: Infectious Papillomavirus in the vapor of warts treated with carbon dioxide laser or electrocoagulation: detection and protection. J. Am. Acad. Dermatol. 21: 41-49; 1989.

Sliney, D.H. et al.: Semitransparent curtains for control of optical radiation hazards. Appl. Opt. 20: 2352-2366; 1981.

Smith, J.P., et al.: Evaluation of a smoke evacuator used for laser surgery. Lasers Surg. Med. 9: 276-281; 1989.

Smith, J.P., J.L. Topmiller, and S. Shulman: Factors affecting emission collection by surgical smoke evacuators. Lasers Surg. Med. 10: 224-233; 1990.

Sosis, M.: Polyvinylchloride endotracheal tubes are hazardous for CO2 laser surgery (letter); Pashayan, A.G. et al. (reply). Anesthesiology 69: 801-802; 1988.

Sosis, M.B. and F.X. Dillon: Comparison of CO2 laser ignition of the Xomed plastic and rubber tracheal tubes. In Proceedings of the 1992 International Laser Safety Conference. Orlando, FL: Laser Institute of America, 4M-13 - 4M-16; 1993.

Streifel, A.J. and D. Akale: Evaluation of methods for limiting exposure to laser plume. In Proceedings of the 1992 International Laser Safety Conference. Orlando, FL: Laser Institute of America, 4M-25; 1993.

Troutman, K.R.: Ventilation system design for industrial laser operation. In Proceedings of the International Laser Safety Conference. Orlando, FL: Laser institute of America, pp. 3-55 - 3-67; 1991.

Willeke, K. et al.: Penetration of airborne microorganisms through a surgical mask and a dust/mist respirator. Am. Ind. Hyg. Assoc. J. 57:348-355; 1996.

Wollmer, W.: Protection measures against the influences of laser plume in medical applications. In Proceedings of the International Laser Safety Conference. Orlando, FL: Laser Institute of America, pp. 372-382; 1997.

Yeh, C.R.: New capture and collection technology - assures removal of surgical smoke. In Proceedings of the International Laser Safety Conference. Orlando, FL: Laser Institute of America, pp. 393-395; 1997.

Table F1a. Laser Generated Air Contaminant (LGAC) Thresholds

Approximate LGAC Thresholds and Guide to the Determination of Air Monitoring

Irradiance ($W \cdot cm^{-2}$)	Plastic	Composites	Metals	Skin
$> 10^7$	X	X	X	X
10^3 to 10^7	X	Δ	Δ	Δ
$< 10^3$	O	O	O	O

Notes:

X - can exist

Δ - may exist

O - probably do not exist

Table F1b. Laser Generated Airborne Contaminants

Operational Parameters	Decomposition Products	Comment	Reference
Industry and Research			
15 to 25 W CO_2 on PVC, nylon & PMMA	PMMA: methyl methacrylate monomer; PVC: HCl, benzene, toluene, styrene, PAHs; nylon: volatile amides	Analyzed gaseous material	Rockwell et al., 1976
1.6 kW CO_2 on PVC; shield gas: air or Ar	Benzo(a)pyrene, pyrene, fluoranthene, o-terphenyl pyrolsates, 1-methylpyrene, more	Condensed-phase material	Kokosa & Doyle, 1985
2.5 kW CO_2 on Kevlar; shield gas: He	Benzene, styrene, pyrene, benzo(k)fluoranthene, chrysene/benz(a)anthracene, biphenyl, fluorene, other PAHs	Between 0.25 & 0.062 mg of benzene per inch of cut material	Doyle & Kokosa, 1986
10 kW CO_2 on steel and concrete	Cr, Ni, Fe	SS 304; evaluated aerosols	Tarroni et al., 1986
CW CO_2 on PVC, polyester, Kevlar, leather, mild steel	Typically < 90% of aerosol is smaller than 1 μm; SS 347: Cr & Ni oxides; galvanized steel: Fe & Zn oxides; nonmetals: CO, benzene, toluene, others	Includes discussion of exhaust ventilation	Ball et al., 1988
1 kW CO_2 on graphite composite materials; shield gases: air or Ar	Aniline, cresols, quinoline, 1,1-biphenyl, dibenzofuran, phenanthrene, many more	Base materials were epoxy & polyimide-based	Kwan, 1990
350 W CO_2 on Kevlar & Kevlar-graphite	CO, HCN, NO, NO_2, 1,1,1-trichloroethane, ethyl acetate; methyl isobutyl ketone	Workplace survey; no overexposures found	Moss & Seitz, 1990

Table F1b. Laser Generated Airborne Contaminants (cont.)

Operational Parameters	Decomposition Products	Comment	Reference
600 W CO_2 on fused quartz, PMMA, ABS	Fused silica from quartz; ethyl acrylate from polymers	Personal & area samples	Fleeger & Moss, 1990
2.5 kW CO_2 on Al, carbon steel, SS, PMMA-plastics	C-steel: Fe oxides; SS: Cr oxides, others; plastics: benzene, pyrene, toluene, PAHs	Identified hexavalent Cr from SS	Hietanen et al., 1992
900 W CO_2 on mild steel & SS	SS: Fe > Fe_2O_3 > Cr > Cr_2O_3 > Ni > NiO	Diameter of projected particles ranged in size from 50 to 500 μm	Powell et al., 1993
25.9 W CO_2 on felt, woven fabrics, PVC, PMMA, acrylic, Formica	Felt: formaldehyde, HCN, acrylonitrile, acetonitrile, acrolein; Fabric: formaldehyde, HCN, benzene, styrene; Formica: formaldehyde, HCN, methanol, acetonitrile, furan; others	Area air samples: CO levels low (≤ 2 ppm) for all materials	Kiefer & Moss, 1997
2.6 kW CO_2 on SS; assist gas: N_2 or O_3	Operational parameters related to highest fume concentration: N_2: speed; O_2: power	2 mm thick SS	Siggard & Olsen, 1997
750 W CO_2 on carbon steel, galvanized steel and SS	Generally, 75-80% of particles < 3 μm in diameter	Concentration of airborne samples can exceed magnitude of exposure limits	Pena et al., 1998
280 to 300 W Nd:YAG; 2.2-5 kW CO_2; both on SS & Zn-coated steel	Respirable dust concentrations 0.12-0.76 mg/m^3 (Nd:YAG) & 0.22-2.30 mg/m^3; airborne metals: Fe, Zn, Mn, Cr, Ni	Exposure limits not exceeded for dust or elements	Klein et al., 1998
Degradation of ZeSe infrared optical components	Possibly ZnO, SeH_2, SeO_3 or H_2SeO_3; Th compounds may be released	Laser-induced degradation & damage	Dahmen et al., 1995
2.5 kW CO2 welding on steel and Al; shield gas: Ar	Steel: 0.21 mg/s O_3 & 0.88 mg/s NO_x; Al: 0.72 mg/s O_3 & 3.62 mg/s NO_x	O_3 concentration quickly increased above exposure limit	Schroder et al., 1997
Pulsed KrF excimer (248 nm) on polymer-based thin films & unfired ceramics	Polymer-based films: majority of particles < 0.1 μm; ceramic: particle diameters between 0.5 and 5 μm	Analyzed by scanning electron microscopy and shadow photography	Thomas & Scott 1995
Health Care			
1 kJ Nd:glass on animal tumors	Projectile particulate matter may reach an initial velocity of 5000 feet per second	Discusses control measures	Wilkinson, 1969

Table F1b. Laser Generated Airborne Contaminants (cont.)

Operational Parameters	Decomposition Products	Comment	Reference
KrF, XeCl & CO_2 on atherosclerotic plaque	Liquid or fibrous plaques: lipids, proteins, diene & triene hydroperoxides of fatty acids, water: main product for UV lasers	*In vitro* experiment	Furzikov et al., 1987
5 to 30 W CW Nd:YAG & 10 to20 W CO_2 (pulsed) on pig tissue	Aerosol concentration highest 20 cm above surgical site; VOCs: toluene, styrene, ethylbenzene, benzaldehyde, 2-butanone, pyrrole/pyridine, others	VOC concentrations relatively low; aerosol concentration relatively high	Wasche & Albrecht, 1988
300 W CO_2 on beef liver 30 W Nd:YAG	Benzene, smoke, acrolein, formaldehyde, PAHs Composition similar to CO_2 laser, above	Irradiance as low as 380 W/cm^2 produce LGAC	Kokosa & Eugene, 1989
30 W CO_2 on pork chop 38 to 74 W Nd:YAG on pork chop 4 W CO_2, 2.5 W Ar laser	Acetone, isopropanol, toluene, cyclohexane, alkanes, formaldehyde, HCN, Ethanol, isopropanol, cyclohexane, toluene, alkanes, methyl isobutyl ketone, formaldehyde Formaldehyde	Laboratory evaluation Laboratory evaluation Procedure on patient	Moss et al. 1990
CO_2 & XeCl on pig tissues	Ethene, propene, benzene, methyl-1-propene, toluene, cis-2-butene, acetonitrile, 2-propenenitrile, others	*In vitro* experiment	Weigmann et al., 1996
200 mJ Er:YAG, 40 mJ XeCl, 10 W CO_2 & 20 W Nd:YAG on dental materials, pig tissue, and agar gels	Particle velocities on the order of hundreds of m/s for pulsed ablation; some m/s for CW ablation	Size distribution & morphology depend on laser type & material	Treffler et al., 1996
6-45 W CO_2 on agar targets seeded with 2 bacteria	Viable *Escherichia coli* & *Staphylococcus aureus*	*In vitro* experiment found *S. aureus* to be more resistant to laser thermal effects	Byrne et al., 1987
Er:YAG on agar target	Viable bacteriophage ΦX174 transported in the plume	*In vitro* experiment	Ediger & Matchette, 1989

Table F1b. Laser Generated Airborne Contaminants (cont.)

Operational Parameters	Decomposition Products	Comment	Reference
10 W CO_2 on (HPV) plantar warts on patients & bovine warts (BVP)	Viral DNA found in plume but infectivity not ascertained	Procedure on patient (HPV); *in vitro* experiment (BPV)	Sawchuk et al., 1989
CO_2 on genital HPV infections	Viral DNA dispersed by laser therapy	Procedure on patients	Ferenczy et al., 1990
20 W CO_2 on HIV-infected cells in Petri dish	HIV pro-viral DNA	*In vitro* experiment	Baggish et al., 1991
4.3 W CO_2 & 1.2-6.8 W Ar laser on agar bacteriophage substrate	Dispersion of viable bacteriophage ΦX174 with airborne particles that settle within 100 mm of beam interaction site	*In vitro* experiment	Matchette et al., 1991
5 W CO_2 on agar-bacteriophage substrate	Viable bacteriophage ΦX174 contained in the plume	*In vitro* experiment	Matchette et al., 1993
0.5 J/cm^2 CO_2 laser on skin (resurfacing)	5 of 13 cultures were positive for *Staphylococcus*; 1/5 had growth of *Corynebacterium* & 1/5 had growth of *Neisseria*	Plume & debris from 13 patients receiving laser resurfacing	Capizzi et al., 1998
60 mJ, pulsed Er:YAG on supernatants from a cell line producing retroviruses carrying a marker gene	Viral marker gene detected in 16% of samples at distances of 5.0-6.3 cm and 59% of samples 0.5-1.6 cm from laser impact	*In vitro* experiment	Ziegler et al., 1998

Abbreviations: ABS – acrylonitrile-butadiene-styrene; Al – aluminum; Ar – argon; BVP – bovine papillomavirus; Fe – iron; CO – carbon monoxide; CO_2– carbon dioxide; Cr – chromium; DNA – deoxyribonucleic acid; Er:YAG – erbium:YAG; He – helium; HCN – hydrogen cyanide; HIV – human immunodeficiency virus; HPV – human papillomavirus; KrF – krypton fluoride; mg – milligrams; Mn – manganese; N_2 – nitrogen; Nd:YAG – neodymium:YAG; Ni – nickel – NO – nitric oxide; NO_2 – nitrogen dioxide; O_3 – ozone; PAHs- polycyclic aromatic hydrocarbons; PMMA – poly(methyl methacrylate); ppm – parts per million; PVC – poly(vinyl chloride); SS – stainless steel; Th – thorium; VOCs – volatile organic compounds; XeCl – xenon chloride; Zn – zinc; ZeSe - zinc selenide.

Table F1c. Control Measures for Laser Generated Air Contaminants (LGAC)

IRRADIANCE ($W \cdot cm^{-2}$)	POTENTIAL BIOLOGICAL EFFECTS	POSSIBLE CONTROL MEASURES
$> 10^7$	Air contaminants assoc. with chronic effects	Process isolation Local exhaust ventilation Training and education Limit worker access Robotic/manipulators Housekeeping Preventive maintenance
10^3 to 10^7	Air contaminants assoc. with acute effects; noxious odors; visibility concerns	Local exhaust ventilation Respiratory protection Personal protective equip Preventive maintenance Training and education
$< 10^3$	Potential for light odors	Adequate building ventilation Information

Appendix G
Biological Effects of the Eye and Skin

G1. Minimal Biological Effects of Laser Radiation on the Eye

G1.1 General. The majority of the work in arriving at the MPEs in Section 8 of this standard has been concerned with how to compare and weigh the data or damage thresholds from various laboratories. Among different laboratories, some differences in standardization and calibration probably exist. This has introduced a certain spread among the data. Where regression lines were available, they indicate that a factor of 10 below the 50% damage level gave a negligible probability of damage. Whenever possible, these regression lines formed the basis for the level selected for any particular MPE. If the data indicated a steeper regression line, a factor less than 10 was used.

G1.2 Corneal Damage. For the purposes of this standard, a minimal corneal lesion is a small white area involving only the epithelium and whose surface is not elevated or swollen. It appears within 10 minutes after the exposure. Very little or no staining results from fluorescein application. A minimal lesion will heal within 48 hours without visible scarring.

G1.2.1 Infrared (1.4 to 1000 μm). Excessive infrared exposure causes a loss of transparency or produces a surface irregularity in the cornea. The MPE is well below the energy or power required to produce a minimal lesion. These observations are based on experiments with CO_2 lasers; extrapolation to wavelengths other than 10.6 μm must be made with care.

Damage results from heating resulting from absorption of the incident energy by tears and tissue water in the cornea. The absorption is diffuse, and simple heat flow models appear to be valid. The identity of the sensitive material or protein in the cornea is not known. Although the exact critical temperature threshold value has not been found, it does not appear to be much above normal body temperature, and there are many indications that it is a variable function of exposure duration.

G.1.2.2 Ultraviolet (0.18 to 0.4 μm). Excessive ultraviolet exposure produces photophobia accompanied by surface redness, tearing conjunctival discharge, and corneal surface exfoliation and stromal haze. The MPE is well below the energy required to produce any of the changes named. The adverse effects are usually delayed for several hours after the exposure but will occur within 24 hours.

Damage to the epithelium by absorption of ultraviolet light probably results from photochemical denaturation of proteins or other molecules in the cells. Some of the most important molecules are the deoyribonucleic acids (DNA) and ribonucleic acids (RNA). The absorption is probably by selective sensitive portion of single cells. The action of the ultraviolet radiation is photochemical rather than thermal, since the temperature rise calculated for experimental exposure is negligible.

G1.3 Retinal Damage (0.4 to 1.4 μm). In the visible and near infrared region, 0.4 to 1.4 μm, the MPE is well below the exposure required to produce a minimal (or threshold) lesion. For the purposes of this standard, a minimal retinal lesion is the smallest ophthalmoscopically visible change in the retina. This change is a small white patch (apparently coagulation which occurs within 24 hours of the time of exposure). At threshold, the lesion is probably the result of local heating of the retina subsequent to absorption of the light and its conversion to heat by the melanin granules in the pigment epithelium. The most serious effects on vision will occur for damage in the central portion of the retina, the macula, and especially in the fovea.

Extended exposure lasting several minutes for a retinal image that is very small is difficult to accomplish, except by stabilized image optics. Thus, there exists no experimental data for long exposures and small spot sizes. However, accidental retinal exposures which combine long periods of time and small spot sizes are very unlikely.

G1.4 Other Ocular Damage. There are two transition zones between corneal hazard and retinal hazard spectral regions. These are located at the wavelength bands separating the ultraviolet and visible regions and separating near infrared and infrared. The transition wavelengths are not precise, and in these transition regions, there may be both corneal and retinal damage. Also, damage to intermediate structures, such as the lens and iris, can occur.

Gl.5 References. The most important references are cited in this section. They cover the major portion of the data used in deriving this standard. Several of the references are review articles; their bibliographies should be used as a source of additional references. The most comprehensive and up-to-date bibliography of laser effects on the eye and skin is Laser Hazards, Bibliography published by the U.S. Army Environmental Hygiene Agency, Aberdeen Proving Ground, MD 21010-5422, and the latest version should be consulted.

Adams, D.O., Beatrice, E.S., and Bedell, R.B. Retinal Ultrastructural Alterations Produced by Extremely Low Levels of Coherent Radiation, Science, 177(4043):58-60; 1972.

Allen, R.G., Thomas, SJ., Harrison, R.F., Zuclich, J.A., and Blankenstein, M.F. Ocular Effects of Pulsed Nd Laser Radiation: Variation of Threshold with Pulse Width, Health Physics, 49(5):685-692; 1985.

Bimgruber, R., Hillenkamp, F., and Gabel, V.P. Theoretical Investigations of Laser Thermal Retinal Injury, Health Physics, 48(6):781-796; 1985.

Birngruber, R., Puliafito, C.A., Gawande, A., Lin, W., Schoenlein, R.T., and Fujimoto, J.G. Femtosecond Laser Tissue Interactions: Retinal Injury Studies, *IEEE Journal of Quantum Electronics,* QE-23(10):1836-1844; 1987.

Cain, C.P., Toth, C.A., DiCarlo, C.D., Stein, C.D., Noojin, G.D., Stolarski, D.J., Roach, W.P., "Visible Retinal Lesions from Ultrashort Laser Pulses in the Primate Eye", Investigative Ophthalmology and Visual Science 36: 879-888; 1995.

Cain, C.P., Toth, C.A., Noojin, G.D., Carothers, V., Stolarski, D.J., and Rockwell, B.A., "Thresholds for Visible Lesions in the Primate Eye Produced by Ultrashort Near infrared Laser Pulses", Invest. Ophthal. and Visual Science 40: 2343-2349; 1999.

Clark, A.M. Ocular Hazards From Lasers and Other Optical Sources, *Critical Review in Environmental Control,* (3):307-339; November, 1970.

Courant, D., Court, L., Abadie, B., and Brouillet, B. Retinal Damage Thresholds from Single-Pulse Laser Exposures in the Visible Spectrum, *Health Physics.,* 56(5):637-642; 1989.

Docchio, F., and Sacchi, C.A. Shielding Properties of Laser Induced Plasmas in Ocular Media Irradiated by Single Nd:YAG Pulses of Different Durations, *Invest. Ophthalmol. Vis. Sci.,* 29(3):437-443; 1988.

Farrer, D.N., Graham, E.S., Ham, W.T. Jr., Geeraets, W.J., Williams, R.C., Mueller, H.A., Cleary, S.F., and Clarke, A.M. The Effect of Threshold Macular Lesions and Subthreshold Macular Exposures on Visual Acuity in the Rhesus Monkey, Am. *Ind. Flyg. Assn. J.,* 31(2):198-295; 1970.

Gabel, V.P. and Birngruber, R.A. Comparative Study of Threshold Laser Lesions in the Retina of Human Volunteers and Rabbits, *Health Physics.* 40:238-240; 1981.

Ham, W.T. and Mueller, H.A. Photopathology and Nature of Blue Light and Near UV Retinal Lesions Produced by Lasers and Other Optical Sources. pp. 191-246. In: *Laser Applications in Medicine and Biology,* M.L. Wolbarshi4 ed., Plenum Publ. Corp., New York; 1989.

Hansen, W.P. and Fine, S. Melanin Granule Models for Pulsed Laser Induced Retinal Injury, *Applied Optics,* 7(l):155-159; 1968.

Hayes, J.R. and Wolbarsht, M.L. Thermal Model for Retinal Damage Induced by Pulsed Lasers, *Aerospace Medicine,* 39(5):474-480; 1968.

Laser Health Hazards Control, U.S. Department of the Air Force Manual AFM-161-32; April 20, 1973. Available from National Technical Information Service, Springfield, VA 22161.

Lund, D. and Beatrice, E.S. Near Infrared Laser Ocular Bioeffects, *Health Physics.,* 56(5):631-636; 1989.

Marshall, J., Trokel, S., Rothery, S., and Schubert, H. An Ultrastructural Study of Corneal Incisions Induced by Excimer Laser at 193 nm, *Ophth.,* 92(6):749-758; 1985.

Ness, J.W., Zwick, H, Stuck, B.E., Lund, D.J., Lund, B.J., Molchany, J.W. and Sliney, D.H. "Retinal Image Motion during Deliberate Fixation: Implications to Laser Safety for Long Duration Viewing", Health Physics 78(2): 131-142; 2000.

Roach, W.P., Johnson, T.E., and Rockwell B.A., "Proposed Maximum Permissible Exposure Limits for Ultrashort Laser Pulses", Health Physics 76: 349-354; 1999.

Rockwell, B.A., Hammer, D.X., Hopkins, R.A., Payne, D.J., Toth, C.A., Roach, W.P., Druessel, J.J., Kennedy, P.K., Amnotte, R. E., Eilert, B.G., Philips, S., Noojin, G.D., Stolarski, D.J., and Cain, C.P., "Ultrashort laser pulse bioeffects and safety," Journal of Laser Applications 11: 42-44; 1999.

Rockwell, R.J. Jr., Marshall, W.J., Wolbarsht, M.L., and Sliney, D.H. An Overview of the Proposed Changes to the American National Standard Institute Z-136.1 for the Safe Use of Lasers, *Journal of Laser Applications*; 1992.

Sliney, D. H., Aron-Rosa, D., DeLori, F., Fankhauser, F., Landry, R., Mainster, M., Marshall, J., Rassow, B., Stuck, B., Trokel, S., West, T. M., and Wolffe, M. "Adjustment of guidelines for exposure of the eye to optical radiation from ocular instruments: statement from a task group of the International Commission on Non-Ionizing Radiation Protection (ICNIRP)", *Applied Optics* 44(11): 2162 – 2176(2005).

Sliney, D.H. and Wolbarsht, M.L. *Safety with Lasers and Other Optical Sources,* New York, Plenum Publishing Company; 1980.

Sliney, D.H., Doich, B.R., Rosen, A., and DeJacma, F.W. Jr. Intraocular Lens Damage from ND:YAG Laser Pulses Focused in the Vitreous. Part 11: ModeLocked Lasers, *J. Cataract Refract. Surg.*.14(5):530-532; 1988.

Sliney, D.H. Interaction Mechanisms of Laser Radiation with Ocular Tissues, pp. 64-83. In: *Lasers et Normes de Protection, First International Symposium on Laser Biological Effects and Exposure Limits,* Court, L.A.,

Sliney, D.H. Development of Laser Safety Criteria. In: *Laser Applications in Medicine and Biology,* M.L. Wolbarsht ed., vol. 1, New York, Plenum Press, pp. 153-238; 1971.

Stuck, B.E., Lund, D.J., and Beatrice, E.S. Ocular Effects of Holmium (2.06 μm) and Erbium (1.54 μm) Laser Radiation, *Health Physics.,* 40:835-846; 1981.

Taboada, J., Mikesell. G.W., and Reid, R.D. Response of the Comeal Epithelium to KrF Excimer Laser Pulses, *Health Physics.* 40(5):677-683; 1981.

Threshold Limit Values for Chemical Substances and Physical Agents in the Workroom Environment with Intended Changes for 1992, American Conference of Governmental Industrial Hygienists; Cincinnati, 1991-92.

Toth, C.A., Narayan, D.G., Cain, C.P., Noojin, G.D., Winter, K.P., Rockwell, B.A., and Roach, W.P., "Pathology of Macular Lesions from Subnanosecond Pulses of Visible Laser Energy" Invest. Ophthal. And Visual Science 38(11): 2204-2213, 1997.

Vassiliadis, A. Ocular Damage From Laser Radiation, pp. 125-162. In: *Laser Applications in Medicine and Biology,* M.L. Wolbarsht, ed., vol. 1, Plenum Press, New York; 1977.

Vos, JJ. A Theory of Retinal Burns, *Bulletin of Mathematical Biophysics,* 24:115-128; 1962.

White, TJ., Mainster, M.A., Tips, I.A., and Wilson, P.W. Chorioretinal Therffial Behavior, *Bulletin of Mathematical Biophysics,* 32(9):315-322; 1970.

Wolbarsht, M.L. Cataract from Infrared Lasers: Evidence for Photochemical Mechanisms, Lasers *Light Ophthamol.* 4:91-96; 1992.

Wolbarsht, M.L. and Sliney, D.H. Historical Development of the ANSI Laser Safety Standard, *Journal of Laser Applications,* 3(5):5-11; 1991.

Zuclich, J.A. Ultraviolet Laser Radiation Injury to the Ocular Tissues, pp. 256-275. In: *Lasers et Nornes de Protection, First International Symposium on Laser Biological Effects and Exposure Limits,* Court L.A., Duchene, A., and Courant, D., eds., Fontenay-aux-Roses: Commissariat al'Energic Atomique, Departement de Protection Sanitaire. Service de Documentation; 1988.

G2. Biological Effects of Laser Radiation on the Skin

G2.1 General. The large skin surface makes this body tissue readily available to accidental and repeated exposures to laser radiation. The biological significance of irradiation of the skin by lasers operating in the visible and infrared regions is considerably less than exposure of the eye, as skin damage is usually reparable or reversible. Effects may vary from a mild reddening (erythema) to blisters and charring. Depigmentation, ulceration, and scarring of the skin and damage to underlying organs may occur from extremely high-power laser radiation.

Outside of the UV region, latent and cumulative effects of laser radiation to the skin are not known at this time. The possibility of such effects occurring, however, should not be ignored in planning for personnel safety in laser installations.

Little or no data is available describing the reaction of skin exposed to laser radiation in the 0.2 to 0.4 μm spectral region, but chronic exposure to ultraviolet wavelengths in this range can have a carcinogenic action on skin as well as eliciting an erythematous response.

On the basis of studies with noncoherent ultraviolet radiation, exposure to wavelengths in the 0.25 to 0.32 μm spectral region is most injurious to skin. Exposure to the shorter (0.2 to 0.25 μm) and longer (0.32 to 0.4 μm) ultraviolet wavelengths is considered less harmful to normal human skin. The shorter wavelengths are absorbed in the outer dead layer of the epidermis (stratum corneum), and exposure to the longer wavelengths has a pigment darkening effect. However, the sensitivity of skin to the longer wavelengths may be increased by known or inadvertent usage of photosensitizers.

G2.2 References. The most comprehensive and up-to-date bibliography of laser effects on the eye and skin is *Laser Hazards Bibliography* published by the U.S. Army Center for Health Promotion and Preventative Medicine, Aberdeen Proving Ground, MD 21010-5422, and the latest version should be consulted.

Anderson, R.R. and Parrish, J.A. The Optics of Human Skin, *J. Invest. Dermatol.,* 77:13-18; 1981.

Buchanan, A.R., Heim, H.G., and Stilson, D.W. *Biomedical Effects of Exposure to Electromagnetic Radiation - Part I: Ultraviolet.* Air Development Center Technical Report 60-376, AD 244 786; May, 1960. Available from National Technical Information Service, Springfield, VA 22161.

Goldman, L. and Rockwell, R.J. Jr. *Lasers in Medicine,* New York: Gordon and Breach Science Publishers; 1971.

Kochevar, I.E. Photoallergic to Chemicals, *Photochem. Photobiol,* 30:437-442; 1979.

Lane, RJ. Linskcr, R., Wynne, JJ., Torms, A., and Geronemus, R.G. Ultraviolet - Laser Ablation of Skin, *Archives of Dermatology,* 121:(609-617); 1985.

Laor, Y., Simpson, C., Klein, E., and Fine, S. Pathology of Internal Viscera Following Laser Radiation, *American Journal of the Medical Sciences,* 257(4):242-252; 1969.

Parr. W.H. Skin Lesion Threshold Values for Laser Radiation as Compared with Safety Standards, U.S. Army Medical Research Laboratory Report 813, AD 688 871; 1969. Available from National Technical Information Service, Springfield. VA 22161.

Parrish, J.A., Zaynoun, S., and Anderson, R.R. Cumulative Effects of Repeated Sub-Threshold Doses of Ultraviolet Radiations. *J. Invest.* Dermatol., 76(5):356-8; 1981.

Svaasand, L.O, On the Propagation of Thermal Waves in Blood Perfused Tissues, *Lasers in the Life Sciences,* 2(4):289-311; 1988.

Tan, O.T., Motemedi, M., Welch, A.J., and Kurban, A.K. Spotsize Effects on Guinea Pig Skin Following Pulsed Irradiation, *J. Invest. Dermatol.,* 90(6):877-878; 1988.

Threshold Limit Values for Chemical Substances and Physical Agents in the Workroom Environments with Intended Changes for 1992, Cincinnati: American Conference of Governmental Industrial Hygienists; 1991-92.

Tong, A.K., Tan, O.T., Boll, J.J., Parrish, J.A., and Murphy, G.F. Ultrastructure: Effects of Melanin Pigment on Target Specificity Using a Pulsed Dye Laser (577 run), *J. Invest. Dermatol.,* 88(6):747-752; 1987.

Urbach, F., ed. *The Biological Effects of Ultraviolet Radiation (with Emphasis on the Skin), Proceedings of the First International Conference, 1966,* New York, Pergamon Press; 1969.

Urbach, F. and Wolbarsht, M.L. Occupational Skin Hazards from UV Exposure, pp. 21-35. In: Ocular Effects of Non-Ionizing Radiation (M.L. Wolbarsht and D.H. Stiney, eds.), *Proc. Soc. Photo. Inst. Eng. (SPIE),* vol. 229, Bellingham, WA; 1980.

Van der Leun, J.C. Interactions of Different Wavelengths in Effects of UV Radiation on Skin, *Photodermatology,* 4:257-264; 1986.

Van Gemert, M.J.C., de Kelijn, WJ.A., and Hulsbcrgcn Henning, J.P. Temperature Behavior of a Model PoTt-Wine Stain During Argon Laser Coagulation. *Phys. Med. Biol..* vol. 27, no. 9:10891104; 1982.

Watanabe, S., Flotte, TJ., McAuliffe, DJ. and Jacques. S.L. Putative Photoacoustic Damage in Skin Induced by Pulsed ArF Excimcr Laser, *J. Invest. Dermatol.,* 90(5):761-766; 1988.

Zhac-Zhang, L., Jin-Nu, W., Kang, G., and Yan, Z. Ultraviolet Erythema of laser Radiation, *Lasers in the Life Sciences,* 2(2):91-101; 1988.

Appendix H
Laser Products Classified Under Previous Standards

The earlier standards differed slightly from the criteria currently in use in this and other current laser safety standards. However, the impact upon safe use is normally minimal. Products most likely affected are 1-5 mW laser pointers, expanded beam laser products (e.g., as used in optical communications) and those with highly diverging beams (e.g., some diode laser products). Any laser product previously labeled as a Class 3a product can safely be treated as Class 3R if the beam diameter is less than 7 mm. This appendix provides background information for the laser user on these changes.

The ANSI Z136 committee has always strived to have classification guidelines and requirements identical, or as closely harmonized as possible, with the Federal Laser Product Performance Standard (FLPPS) and the international standards for laser safety issued by the International Electrotechnical Commission (IEC 60825 series). On July 26, 2001 the FLPPS issued Laser Notice No. 50, which provides guidance to laser product manufacturers on the conditions under which IEC 60825-1 can be used as an alternate to the FLPPS.

In the past, the FLPPS issued by CDRH and the ANSI standards did not always consider optically aided viewing of a highly diverging beam--as from a diode laser or fiber pigtail source. Such a highly diverging beam could be collected by an eye loupe and rendered more hazardous. This concern was not previously considered in the development of earlier ANSI standards except in ANSI Z136.2-1997, Safe Use of Optical Fiber Communications Systems (OFCS). Laser products previously classified as Class 3a are now Class 3R unless the emergent beam diameter exceeded 7 mm, in which case they could be Class 1M or 2M if reassessed. **There is no requirement to reassess lasers that were previously classified. However, a laser product with a highly diverging or greatly expanded beam that may have been "over-classified" by the old system can be reclassified in accordance with this updated classification scheme.**

Products that were previously in Class 1 remain in Class 1. A few products previously in Class 3B or 3a could now be Class 1M. In some current standards, Class 1 has been termed "eye safe"[29] and this applies even under worst-case conditions with optically aided viewing. Likewise, Class 1M has been referred to as "eye safe" except with optical aids. All lasers of low risk emitting visible (0.4 to 0.7 μm) radiation are in Class 2 or 2M, due to the aversion response. In all previous standards, Class 2 referred to those lasers emitting visible radiation that were safe for momentary viewing under all conditions; but some of these laser products emitting less than 0.4 mW may now be Class 1. Class 2M did not previously exist, but some lasers that were safe for momentary viewing only without optical aids were in Class 3a and had a Caution label; these would now be Class 2M.

---

[29] *Note: The term "eye safe" in reference to laser use and application is used by the IEC to connote Class 1. Because this term has frequently been misused in the US to refer to "eye-safe" laser wavelengths in the middle infrared spectrum and not solely to Class 1, the ANSI Z136 committee avoids the use of this term when discussing lasers and potential laser hazards at this time.*

The transitional-zone Class 3R ("R" for Reduced Requirements) is largely composed of lasers formerly in ANSI 3a, CDRH Class IIIa, and IEC Class 3B emitting less than 5 mW. Although these differences appear to be substantial, very few laser products actually have different control measures. Virtually all class 2 lasers (i.e., with small beam diameters) remain Class 2 and virtually all Class 1 products remain Class 1. Almost all current Class 3a lasers become 3R. Only products with highly diverging beams or greatly expanded beams are affected.

The advantages of the IEC revision in 2001 were that the same classification time base is now used within each group, and the revised classification scheme became more versatile for application (vertical) standards where controls may differ based upon risk. Additionally common risk concepts are applied for each class, and the revised scheme became easier to teach in laser safety classes. It is re-emphasized that the impact of the new laser safety classification scheme was minimal. Despite the appearance of major changes, the actual impact on existing products will be minimal:

- All former Class 1 are now Classes 1 and 1M.
- Most former Class 2 are now Class 2 (or 2M if a highly diverging beam, e.g., a diode laser).
- All former products labeled as ANSI Class 3a (IEC 3B) with a "Danger" logo, such as most laser pointers were renamed Class 3R.
- Class 3a expanded-beam lasers were rare outside military applications and are now Classes 1M and 2M.

Table H1. Diameters of the Measurement Apertures and Minimum Distance from Apparent Source Used in IEC 60825-1: 2001

Wavelength (μm)	For values expressed in power (W) or energy (J)				For irradiance (W/m^2) or radiant exposure (J/m^2)	
	Condition 1		Condition 2			
	Aperture (mm)	Distance (mm)	Aperture (mm)	Distance (mm)	Aperture (mm)	Distance (mm)
< 0.302 μm	-	-	7	14	1	0
≥ 0.302 μm to 0.4 μm	25	2000	7	14	1	100
≥ 0.4 μm to 1.4 μm	50	2000	7	14-100 depending on source size	7	100
≥ 1.4 μm to 4 μm	25	2000	7	14	*	100
≥ 4 μm to 10^2 μm	-	-	7	14	*	0
≥ 10^2 μm to 10^3 μm	-	-	7	14	11	0

* 1 mm for $t \leq 0.3$ s
1.5 $t^{3/8}$ for $0.3\ s < t < 10$ s
3.5 mm for $t \geq 10$ s.

Note 1: In cases where the apparent source is not accessible by virtue of engineering design (e.g., recessed) the minimum measurement distance would be at the closest point of human access but not less than the specified distance.

Note 2: The measurement distances referring to the apparent source are measured from the apparent source irrespective of any optical element placed between the source and the measurement aperture.

Table H2a. Comparison of National and International Standards for Classification

Class	IEC 60825 (Amend. 2)	U.S.: FDA/CDRH	ANSI-Z136.1
Class 1	Any laser or laser system containing a laser that cannot emit laser radiation at levels that are known to cause eye or skin injury during normal operation. This does not apply to service periods requiring access to Class 1 enclosures containing higher-class lasers.		
Class 1M	Not known to cause eye or skin damage unless collecting optics are used.	N/A	Considered incapable of producing hazardous exposure unless viewed with collecting optics
Class 2a	N/A	Visible lasers that are not intended for viewing and cannot produce any known eye or skin injury during operation based on a maximum exposure time of 1000 seconds.	N/A
Class 2	Visible lasers considered incapable of emitting laser radiation at levels that are known to cause skin or eye injury within the time period of the human eye aversion response (0.25 seconds).		
Class 2M	Not known to cause eye or skin damage within the aversion response time unless collecting optics are used.	N/A	Emits in the visible portion of the spectrum, and is potentially hazardous if viewed with collecting optics.

Table H2a. Comparison of National and International Standards for Classification (cont.)

Class	IEC 60825 (Amend. 2)	U.S.: FDA/CDRH	ANSI-Z136.1
Class 3a	N/A	Lasers similar to Class 2 with the exception that collecting optics cannot be used to directly view the beam Visible Only	N/A
Class 3R	Replaces Class 3a and has different limits. Up to 5 times the Class 2 limit for visible and 5 times the Class 1 limits for some invisible.	N/A	A laser system that is potentially hazardous under some direct and specular reflection viewing condition if the eye is appropriately focused and stable.
Class 3B	Medium-powered lasers (visible or invisible regions) that present a potential eye hazard for intrabeam (direct) or specular (mirror-like) conditions. Class 3B lasers do not present a diffuse (scatter) hazard or significant skin hazard except for higher powered 3B lasers operating at certain wavelength regions.		
Class 4	High-powered lasers (visible or invisible) considered to present potential acute hazard to the eye and skin for both direct (intrabeam) and scatter (diffused) conditions. Also have potential hazard considerations for fire (ignition) and byproduct emissions from target or process materials.		

Index

W

NOTES

NOTES

NOTES

NOTES

NOTES

NOTES